DATE DUE

Pritikin:
The Man Who Healed America's Heart

by Tom Monte
with Ilene Pritikin

Rodale Press, Emmaus, Pennsylvania

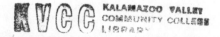

Printed in the United States of America on recycled paper containing a high percentage of de-inked fiber.

Book design: Acey Lee
Photographs: courtesy of Ilene Pritikin

Library of Congress Cataloging-in-Publication Data

Monte, Tom.
    Pritikin, the man who healed America's heart.

    Includes index.
    1. Pritikin, Nathan.   2. Nutritionists–United States–Biography.   3. Health reformers–United States–Biography.   I. Pritikin, Ilene.   II. Title.
    RM214.62.P75M66   1988   613.2'092'4 [B]   87-24321
    ISBN 0-87857-732-7   hardcover

    2   4   6   8   10   9   7   5   3   1   hardcover

Notice

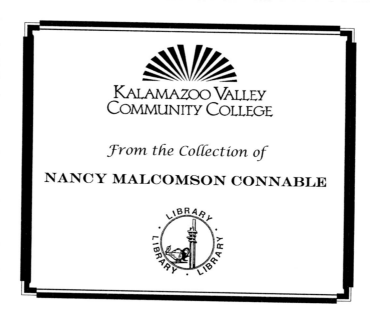

Dedication

*T*o the memory of Nathan and the health of the world's children

Contents

Foreword

*A*s Nathan Pritikin's wife and life partner, it was my great privilege and adventure to watch and help him emerge as an influential nutritional scientist, reformer, and advocate of a lifestyle that profoundly benefited the health of many thousands of people.

For much of the almost four decades that Nathan's life was my life, we enjoyed relative privacy. This began to change after 1976 when he started his first Longevity Center, and especially after the publication in 1979 of his book, *The Pritikin Program for Diet and Exercise*, which had millions of readers in many countries. As he gained the public's attention, the world's claim on him grew progressively greater.

It was my joy, and his, that his perseverance and hard work had an impact on the lives of so many. Before his 65th birthday in 1980, almost five years before his death, I prepared to commemorate the day in the most appropriate way I could conceive. I wrote to all of the people who had been patients at the Pritikin Longevity Centers, suggesting that they send Nathan a birthday letter telling him how their health had changed as a result of following his diet and exercise program. There was an avalanche of heartwarming letters, as I expected. One grateful writer put it this way: "When one man is responsible for saving another man's life, it seems only fitting that he should know about it."

Now, after Nathan's death, it's time that everyone should know about it. To me, he belonged not only to the family that loved him but to the thousands he helped–and to the world, too.

The choice of Tom Monte as Nathan's biographer seemed a logical one. Tom, a journalist and author, had interviewed Nathan many times over the years. Tom admired Nathan and understood his goals. Nathan, for his part, liked Tom, and felt the young writer had a fine grasp of the issues Nathan was promoting. In 1984, a year before Nathan's death, Tom approached him on the matter of being his biographer. Nathan had an interest, but felt a biography was premature. He wanted his large study–the "plasmapheresis study"–to be completed first. That project is now well on its way, and the story is told in these pages.

Working with Tom in putting Nathan's life together on paper so soon after Nathan's death has not been an ordeal for me. Rather, it has given me serenity and gratification. In the process, the meaning of Nathan's life has more clearly emerged. Nathan's complex personality included shortcomings, but to a remarkable degree he possessed insight, courage, vision, and determination. From his callow youth through his demanding life, he grew in character in a way that can be an inspiration to any of us.

His is an incredible story–a lone, nonprofessional believer who captured the attention of physicians, medical scientists, government leaders, and the general public around the world. More so than any other individual before him, he changed the nutritional habits of multitudes of people in the United States and abroad. The consequence in saved or improved lives can only be guessed.

Nathan's legacy is his program. Even in death his influence continues, reaching larger and larger circles, much in the manner of pebbles spreading ever-widening concentric patterns when thrown into a pond.

It was with love and pride that I participated in the telling of Nathan's remarkable story. And it is with the deepest heartfelt gratitude that I take this opportunity to thank the many people who believed in Nathan's dream, working beside him over the years. Whether individually named in these pages or not, all of them are truly part of his story.

Ilene Pritikin
Santa Barbara, California
March, 1987

PART 1

Pritikin—The Man

CHAPTER 1

A Moment of Glory

On a sunny day in April 1984, a thin, wiry man, no more than five feet, eight inches tall, with wavy black hair and a tight, serious face, hurried to the podium at New York City's Mount Sinai Medical School and prepared to speak. His audience, composed of nearly 400 doctors, scientists, and other health professionals from all over the nation, shifted about, many of them still amazed that the prestigious Mount Sinai would deign to cosponsor a medical conference with the man they were about to hear. He was, after all, a layman. More importantly, he was the creator of a health program that treated serious and life-threatening illnesses, not with conventional methods, but with a diet and exercise regimen that had been credited with literally thousands of "miracle" cures. It was the same program he had used to successfully treat his own heart disease.

For much of the past decade, he had carried on a very public battle with the leading government and private health agencies, as well as with the American Medical Association, in an effort to change the way serious diseases were treated. Between 1976 and 1984, he had developed a large and influential following that included a growing number of medical doctors and scientists. As his influence grew, he became as controversial as the message he tried to spread: that diet was both the cause and the cure for many of the most widespread diseases of modern times. The vast majority of physicians and scientists were still not ready to accept that premise, despite the ever-increasing scientific evidence that supported it. Indeed, many of the doctors and scientists present in this room had long regarded him as an enemy of establishment medicine.

And yet, here he was in the Stern Auditorium at Mount Sinai, looking at his audience with that familiar expression of impassive, unshakable confidence, focused only on his message, which had carried him through a gauntlet of criticisms and personal attacks to his current status as the leader of the diet and health revolution.

For Nathan Pritikin, it had been a long and remarkable journey.

Chicago Tribune reporter Jon Van, who was present at the conference, asked the venerable Dr. Jeremiah Stamler about the significance of Mount Sinai's willingness to work with Nathan Pritikin. As chairman of the Department of Community Health and Preventive Medicine at Northwestern University in Chicago, Stamler—who was also one of the conference speakers—was regarded as one of the leading figures in cardiovascular disease research.

"It's extraordinary that Pritikin has become accepted," Stamler told Van. "It's a good sign that Mount Sinai joined Pritikin in sponsoring this conference."

Mount Sinai's willingness to work with Pritikin was indeed a sign, if not a statement to the scientific world, for Pritikin was highly critical of many current medical therapies. He questioned medicine's reliance upon drugs and surgery and maintained that, in most cases, his program should replace existing medical therapies as a treatment for heart disease, high blood pressure, adult-onset diabetes, gout, and other serious disorders. Such illnesses afflict more than 50 million Americans. Pritikin maintained conventional medical treatment failed to get at the root causes of these diseases and, in addition, had severe side effects.

He had struck at the very heart of orthodox medicine, and offered an alternative to the therapies medical science was most proud of. Accepting him into the brotherhood of the scientific community was tantamount to acknowledging both Pritikin's accomplishments and the legitimacy of his criticisms.

For many, this was a particularly bitter pill because Pritikin was a self-trained scientist with only two years of college at the University of Chicago. His study of health began as a hobby while he was in high school. He had trained himself in medicine and nutrition during 40 years of intensive study. But his lack of formal credentials made him an anathema to the medical community. Many doctors wondered how Pritikin had the audacity to address the medical profession at all, much less come up with an alternative therapy and then apply it openly to thousands of severely ill people. To many physicians, he was an outlaw.

But Pritikin had a genius for moving into complex and technical fields and solving intractable problems. Long before he had started his formal career as a nutritionist and health proponent, Pritikin had flourished in the fields of electronics and engineering. He held more than two dozen patents in electronics, engineering, physics, and chemistry. He added to or reshaped every field he entered. And yet he had no formal training in any of these areas.

When Mount Sinai agreed to cosponsor a medical conference with Pritikin, the prestigious institution was acknowledging what many leading scientists already knew: Nathan Pritikin had become too important a figure to ignore.

Pritikin had spoken in front of hundreds of large audiences at major universities, but he had never before been asked to participate in a medical forum with highly credentialed people. This medical conference was the equivalent of his being admitted to an elite club. Still, Pritikin was by no means ready to play by the club's rules.

The speech he was about to give was not the one that had been approved by Mount Sinai's conference chairman, Dr. Virgil Brown. Brown had given his approval to a speech on diabetes Nathan had submitted for approval weeks before. This was the speech that had been announced on the conference program, and the one his audience expected to hear. But Nathan had no intention of delivering that talk. He had some of the leading scientists in the country in front of him and he was not about to waste the opportunity. Pritikin was about to launch yet another stinging attack on the scientific establishment, including the American Heart Association, for which Brown served as chairman of its Committee on Nutrition. In the past, Pritikin had attacked the scientific community for pouring millions of dollars into the search for a pharmaceutical solution to illness, when a dietary one already existed.

In 1984, there was little question among most leading scientists that a low-fat, low-cholesterol diet–such as the one advocated by Pritikin–could prevent heart disease, as well as other major illnesses. There was even considerable evidence that such a diet could be effective as a therapy against certain diseases, including heart disease. One piece of the puzzle remained in doubt, however: No one had ever shown that the fat and cholesterol deposits in the coronary arteries of humans actually regress on a low-fat, low-cholesterol diet. Such a study had never been done. These deposits, known as atherosclerosis, are the major cause of heart attacks and strokes. Reversal of atherosclerosis using a low-fat, low-cholesterol diet had been found in the coronary arteries of monkeys, and many researchers already believed that reversal was taking place in humans on Pritikin's diet. But no study had been done as yet to prove it.

Unbeknownst to his audience, Pritikin already was attempting to provide such proof. He had been working quietly with a group of scientists at a major university hospital in an effort to prove that a low-fat, low-cholesterol diet reverses atherosclerosis in the coronary arteries of humans. He hoped to have preliminary results sometime in 1985 or 1986. If his research revealed what he had predicted, the leading health agencies would be forced to recommend a low-fat, low-cholesterol diet as the treatment of preference in many cases of heart disease. Drugs and surgery would be regarded as secondary approaches for most people. This would open the way for diet as a treatment for other illnesses. He was already using diet effectively to treat high blood pressure, angina, adult-onset diabetes, gout, and other degenerative diseases, and he believed it could be effective in the treatment of certain types of cancer. In any event, his study would surely change the way heart disease was treated. When that happened, he would have defeated cardiovascular disease, and also would have given proof to those remaining in the scientific community who resisted his message: that diet was both the cause and the cure of the leading killer disease in the Western world.

But, he wondered, did he have the time? He had never felt the press of time at his back as he did now. He had only to look at his white fingernails or feel the discomfort caused by his swollen ankles to be reminded of the disease that was raging in his bloodstream.

In 1976, just months after he had opened his Longevity Center in Santa Barbara, California, a physician in Los Angeles had diagnosed the presence of an uncommon form of leukemia, a condition he had kept secret from all but his family. The origins of the disease went back to 1957, the year he had allowed himself to undergo x-ray treatments for a chronic skin problem. His white blood cell count had never been quite right since. But it was nearly 20 years before the diagnosis would be made.

For the next eight years, the illness remained under control with only occasional medical intervention. But in the early part of 1984 it struck again, with a vengeance. His red blood cell count began dropping rapidly, causing anemia and chronic weakness. He struggled with increasingly uncomfortable edema, and the swelling prevented him from running or even staying on his feet too long. Nathan realized he would need blood transfusions soon if he and his medical consultants did not come up with an effective treatment for his illness.

There was so much for him to be attending to now. He had achieved worldwide recognition, but the consequence of fame was that there were demands made upon him every minute of every day. He was moving at a frightening pace, enough to bring down a healthy man, much less one who was battling cancer. Was there time to accomplish all that he hoped for and still find an answer to the leukemia?

Nathan looked out at his audience and then at his speech. The message was as familiar to him as an old friend.

"The major cause of death in the United States is food poisoning," he began in that sonorous voice, deep, rich, and masculine. "It is not the kind of food poisoning you usually think about. Our food poisoning comes from the normal foods in the diet that we eat. . . ."

Nathan had forgotten his personal concerns, as he always did. The joy and the challenge of the mission had overtaken him once again.

CHAPTER 2

The Early Years

*N*athan Pritikin–inventor, businessman, and medical pioneer–was a person of enormous paradox. To those who came to him seeking health advice, Pritikin was the consummate healer: kind, compassionate, infinitely tolerant, a man who possessed an encyclopedic knowledge of many subjects in health and medicine and an equally remarkable memory. For those who watched him spread his message on television or saw him give public lectures, he often appeared angry, relentless, even arrogant. He possessed a warrior's courage and love of a fight. In business, Pritikin presented yet another personality: reticent, elusive, and supremely independent. He was a man who kept his own counsel–his associates rarely knew what he planned to do next–and he seemed to be able to miraculously bounce back no matter what the crisis or obstacle that stood in his way.

Because Pritikin was so different in each milieu, people who knew him only in business found it hard to understand how thousands of men and women so loved or admired him. Those who saw him on television as he attacked the medical establishment had trouble picturing his compassion. And those who witnessed his selfless service and broad understanding of health had difficulty envisioning the hard-driving businessman who was also Nathan Pritikin.

And yet, he was all these things in full bloom, changing roles as the situation demanded.

Beneath these public personas existed a gentle, private man. He loved puns and little plays on words. He was remarkably detached from those who worked with or for him, affording them the same freedom and privacy he sought for himself. At the same time, he was possessed by an enormous ambition and a driving need to be in control of his life. He refused to let experts in any field–medicine, business, or engineering–have control over his judgment. He guarded his vision as his most prized possession. And with it, he changed every field he entered.

The roots of these seemingly disparate qualities can be traced in part to his childhood and family life. Pritikin was the progeny of distinctly different parents and thus inherited and adopted characteristics of both.

Nathan was born on August 29, 1915. He was the oldest of Jacob and Esther Pritikin's three children. His birth was distinguished by the fact that he emerged into the world with his head covered by the amniotic sac that had been with him in the womb. Jewish tradition sees this as a good omen, a sign from God, to signify the birth of a special personage. His brother Albert was two years younger than Nathan; his sister Ruth was seven years his junior. All three children were born and raised on Chicago's West Side.

Jacob and Esther were Eastern European Jews who had come to the United States as infants with their parents. Jacob's family arrived from Kiev, Russia, in 1891, when he was one; Esther's family arrived from Poland two years later when she, too, was a year old. Both families settled in Chicago, in predominantly Jewish neighborhoods.

Jacob Pritikin was a timid, hard-working man who, through years of dedication, managed to become a highly successful salesman.

In 1901, when hard times hit his family, Jacob–at the age of 11–was forced to leave school and sell newspapers and shine shoes on the streets of Chicago. As a young teenager, he worked all day and attended night school to learn bookkeeping, typing, shorthand, and business law. At the age of 19, he went to work for General Outdoor Advertising, Inc., and stayed with the company for the next 46 years, retiring in 1955 after becoming one of the most successful salesmen in the company's history.

During the Depression, Jacob had sizable savings and owned two small apartment buildings in Chicago and a house in Maywood, Illinois, a Chicago suburb. Jacob underwrote all of Nathan's early ventures in photography and engineering, the first two fields he entered. At one point, when Nathan was just starting out in engineering, Jacob loaned him $68,000 to purchase equipment and tools and to rent a factory. Nathan paid back every penny his father loaned him.

Jacob's parents and three of his five sisters, who lived in the same apartment building where he and Esther lived, exerted an inordinate amount of influence over Jacob and his young family.

Each day after work Jacob would go first to his parents' apartment and discuss with them the day's events before going home to his wife and children. His parents had to be consulted on virtually every decision he and Esther made, including when to purchase new shoes or clothing for their three children.

Jacob maintained a deep fear and distrust of authority figures. He worked for decades under a man who was a staunch anti-Semite; his employer often referred to him as "that damned Jew." Jacob tolerated it because he was afraid of losing his job and being unable to find another one. Later in life, he became cynical about powerful people and institutions and frequently told his children to "trust no one."

Jacob worked long hours and spent a great deal of time away from his family. His cool demeanor and preoccupation with his job made him a rather remote figure to his children. He worked hard, had strong ideas about integrity, justice, and responsibility, and frequently lectured his children on these subjects.

Jacob was short and slender–five feet, five inches tall and 140 pounds– with a dignified bearing and an explosive temper. He possessed a strong sense of right and wrong which, when violated, touched off an emotional tirade that could not be appeased until it had run its course. In the early years of his marriage, he would occasionally lose all control of himself and throw dishes about in a rage. Nathan would recall the time he and his mother hid behind a closed door as his father threw dishes at them from the other side.

And yet Jacob loved his family and wanted to provide them with as much material comfort and security as he could. He compensated for his inability to convey warmth by his willingness to loan money and to help people find work.

Of all the people Jacob supported and cared about, Nathan was clearly his favorite. As Nathan got older, Jacob came to realize his oldest son had both courage and ambition, traits Jacob admired in anyone, but almost idolized in his son.

A letter from Jacob to Nathan written in late 1944, when Nathan was 29, reveals Jacob's high ambitions for Nathan, and Jacob's desire to claim for himself some of his son's better qualities. Nathan had just paid back the final installment on a loan from his father, which Nathan had used to invest in his photography business, called Flash Foto.

> I just received a check for $2,260 to pay balance of loan of $3,400 ($1,140 paid 11/3). You can be assured that this is the greatest happiness in my life–as I thought this is another loss–you sure surprised me. But I know that you inherit the great work of a hard worker and a go-getter. You can be sure I am in back of you of every dollar I own to assure your success, Nate. I want to take off my hat to you. You are a go-getter. My investment in you is really drawing dividents [*sic*]. . . . I assure you, you are on the way up. At least one of my children will make me happy. I wish you great happiness and

prosperity and hope you [have] great success. Don't forget I am always thinking of you. God bless you and give you good health and success to you my hard working son–your wife and our dear grandson. . . .

Mother and Dad

As the years went by, and Nathan became more successful, his father would increasingly live vicariously through Nathan's business ventures and success.

Nathan saw his father as an honest and capable man who was kept from realizing his fullest potential by his own timidity and by people in higher places. He attributed his father's tyrannical outbursts to the pressure he was under at work and to the abuse he regularly received from his bigoted employer.

Nathan, too, came to distrust people in positions of power, an attitude heightened by the fact that he grew up in Chicago during the 1920s, 1930s, and 1940s, when organized crime controlled many government officials and virtually ruled the city. During the twenties and thirties, Al Capone–one of America's most famous gangsters–turned Prohibition into a profit-making industry, and Chicago was widely recognized as the capital of organized crime.

In the fall and winter of 1930, Pritikin kept a journal as a high school class assignment. In it he recorded many of his inner thoughts and ambitions. To the 15-year-old Pritikin, Chicago looked like a grim place to make a living. On October 13, 1930, Nathan wrote:

I wonder if Judge Shulman will be elected this year. I personally don't thin[k] so, because of all the crooked things he's [done] already. Even the chief of police and the mayor and ever[y] high official is crooked. What chance has an honest man in Chicago?

During Pritikin's youth, every major institution was under attack. Charles Darwin's theory of evolution made inroads into the school systems, resulting in the famous trial of John T. Scopes, who was arrested for teaching evolution to school children in Dayton, Tennessee. As if Darwin's theories were not enough to undermine many religious convictions, Sigmund Freud's investigations into the psyche caused further erosion of long-held religious beliefs. In 1927, Arthur H. Compton of the University of Chicago won the Nobel Prize for his advancement of x-ray technology as a diagnostic device. By the 1930s penicillin had been discovered, signaling the rise of antibiotics and the notion that, within the near future, physicians would have a pharmaceutical panacea to most of human sickness. Science, not religion, promised to answer humanity's questions.

Nathan learned early in life that a degree did not necessarily confer infallibility, however. Pritikin was 13 years old when his grandfather,

Samuel Pritikin, fell gravely ill. Nathan joined his family in prayer vigils for the divine restoration of his grandfather's health. Meanwhile, a doctor was summoned to the house and, after examining and treating the old man, he announced that the patient would soon be well. Several days later, Sam Pritikin died.

For Nathan, the death of his grandfather was a profound experience. Doctors, he realized, weren't infallible, a thought that stayed with him for the rest of his life.

Nathan's mother was every bit as soft and nurturing as his father was cool and exacting.

Esther Pritikin was the third of six children born to Nathan and Yetta Leavitt. The Leavitts were Orthodox Jews who observed the kosher dietary laws.

Esther, who was called Kitty throughout her life because of her fondness for cats, had large brown eyes, dark wavy hair, and a full figure. She was warm and compassionate, and followed her traditional upbringing by taking a submissive and dutiful role in her relationship with Jacob, whom she married in 1914 at the age of 21.

Perhaps her most striking characteristic was her simplicity. Many years later, after Nathan had become an adult, he would say his mother's intellectual development had stopped when she was a teenager. From that point on, her life was devoted to keeping the peace in her home. She rarely uttered a critical word to anyone. She managed to find reasons–and excuses when necessary–for the worst kinds of behavior.

Her submissive and retiring exterior was only one side of her personality. Away from home, she blossomed. She loved to dance and participate in all types of social gatherings. At weddings and parties she would come alive, dancing for hours–mostly with her sons and other relatives. In contrast, her husband would retire to a safe part of the room or simply tolerate the events until the end of the night. Beneath her submissive exterior, Kitty had a simple zest for living. She was something of a dreamer who fantasized about living a more challenging and adventurous life.

In the 1920s, a doctor told Kitty that whole grains, whole grain flours, and fruit were better for one's health than refined foods and white sugar. She took the advice to heart, and used whole grains in her cooking, and raisins to sweeten her desserts. She subscribed to magazines that touted health food recipes and later, before Nathan became a famous nutritionist, was an ardent supporter of Adelle Davis, one of the pioneers of nutrition education whom Nathan would later repudiate for her many unscientific claims.

Nathan took an extremely protective role toward his mother. Jacob's sisters often criticized Kitty, which at times brought her to tears. Young

Nathan's response to such events was to run upstairs to his aunts' apartments and fiercely scold them. He saw his mother as vulnerable and threatened and sought to protect her against such attacks. At a young age he was cast in the role of protector of the weak, a characteristic that would remain a fundamental part of him.

As a young man, Nathan already was independent and distrustful of authority figures and powerful institutions. He felt compassion for those weaker than he was, and vowed to always be his own person. In fact, he was never employed by anyone but himself during his entire life.

Science an Early Interest

Jacob, Esther, and their three children lived on the West Side of Chicago in the apartment building they owned until 1929, when they bought a home in Maywood, a suburb of Chicago. The family took up residence in the small, three-bedroom white stucco house that had a one-car garage and a small backyard. Nathan was 14 years old and began attending Proviso High School in Maywood. It was during these years that many of the traits that seemed so characteristic of him later in life began to emerge.

Pritikin was a good but selective student in high school. He got As and Bs in all the physical sciences, mathematics, and Latin. He enjoyed technical subjects, and his singular love outside of school was photography.

In his early teens, he took an interest in health and anatomy and taught himself the names of all 206 bones in the human body. He enjoyed going to Chicago's Field Museum of Natural History and would spend hours studying the exhibits. He belonged to the science, Latin, and photography clubs at school, and served as the president of the photography club during his junior and senior years.

On September 30, 1930, at the age of 15, Nathan summarized in his journal the three areas of his budding intellectual life that especially gave him pleasure:

> Not a bad day in my studies. The more I take geometry the more I like it. It seems so easy. It's too bad Mr. Davis wouldn't go a little faster. I looked through a microscope for the first time in my life. What a thrill! I saw . . . a grasshopper's eye. The "Popular Mechanic" magazine is pretty good. Especially about taking pictures from the air. The science books as a rule are always good reading matter.

He discovered early in life that hard work tended to make things easier. As he noted on October 6:

> It seems that in any easy subject, there are many failures; but, in a subject that is hard, there aren't many failures.

On October 9:

> If I miss a day or two of Latin, it all seems very hard. But if I keep up with my work everything is easy.

Even at 15, Pritikin was highly ambitious and eager to learn. He saw that knowledge and hard work had many fringe benefits. On October 8, 1930, he confided to his journal:

> It seems funny that only one half year ago, I was popular for my dum[b]ness. When I transferred to Proviso, a new change came over me. I decided that I had neg[l]ected my lessons long enough. Taking a new interest in my studies, I began to learn the secret of popularity. Hard work! After becoming known in every class, I found that any person, if willing to do a little home and brainwork, can be well liked around the school.

He expected his hard work to pay off, but when the results did not live up to his expectations, he refused to throw up his hands in defeat. On October 21, after finding out his grades at school, he wrote:

> I'm almost disgusted. Only honorary mention. I expected to be an honor student, sure! But that's what happens when you get too much confidence in yourself. What was worrying me all the time was the mark I was to get in zoology. I'll have to raise my mark to a 1 [the equivalent of an A in most schools], and surprise Miss Shepard. I'm going to study "from dawn of day till night" . . . I'll use the old motto, "I never fail if I try."

Nathan was a serious and ambitious student in the areas he enjoyed, but devoted minimal attention or energy to those subjects he cared little about. He barely got by in English and the social sciences. On his college entry examinations he scored a B in biological sciences, a C in the social sciences, and a D in English.

His high school grades and test scores accurately reflect the sharply contrasting aspects of his nature. Throughout his life, he had little interest in the "soft" sciences like sociology and psychology. He had a passion for history and politics, but rarely read fiction and maintained only a distant appreciation of the arts. He enjoyed popular music, loved rhythmic songs that he could dance to, and once claimed Spike Jones–the musician who used everything from kitchen paraphernalia to foghorns as instruments–as one of his favorite entertainers. As he got older, however, his taste in music matured, and an aria from *Turandot* could bring tears to his eyes. Nathan regarded the arts as a world unto themselves, a world he respected but did not understand.

As a youth, Pritikin loved many individual sports, including running, swimming, and some track and field events, but had no interest in team competition. He once jokingly described baseball to his son Ken as "a game in which one team throws a ball to a second team, which tries to hit the ball as far as it can, forcing the first team to run after the ball. After they've finally caught up to it, they throw it back to the second team, which hits the ball again. Hasn't anybody learned anything?"

Pritikin was introverted and self-aware. Though he was well liked in high school, he kept a certain part of himself inaccessible, as he did for the rest of his life. As his brother, Albert, put it, "Nathan was friendly without being personal."

Even as a child, Nathan rarely, if ever, dwelled on emotional issues. His response to virtually every problem was to turn his attention to some intellectual challenge.

"The way I cheer myself up is to solve some geometry problems," he wrote in his journal at the age of 15. "After twenty minutes in Mr. Davis['] room I [am] filled with life and forget about the boy who deposited his oranges and waste paper in the basket of my bike."

When he wanted to escape, he read books or went to the movies. Despite the seriousness of his personality, or perhaps because of it, Nathan's favorite films were comedies. As a boy, he loved Buster Keaton–calling him the "most comical, most ingenious, best, funny faced, dishpanned comedian on the market of shows today"–and later, as an adult, enjoyed musical comedies and anything starring Danny Kaye.

Nathan had an excellent sense of humor, which he used effectively to lighten the mood during a crisis or to deflect personal questions about himself or others. He could turn what initially appeared to be a grave matter into an ingenious witticism in an instant. Family therapist Jeanne Rand Green, a close friend of Nathan's wife during the last 20 years of his life, believed he used his sense of humor to keep from dealing with his emotions, which he kept to himself.

Pritikin was not without strong feelings; he cried openly at joyous occasions, such as his daughter's marriage, or at sad or moving events. Even emotional films would bring tears to his eyes. His son Robert said his father was very sentimental, but could not express it in words. He rarely told anyone of his appreciation for them, and never expressed his love for people in words. Once, when Robert was a small boy, Nathan sent him a postcard while on one of his trips. He concluded the postcard with just the words, "Goodbye, Daddy." Pritikin had a mental block about using the word love to anyone, including his children or his wife Ilene.

He once sent Ilene a dozen roses–for Nathan, an unusual gesture in itself–with a card signed only, "From a secret admirer."

Despite his inability to convey his love in words, people came away from him having felt his compassion and kindness. Like his mother,

Nathan projected a patient and caring personality. But like his father, he could only express it in silent acts of generosity.

Even with his children, Pritikin could be mysterious and inaccessible at times. They had to draw him out of his world and into theirs. But once they drew him out, he gave them his full attention. "Dad could block out everything and concentrate all his attention on whatever was in front of him," said Ken. "Whether it was a problem brought to him by one of his children, or something he was working on, it seemed like nothing else mattered at that moment. My father was not the kind of man who talked about himself, though. If you asked him a question about himself, he'd answer it, but he didn't volunteer. He was very project-oriented; his thoughts were on whatever problem he was dealing with at the time."

Nathan flatly rejected his father's violence and temper, however. Throughout his life, he refused to raise his voice in anger or demonstrate any loss of temper. By the time he was 18, Nathan had adopted a philosophy of nonviolence and took a pacifist's view toward world affairs. His journal reveals his change of heart between the ages of 15 and 18. On October 17, 1930, when he was 15, Pritikin noted the growing tensions and hostilities arising in Germany. He wrote:

> I happened to read about the German country trying to exile the Jewish People. I think it is a shame! I don't see any reason for such a [prejudice] against the Jewish nation. I'd like to put a bomb under him [Hitler] or them [the German leadership].

Three years later Pritikin reviewed his journal and, in an addendum, recorded his changed attitude toward his earlier expression of violence.

> A prologue for the Nazis–however, I have grown more tolerant and worldly. If confronted with the same problem today, my verdict would be either reversed or neutral, but not forceful.

As he got older, Nathan came to see his father's periodic losses of temper or violent outbursts as Jacob's personal failures. His father had lost control of himself, something Nathan had decided early in life never to do.

Rational behavior and mastery over his body were central themes in Pritikin's life. He came to believe most behavior is learned, and therefore could be relearned. Taste for food, for example, was more a matter of culture and early training than biological necessity. With a little time and patience, he believed, a person could learn to enjoy new and unfamiliar foods just as much as the old ones. (Years later, he would convince thousands of others to believe the same thing.)

As a youth, Nathan's desire to control his life began by controlling his emotions. Years later, after he was married and had a family, his children would marvel at (and were sometimes frustrated by) the fact that Nathan would never lose his temper or raise his voice in anger. "A bomb could go off in the living room, four of us could be involved in a rumble in the middle of the dining room, and dinner could be burned to a crisp, and Dad would be cool as a cucumber, off reading a medical journal in his study," recalled his son Ralph. "You couldn't get that guy angry, no matter how hard you tried."

Nathan's driving need to control himself would dictate the kind of life he led, as well as the kind of death he would later experience.

A Closeness with Nature

Pritikin joined the Boy Scouts when he was 12 years old and was introduced to the wonders of nature and the joy of achievement.

Each summer, his scout troop would go to Camp Owasippi, Michigan, where Nathan reveled in the beauty and wonder of nature. In the same verdant country that inspired Ernest Hemingway's "Big Two-Hearted River," Nathan learned to swim, hike, tell stories by the campfire, and track animals. He got the chance to test himself against the elements–his brother Albert remembers the time he rowed a boat next to Nathan, who was swimming five miles just to see if he could do it–and to fall in love with the stars. As with all aspects of nature, Nathan was fascinated by the heavens. His son Jack remembers Nathan's joy at getting up with him on several occasions at 4:00 A.M. to gaze through a telescope and watch Mercury rise. When Jack wanted to photograph the moon during an eclipse, Nathan purchased a large binocular telescope, and together they tracked the eclipse through the night.

Pritikin would come to see nature as the ultimate truth. Every important idea he had as an adult he held up to nature to see if it corresponded to his view of natural law. As far as he was concerned, nature held all the secrets. Science made nature accessible.

But the wonder of nature did not necessarily give evidence of the existence of God, Pritikin believed. Such questions as the existence of God were unknowable, he maintained, and were thus irrelevant to his thinking. To understand human existence, one need study only nature, Pritikin said.

In 1983, Paul Rifkin, author of *The God Letters*, a book that espoused atheism, wrote to Nathan posing as a 13-year-old Massachusetts high school student. Rifkin asked Pritikin whether he believed in God. Nathan wrote the following reply:

Dear Paul,

When I was a boy, I believed in God and continued my belief until I was 13 years old, when I was in my first year in high school and was introduced to the theory of evolution. Seeing the evidence as to how man has evolved from fish-like creatures and earlier from a single cell impressed me. But what convinced me was the growth of a human from a single cell to full development. During one stage of this development, the fetus has gills just like a fish. In a more advanced state, the fetus has a tail like a monkey.

One can trace the entire evolution of man from a single cell, through the fish and mammals, and finally to man, by studying the development of a human child before it is born.

Once I understood this, I no longer required the explanation of a supernatural being to explain the origin of life.

There are many mysteries that remain. But if you believe in a god, you need to ask who made god, and who made the being that made god? Believe only what can be observed or proven.

With all good wishes,
Nathan Pritikin

While he did not believe in a supreme being, Pritikin nonetheless left open the question of whether nature, as the origin of life, or the "who" that made man, had a divine status. Nathan's brother Albert indicates that Nathan held nature in such awe that his appreciation for it approached a kind of pantheism.

For Nathan, nature was the realm in which science and art became one. Plants had evolved to their present form for a functional purpose: to facilitate life. Trees and flowers not only were beautiful and inspiring forms, but also were living systems designed to promote life in the most efficient way possible.

Nathan was mentor to a number of young men who later went on to become doctors or scientists. One of them was his nephew, Dr. Stephen Kaye, who would later help Pritikin start the Longevity Center in Santa Barbara. Kaye once asked Nathan whether he believed in God. Pritikin's answer was, "If there is a God, then God is nature, or natural phenomena."

Pritikin believed that truth was an unfolding process of nature. He saw that this process had an inevitability and a power. "You get an inner strength by knowing you have the answer," Pritikin told Kaye.

This was certainly Nathan's attitude later in life when experts everywhere were telling him that his ideas about diet and health were wrong.

Pritikin's views included a deep social responsibility toward people. In fact, he associated characteristics such as generosity, honesty, and unselfishness with saintliness.

Pritikin greatly admired Ilene's parents, Nathan and Rose Robbins, who seemed to embody many of the characteristics Pritikin respected most. He was especially fond of Ilene's father, who late in life achieved success as a building contractor in Chicago. Nathan Robbins was a kind and wise man whom Nathan sought out for advice and who came to Pritikin's aid many times.

In a rare display of appreciation, Nathan wrote to his parents-in-law on December 26, 1970, expressing his gratitude and love for them.

Dear Mother and Dad,

At the end of an old year, one sits back and reflects on the events of the past months. The good times, the sadness, the joys, the sorrows, your friends, and your family all go through your thoughts. Today, as I think about these things, my mind goes back many years. I have never written to you before, but don't feel badly, I have never written to Ilene either. I'm not in the habit of writing, but a letter can express your thoughts better than a conversation.

When I think about you and Dad, and the relationship we have had all these years, I find it hard to believe that parents like you exist in this world. Your kindness, consideration, thoughtfulness in every action mark you as religious saints who devote their lives to helping humanity. Except that you do these generous acts not because of religion but out of the goodness of your hearts.

Of course, I appreciate your many gifts of money and material things, but more than that your concern and interest in all of our well being is something that cannot be measured. Your lives are devoted to helping and being concerned with the problems of others, done many times by sacrificing your own enjoyments.

My good luck in having you as in-laws is the best thing that could have happened to me. I hope both of you stay well and happy with your family and children for next year and many years to come. We all appreciate you. Happy New Year.

Nathan (& Ilene & all of the children)

Even as a youth, Pritikin was ambitious and struggled for achievement, and the Boy Scouts provided him with an outlet for his yearning to distinguish himself. He joined the scouts at the age of 12, and by 15 had achieved the rank of Eagle Scout, the highest honor available to boys in scouting. Most scouts never attain this rank after many years in scouting; Pritikin was able to do it in near-record time.

Scouting gave Nathan clearly defined tasks and, in its merit badges and levels of achievement, a well-delineated ladder to success. Pritikin regarded scouting as a good credit on his record. He was eager for experience and the chance to make a name for himself.

In a letter to his parents dated August 10, 1931–19 days before he turned 16–Nathan appealed to his parents to change their decision and let him stay at camp for another session. He wrote:

Dear Parents:

Our [news]paper, "The Blackhawk Flash," has been copied into 500 copies and has been sent out to every scout executive in the city that means anything at all in scouting. I wrote out the whole paper myself that day, and Albert drew the cartoon. In short, we wrote out the whole paper ourselves. I am sending an enclosed copy of the first page of the mimiographed [*sic*] sheet that everybody in camp has now, because they have about 30 scoutmasters and officers in camp now. In that way I have a good start in getting a job in camp next summer and staying up free of charge all summer. Albert won first prize in a swimming race, Sunday. Send some money as soon as possible, because we are dead broke, and owe a friend of mine 40 cents for four days now.

Are we going to stay the fourth period? When you decide that we are send two checks to the order of Owasippi Scout Camps for $20 apiece to us in a few days, that is, by Wednesday, or Thursday at the very most. I have written a letter to HERBERT HOOVER, OUR PRESIDENT at WASHINGTON for a job with another Eagle Scout at Blackhawk. We expect to get a job or go on a trip with some famous explorer that goes on any trip worthwhile in the future, because all the men that go on any trip worthwhile use Eagle Scouts exclusively. I am working for the merit badges in nature that are required for such a trip. If I can stay the fourth period, I can do more work in these two weeks than I could in two years at home to achieve the necessary knowledge that such a trip requires. Think of all the publicity one gets when he goes on such trips. He is known all over the U.S. and in that way think of how easy you can succeed in your life's work. Why not give me the opportunity as it is only once in a lifetime that anything happens to come along. As I told you in my last letter, for an adventure which I shall have as soon as I come home, I will receive a gold metal [*sic*]. That's my start, why not let me receive a finished polish on such knowledge, so that when the time shall come, I will be absolutely prepared. In a week, Hoover will send me an answer, and put me on his list for Eagle Scouts that want to be considered on great things done.

RECONSIDER
Nathan

Such fortitude pleased Nathan's father, who placed enormous pressure on his son to succeed. Jacob saw in Nathan the potential to go far beyond his own success and made it clear to his son he wanted Nathan to fulfill his father's ambitions. But Nathan's propensities and his father's ambition for him were in conflict.

When he was 15, it took him a month to save three dollars from his allowance to purchase a crystal radio set. The radio was not only a fascinating device but also a means of listening to people in neighboring cities and states. As he saved his money to purchase the radio, he noted in his journal:

I'm thinking of getting a short wave length set. I['ll] be able to use it in camp, or on hikes. I'd be able to tune in plenty long distance stations too. And that is something not everyone can have.

A few weeks later, Nathan bought the crystal set. When he brought his prize home and proudly displayed it to his parents, his father flew into a rage and threw the radio to the floor, smashing it to bits. He didn't want his son wasting his time on such frivolous pastimes.

Jacob wanted Nathan to be a lawyer, not a scientist. He hoped his son would attend the University of Chicago to study law after he graduated from high school. In the meantime, Jacob made sure that Nathan understood which of Nathan's interests pleased his father and which ones did not.

As Nathan sadly confessed to his journal on November 3, 1930:

> After reading an aviation story, I want to become an aviator. After reading a "buggy" story, I want to become a scientist. But since I know that my parents wouldn't even think of it, I'll never be anything I want to be; but, everything they want me to be.

Nathan was not one to be put off, however. He had tremendous persistence and the kind of mind that refused to be directed by others. He was an unconventional thinker from the start.

"Mr. Davis says it is impossible to trisect a given angle," wrote the young student in 1930, when he was 15. "That doesn't bother me, I'm going to work on it anyhow."

Photography: His First Success

Outside of his schoolwork, the most important thing in Pritikin's life was photography.

He bought his first camera in November 1930, and the months leading up to it were filled with anticipation.

On September 29, he confided to his journal:

> Wonder if I'll ever get my camera. Everyone tells my father this: "He's too young for such a camera," "O, he'll wreck it anyhow." Those blabbermouths, I wi[sh] they would shut up.

Despite his detractors, Nathan was confident he would get his camera and studied everything he could about photography while he saved his allowance. On October 16, he noted in his journal:

> I have passed the $20 mark in a fight for a camera!!! Not bad, but it's little over half the amount anyhow. It shouldn't take me more than two months to save the necessary money. When I get the camera, I'm going to "snap" the teachers in action, I should be able to do it with a 3.5 Wollensak lens. I'll use a 1/200th of a second at a 45 degree angle. Enlarge the picture, and give it to my teachers. Will they be surprised?

He was ready to sacrifice his most cherished pleasures to speed the growth of his savings. On October 26, he wrote in his journal:

> I guess I'll get my camera in two weeks or so. When I get it, I'll be low in funds, but to comply with the old saying, "Save not for fleeting pleasures, but

for everlasting pleasures." I've cut away so many "fleeting pleasures["] that an ice cream soda is something of indefinite rarity, and a thing of the by-gone days. It won't be long now!

As November arrived and his savings grew, Nathan's excitement swelled. On November 1, he wrote:

> Wonders of nature; speed; everything. Next week! And then the world shall be mine. On Saturday, my ambitions shall be fulfilled. Only four dollars between us. Four little . . . measley [*sic*] dollar bills are all. How can I think of anything else? My whole soul is in this enterprise.

He did not fulfill his ambitions until nearly three weeks later, on November 17, when he finally purchased his camera. Just before he went to the camera store that day, he recorded a ditty in his journal that he was singing to himself.

> Wandering down a lane with your breeches full of pain, and a boy's best friend is his mother, his mother. It seems funny that I should be musical today, but I am, yes, and why shouldn't I be. I'm getting my camera. What a dream, what a dream!

The camera purchased was a 35-millimeter Agfa Memo, a small, versatile camera that was a cheaper version of a popular Leica model.

Three years later, when he was 18, Pritikin reread this journal and under several entries wrote short notes that reflect his more mature attitudes and new priorities. Sounding slightly self-conscious, Nathan wrote the following addendum under the November 17, 1930, entry:

> Youthful bubbles of enthusiasm, which I don't think I'll ever experience again. November 17, 1930 was the last time I was ever thrilled except in love.

Despite the dull sound of disillusionment that resonates in this note, photography proved to be one of Pritikin's most generous benefactors. It gave him the means to start a successful business (the first of many that would follow) and the confidence to move into other technical fields, including chemistry, physics, and engineering. Photography was an exciting, endlessly challenging discipline that awakened his inventive genius and formed the technical basis for many of his inventions.

At 18, Pritikin was hard working, determined, and something of a loner. The quote he chose for his high school yearbook captured the things he valued most in himself: "He does his tasks from day to day, and meets whatever comes his way."

Following his graduation, Nathan was given a scholarship to the University of Chicago, where he enrolled in September 1933. That same year, he and his brother Albert opened Pritikin Photographers, specializing in photographing banquets, conventions, baseball teams, and social clubs.

As soon as they opened, Nathan began to design new cameras and alternating lenses to create his desired effects. Albert recalls that long after he retired to bed at night Nathan would still be up, processing film or working with the cameras. The work paid off. Nathan and Albert, still teenagers, were both earning $25 a week, which in 1934 was more than many adults were earning.

That year, Albert left the business, and Nathan hired his friend Leonard Dubin to assist him. Pritikin also renamed the business Flash Foto. While he worked long hours at his photography office, he attended the University of Chicago full time. He had acquiesced to his father's pressure and majored in prelaw with the intent of becoming a lawyer, but he could not keep himself from taking more science courses than anything else. Science and mathematics were the only subjects he excelled in; he failed English composition and, during the 1934 autumn semester, scored Ds in humanities and social science.

In the spring of 1934, Pritikin took seven courses, passing them all. It was his most demanding semester (the typical workload for most students is four to five courses per semester) and seemed to drain him of any enthusiasm for continuing his formal education.

As his business became increasingly demanding, Pritikin began to spend more time at his photography office and less time at his studies. He also was investing his salary back into the business, which made the five dollars a week he was paying for room and board at the university seem like an increasingly unnecessary–and unprofitable–investment. He had no real desire to become a lawyer, and while he could have turned to his father for financial assistance, it would only have meant that he would have to continue pursuing a law degree. Pritikin officially withdrew from school at the end of the 1935 spring semester. He had completed the first two years at the University of Chicago.

Once he left college, Pritikin plunged himself into the business of making Flash Foto a success. The big problem with his business was that he needed more photographers on his staff to increase the number of conventions and banquets he photographed. But he couldn't afford to hire skilled photographers.

Abe Asher, a friend and former employee of Pritikin's at Flash Foto, recalled Nathan's solution.

"Nathan invented a self-focusing box camera that took 12- by 20-inch prints that could be used by anyone walking in off the street. He also formulated a lighting system that was standardized so that anyone could set up the lights. Then he came up with the idea of processing the film in the station wagon that we had parked outside the hotel so that we didn't have to run back to the darkroom. He'd be in the station wagon processing the film, and we'd sell the photographs right there in the hotel."

Soon Pritikin had 15 photographers and salesmen working the banquets and conventions while he drove his "darkroom" from hotel to hotel, processing proofs. It wasn't exactly a Polaroid, but it was fast enough to keep many buyers from having second thoughts.

No job was too risky or too far-fetched for Nathan's tastes. Throughout his life, Pritikin had had an inner ear problem that frequently caused him to be nauseated whenever he rode as a passenger in cars, buses, or Chicago's elevated trains. He had especially strong reactions when he rode in the back of cabs that came to sudden stops. Yet, when an assignment called for aerial photographs of the city, Nathan hired an airplane with an open cockpit and ordered the pilot to fly upside down so that he could get unobstructed shots of the city. Years later, he would comically recall being sick after each snap of the camera. One of his favorite photographs of himself shows him standing tenuously atop a 25-foot ladder, setting up the lights for a high school graduating class photograph.

Pritikin's resourcefulness paid off. Soon, Flash Foto was Chicago's second leading banquet and convention photography service, with orders pouring in to shoot everything from class reunions to medical conferences.

The medical conferences became increasingly appealing to Pritikin. He couldn't afford to pay the high admission fees to such conferences, so he made a practice of arriving through the kitchen doors along with the dining attendants. He took an empty seat in the banquet room and listened intently as the doctors lectured on everything from brain surgery to heart disease to proctology.

More and more, he enjoyed picking up books on medical specialties and health. It was just a hobby then, a diversion, he thought.

In 1936, when he was 21, Pritikin met Roslyn Smith, better known to her friends as Babe. She was a 19-year-old brunette with Hollywood beauty and a lighthearted, adventurous spirit. In love for the first time, the smitten Pritikin grew a thin, dapper mustache–similar to the one worn by Clark Gable at the time–and dressed in smart suits and sports clothes. (Both of these were facts highly uncharacteristic of him in later life. He was always cleanshaven and preferred dress that was the most utilitarian.)

The two carried on an intense romance, much to the dismay of Nathan's parents, who thought that at 21 he was too young to be serious with any one girl. Even Nathan's friends warned him about getting too deeply involved with Roslyn, telling him that they seemed entirely incompatible. He was serious and ambitious and devoted to his work; she was more interested in having fun. Nathan and Roslyn were not to be put off, however, and in April 1937 the two eloped. When they returned, Nathan's parents accepted Roslyn as their daughter-in-law and asked their son to have a formal wedding, which he and Roslyn did on May 22.

The marriage proved to be a disaster. The two were highly incompatible. While Nathan tried to improve upon the small success he and his business had so far achieved, Roslyn complained that he spent too much time at work. Gradually, their interests went in separate directions and they became increasingly divided. In 1941, Roslyn gave birth to a son, Jack, but the marriage continued to decline. As it did, Nathan turned increasingly to his work for escape, spending even longer hours at his office and eventually renting a room nearby where he spent occasional week nights. Roslyn, meanwhile, fell in love with another man. Nathan and Roslyn were finally divorced in 1943, and in an uncontested proceeding, Nathan obtained custody of Jack, who was cared for by Nathan's mother while Nathan was at work.

The divorce devastated Pritikin. He became deeply despondent. Photographs taken of him during this period show him holding Jack as if the two were lost at sea. There is a deep sadness on Nathan's face and more than a hint of resignation. He confided to his brother that his confidence in his judgment of people in general, and women in particular, had been seriously shaken, if not entirely eroded. He felt that he had made a major decision–marrying Roslyn–without looking below the surface. He blamed himself for not seeing what apparently had been obvious to others: he and Roslyn were poorly matched.

For the rest of his life, Pritikin would maintain he was a poor judge of character. Nathan's defense was to guard his emotions and his privacy all the more, and to develop a certain detachment about personal relationships.

Nathan, the Inventor

Following the divorce, Pritikin buried himself in his work. He began to look around for bigger challenges, and when the United States entered World War II in 1941, he found one.

Like his personality, Nathan's attitudes toward the war were complex. He thoroughly despised Adolph Hitler and the Nazi attempt to conquer Europe. But he recognized that the U.S. position toward Germany–especially that of several U.S. industries before the war–was anything but patriotic or anti-Hitler. In fact, it was widely reported Hitler was investing in U.S. companies and trading with many American firms to support the German military buildup before the war. Hitler's "New Plan" in 1934 and his "Four Year Plan" in 1937 gave the Reich the power to nationalize private German investments in the United States and funnel money to the Nazi cause. Moreover, Hitler manipulated investments in the United States and invested in industries that would provide war materiel to the German army. Many American businessmen were knowingly abetting the Nazis, a problem that forced a Congressional investigation in 1940 under Senator Burton K. Wheeler. Nevertheless, Hitler continued to hold majority stock ownership, licensing rights, and trade agreements with U.S. industries–all of which he used to support the German war effort against Europe–until just before the United States entered the war in 1941.

Pritikin was staunchly nonviolent but also politically sophisticated. He realized that for many American businessmen, World War II was not a moral issue so much as a financial one, and that certain American corporations would support Hitler as long as it was economically profitable. When it ceased to be profitable, these corporations would raise the flag and be the most vocal of patriots, Pritikin believed. As a result, Pritikin saw the war as economically motivated, and although there were important moral issues at hand, these were secondary to the profit concerns of many major corporations.

Although Nathan was outraged by the duplicity of these corporations, he wished to do what he could do best to contribute to the elimination of the Nazis. After the United States entered the war, he went to military officials and asked which of the essential war industries were having trouble producing quality products.

He learned that the Air Force was having trouble with a certain vital part of the Nordham bombsight. The part, called a reticle, was a circular piece of glass with parallel engraved lines spaced one-thousandth of an inch apart. By looking through the reticle, the bombardier could judge distances on the ground and thus could sight targets. Reticles also were used in microscopes to determine the size of cells and microscopic particles.

The Air Force officer told Pritikin the reticles being produced were highly inaccurate. No method had been created yet to ensure accurate spacing between the lines at such minute distances. In the early 1940s, reticles were produced by using a stylus to engrave the lines into glass. The process was done mechanically, but because the lines were engraved so closely together, any vibration in the room would affect the stylus and throw off the line. This was partially compensated for by placing the engraving machine on hydraulic supports which absorbed most vibration, but little could be done to truly eliminate all vibration and thus there was a high degree of error in the reticles.

The existing technology was also slow. The most advanced machinery could turn out only four to six reticles at a time.

Pritikin knew nothing about reticles or the technology that was used to produce them. Nevertheless, he feigned confidence and promised the officers that he could produce a superior product in quantities for the Air

Force. He then went home and began to study the subject, which immediately surprised him with its technical difficulty.

Nathan was challenged by the puzzle. The first thing he did was to ask Robert Scott, a photographer who worked for him at Flash Foto, to take over his business in exchange for a percentage of the profits. That freed him from his duties at Flash Foto, and for the next 12 months he studied the reticle and the technology necessary to produce it. Most of his time was spent at the John Crerar Library, now a part of the University of Chicago, which specialized in technical subjects. He pored over books on such subjects as metal and glass etching and engraving, photoengraving, printing, lithography, intaglio, letterpress, rotogravure, electroplating, and metallic deposition. He also became expert in photographic emulsions and the latest techniques in high-resolution photography. When he wasn't studying the material in the library, he was conducting experiments in each of these areas at his Flash Foto office on North Dearborn Street.

Pritikin knew that if he were going to improve upon the existing reticle, he would have to come up with a new way of putting an image on glass. Some altogether new approach was needed. By the end of 1942, he had an idea.

He began by reproducing the exact image of the reticle he wanted on a large six-foot-square piece of paper. At that size he could ensure that the lines were perfectly straight and parallel. He then took a photograph of the image and reduced it to little bigger than a postage stamp, thus bringing the lines within one-thousandth of an inch of each other. (He could change the distance between the lines by changing the original drawing or changing the degree to which the image was reduced.)

The small image was the exact size and pattern of the reticle he wanted to put on glass. He then blackened a sheet of glass with a light-sensitive chemical, called a resist. Any image of light shined upon the resist would be held, or "fixed," in the resist. Pritikin then placed the negative of his reticle over the resist and shined a light through the negative and onto the resist below. This caused the exact image of the reticle to be fixed in the resist-covered glass. He then washed away the portion of the resist not fixed by the light. What was left was a black image of the reticle formed by the resist on the glass.

At this point, Pritikin sprayed a mixture of hydrofluoric and sulfuric acids over the image of the reticle. The acids etched the glass only in the places not covered by the resist, carving tiny opaque lines between the resist-covered lines. Pritikin then washed away the resist entirely, leaving behind a perfect image of the reticle, with a series of clear and opaque lines, each one spaced a thousandth of an inch from another.

This method could ensure accuracy of the lines down to one ten-thousandth of an inch, something unheard of before Pritikin had tackled the problem. Just as impressive was the fact that in the same amount of time it took his nearest competitor to produce six reticles, Pritikin could make a hundred. He was given a lucrative contract from the Air Force and a security clearance that gave him access to classified documents. He was also given exempt status from active military duty. With the help of a loan from his father, he purchased the necessary tools and factory space to produce large quantities of reticles for the Nordham bombsight. He sold Flash Foto and opened Dearborn Photographers, which started turning out reticles in 1943 as quickly as his 50-person staff and factory could produce them.

A Mind for Medicine

Pritikin's desire to explore new fields was not limited to mechanical areas.

In the 1930s, Nathan began to wear glasses to correct his nearsighted-ness. Early in World War II he heard that young men with poor vision were using special eye exercises to improve their eyesight in order to qualify for flight school in the Air Force. The exercises, collectively known as the Bates Method (named for their inventor, Dr. William H. Bates), were being used successfully to restore 20/20 vision. Pritikin began the exercises, practiced them faithfully for several months, and completely restored his sight. By 1942, he had given up his glasses and never wore them again.

Pritikin became very excited about the Bates Method and the regenerative capacities of the eye. He taught himself the physiology of the eye, studied optometry, and could eventually tell the correction of a lens simply by looking at it. (Years later he would write about vision in connec-tion with nutrition.) He also promoted the Bates Method to anyone and everyone he met who was wearing glasses. More than 40 years later Charlotte Dubin, wife of Nathan's employee Leonard Dubin, was still free of her glasses after Pritikin taught her the exercises in 1944. Pritikin also taught the exercises to Daniel Berger, an electrical engineer who worked for him in the 1950s. Berger continued to enjoy good eyesight and freedom from glasses some 30 years after he learned the Bates Method from Pritikin. Charlotte Dubin and Berger stated that in the 1940s and 1950s Pritikin was an ardent proponent of the exercises and had many students. "He would drop everything to teach the exercises to anyone who was interested," recalled Mrs. Dubin.

Nathan's successful use of the Bates Method was his first experiment with his own body. The exercises gave him an awareness of the healing powers of the body, an awareness that would later form the basis of his thinking about health.

The study of the Bates Method and the physiology of the eye came at a time when his interest in the human body was becoming increasingly serious. He seemed driven to know more.

He had studied anatomy in high school and was fascinated by the heart and circulatory system. Through his twenties and thirties, he had become increasingly interested in how the heart became ill. The underlying cause of the disease, scientists believed then, was a "hardening of the arteries" around the heart, which occurred gradually and naturally as one got older. As the arteries grew harder, they closed off the flow of blood to the heart, suffocating it, and causing a heart attack. The condition was complicated by stress, scientists believed. They assumed that the pressure of living in a modern, industrialized society, with its fast-paced lifestyles and intensity, taxed the heart and circulatory system to its limits, causing further degeneration.

In 1942, when he was 27, Pritikin formulated a simple hypothesis. He believed that if aging and stress were the main causes of heart disease, then there should be widespread deaths due to heart disease during World War II. This epidemic, he assumed, would be most severe in Western Europe, where the fighting was most intense. What could be more stressful, he presumed, than regular bombing and the threat of an advancing enemy army.

Pritikin's serious study of heart disease began with this hypothesis. His work on the reticle had provided him with a military security clearance which gave him access to certain classified documents and military records. He had no interest in the classified material, but he did request and receive information on the mortality rates of civilian populations in Western Europe. What he discovered surprised him.

People weren't dying in record numbers from heart disease, as he had assumed would be the case. On the contrary, the mortality rates from heart disease in many of Western Europe's most war-torn nations actually declined, and declined significantly.

In fact, autopsies done on European civilian dead during the war years showed a marked decrease in atherosclerosis, or cholesterol deposits within the coronary arteries leading to the heart. Atherosclerosis is the underlying cause of most heart disease.

Pritikin continued to follow the research during the years immediately following the war and read that heart disease also declined among concentration camp victims who had survived the ordeal.

All of this baffled Pritikin. Despite the ravages of the war and the horrors of the death camps, all of which were among the most stressful events in human experience, heart disease rates actually declined among many civilian and prisoner populations.

It was very puzzling. Pritikin wondered what could have brought about this remarkable decrease in heart disease. As he studied the problem further, he found–as did a handful of other researchers–that heart disease deaths dropped in countries which were put on forced food rationing. Countries such as Austria, Belgium, Sweden, and Norway restricted the diets of their civilian populations by limiting the availability of meat, eggs, and dairy products. These foods were not available in their prewar quantities because farmers had been conscripted into the army. Most of the meat, eggs, and dairy products were fed to the soldiers, while the civilian populations were forced to subsist on their more traditional peasant diets, composed largely of bread, vegetables, potatoes, and grains.

A similar phenomenon occurred among concentration camp victims, who were forced to live on little more than grain porridge during their internment. Those men and women who survived the ordeal had a much lower incidence of heart disease than civilians on unrestricted diets.

The main constituents that meat, eggs, and dairy products have in common, Pritikin learned, are fat and cholesterol. Whole grains and their flour products, vegetables, and fruits are low in fat and free of cholesterol.

Further research seemed to implicate fat and cholesterol as having something to do with the onset of heart disease. Early studies done on animals revealed that as fat and cholesterol intake increased, blood cholesterol became elevated and heart disease rates climbed. The reverse effect also seemed to occur: as fat and cholesterol levels decreased, so too did deaths due to heart disease.

The same thing seemed to be happening in humans during World War II.

During the years 1939 to 1944, Norway experienced a 2 percent drop in deaths due to heart disease for every 2 percent decrease in fat and cholesterol in the civilian diet. In 1944, the decrease in heart disease deaths reached almost 10 percent when, that same year, the fat content of the diet had dropped nearly 10 percent as well.

When the war in Europe ended and food rationing was stopped, the deaths due to heart disease rose steadily at the same rate that the fat and cholesterol content of the diet increased. (Researchers would discover that from 1945 to 1958, there was a 700 percent increase in deaths among Europeans due to heart disease.)

Pritikin realized the World War II data did not support the current scientific theories. He speculated that perhaps heart disease was not a consequence of aging or stress so much as it was a consequence of a high-fat, high-cholesterol diet. He had no idea what he would do with such information, except perhaps to correct his own diet to avoid illness. Yet the whole subject fascinated him. The fact that the World War II evidence did not support the prevailing scientific view greatly excited Pritikin. It was like so many other technical problems he had already encountered: the fundamental ideas seemed incomplete at best, or, perhaps, altogether wrong. He wanted to find out more.

In 1944 Pritikin subscribed to the *Journal of the American Medical Association*, and from that point on he seriously began to study medicine and health.

A New Marriage and a New Beginning

By 1944 Pritikin had emerged as a strongly independent, creative thinker who brought a fresh perspective to the technical problems he confronted. He was also emotionally wounded and left with the responsibility of raising his son Jack, who at four years of age needed a mother. Nathan also needed the companionship of a wife, but was skeptical about his ability to find the right person. By the end of 1944 he had a successful business going, and he began to look for someone to be his second wife.

In the early spring of 1945, he met Ilene Robbins, a 23-year-old graduate from the University of Chicago. The two met at the Jewish People's Institute at the YMCA on Douglas Boulevard in Chicago, where Ilene was presiding over a meeting to raise money for the war effort. At five feet, seven inches, Ilene was nearly as tall as Nathan. Serious and bespectacled, Ilene had dark hair, a slender figure, and a ready smile. She was smart, attractive, and confident–qualities Nathan admired. After the meeting Nathan introduced himself and eventually asked her out.

The two found they had a lot in common. Ilene had a degree in botany, loved nature, and appreciated many of the technical subjects, such as chemistry and biology, that were so much a part of Nathan's world. They had similar social views, but of the two, Nathan was far more unconventional and, at times, even radical.

Ilene came from a very proper and traditional Jewish background. Her father, also named Nathan, had been a carpenter and a cabinetmaker who, together with his son Sidney, created one of the major construction companies in Chicago. Initially, Ilene's parents did not approve of Nathan. At 30, he was seven years older than Ilene, had been divorced, and was responsible for raising a child, facts that did nothing to endear him to Ilene's parents.

Despite her parents' disapproval, Ilene insisted on seeing him. They took long walks along Lake Michigan, where Ilene came to appreciate Pritikin's capacity for clear, logical thinking. His controlled exterior and methodical approach to life revealed his practical nature, and yet his efforts were directed toward his lofty goals and dreams.

To Nathan, Ilene was strong and dependable. She understood his ambitions and could make thoughtful contributions to his work. Ilene was absolutely dedicated to him, but spoke her mind and never was apprehensive about disagreeing with him, sometimes passionately. Ilene got to know Jack, and came to accept the idea of becoming his mother.

By the end of 1946, Nathan was ready to ask Ilene to marry him, but not before he put to rest the last of his doubts about her and his own judgment. So he put her to a test.

On a cold night in the dead of winter in 1946, Nathan drove Ilene to a remote area of town, where he contrived to have the car stall. He made several attempts to start the car, all of which seemed to fail, and then told Ilene that the two of them would have to wait until the car would start or help came. There was no telephone nearby, so they would just have to wait and hope the car would eventually start. The two sat there in the cold for three hours while Nathan observed Ilene's reaction. Ilene, having accepted the situation, tried to make the best of it. A week later, he proposed. They were married on November 1, 1947.

After they were married Nathan's better qualities became apparent to Ilene's parents, and soon Pritikin and his father-in-law became as close as father and son.

When the war ended in 1945, reticles were no longer in high demand and Pritikin had to find other work to keep his factory going.

He changed the name of his business from Dearborn Photographers to Glass Products and expanded into other fields. Using the same photo-resist method he used to make reticles, Pritikin began turning out precision radio dials and edge-lighted glass plates for the radio industry. The glass plates with their engraved numbers were used to show where on the band each radio station could be found. A light was placed behind the plate to illuminate the numbers.

Using the same technology, Pritikin produced printed and inlaid circuits. He also created a commutator, or multicircuit switch, that was used in government weather balloons to record atmospheric information at various altitudes. The device, which was purchased by Bendix Corporation, was still in use in the 1980s. And then, in 1948, he started work on what was for him the most challenging and frustrating engineering project: an improved electrical resistor.

A resistor is a device that controls the voltage of an electrical current. The current that flows from a wall socket to an electrical appliance is usually 110 or 220 volts; however, there are parts within the machine that cannot sustain that many volts without burning out and therefore need a resistor to limit the volts coming into the parts in order to work properly. Resistors are found in most electrical equipment.

In the 1940s, resistors were made of carbon tubing. A wire ran into one end of the carbon tube and out the other. In between, the carbon would lower the voltage by creating resistance. However, the carbon resistor was highly sensitive to heat and humidity and therefore tended to break down under anything but optimal conditions. It was also unreliable in the consistency of its resistance.

Again, Pritikin came up with an altogether new approach.

He began by designing and building an enormous camera, three feet wide and six feet long, capable of high-resolution photography, and of reducing the photographs to precise specifications. He put the camera on a track so that he could move it back and forth easily. He then had a draftsman draw a multiwaved line that resembled a radio wave; the line was drawn according to the exact proportions of thickness and length Pritikin had ordered. He used his camera to take a picture of the wave, and reduced it to the dimensions he desired.

Pritikin then covered a sheet of tin-oxide with a chemical resist, which he had created himself after laboring on it for months. He developed the picture of the wave he wanted, and he placed the negative inside the camera and shined a light through the negative and onto the resist-covered tin-oxide. The light fixed the image of the wave onto the resist. He could repeat the process to produce as many wave-images on the resist as he wanted.

Pritikin was the first to use tin-oxide as a base. The metal was highly conductive and could easily be shaped according to his precise specifications.

Sometimes he electroplated silver or nickel over the tin-oxide wave pattern to improve conductivity. He cut out the wave pattern and embedded it in plastic (Bakelite) or glass. Here was another innovation: he made the wave pattern flush with the glass and then placed another piece of glass over the pattern to serve as insulation.

Working with ceramics engineers, Pritikin made his own glass and furnace in order to make the glass nonconductive. The glass housed the resistor and prevented it from shock or from being contacted by humidity. He then soldered wires to either end of the resistor and it was ready for use.

The thickness and length of the wave caused the amount of resistance Pritikin wanted; the resistance could be altered by changing the thickness and length of the wave image. Because it was made of metal, it was hard, durable, and dependable. Unlike carbon tubing, Pritikin's resistor could withstand all types of environments. As a result, the parts within the electrical device that the resistor served were also more dependable.

In early 1949, Pritikin was advertising his inlaid circuits, commutators, and variable resistors, which had high conductivity, extreme fineness of detail, and firm anchorage in the glass or plastic base. His products were reported in the leading trade publications and Pritikin received a thousand inquiries from manufacturers and consulting engineers throughout the world. In time, his customers would include National Cash Register, General Motors Laboratories, Bendix, Honeywell, and many other major corporations.

The Air Force became interested in Pritikin's design and asked him to produce a resistor that would maintain an even higher degree of stability over a long period of time.

Pritikin hoped to limit the degree of change in resistance to 1 percent, no matter what the environment. Such an accomplishment would give him an exclusive patent on the most superior product available. Yet he was unable to succeed even after consulting the finest minds in the field and pouring seemingly endless time, energy, and money into the search.

The resistor proved to be Nathan's holy grail, an elusive goal that he went in quest of but never captured. It seemed such a simple device on the surface: control the number of volts in a given electrical circuit by creating precise resistance. The compelling simplicity of the idea seemed to draw him in, but the task was far more difficult and frustrating. He seemed to be wrestling perpetually with the problem, even unconsciously. Always a doodler, he now took pencil in hand whenever he was on the telephone and drew configurations curiously like resistors, changing their shapes and playing with new designs, until his doodles looked like ancient markings on megalithic stones. He would draw these intricate patterns for the rest of his life, still pursuing the perfect design long after he had left the electronics field. Eventually, his drawings became so fascinating–like the mysterious drawings of the Incas–that Ilene turned a group of them into a collage, had it framed, and hung it on his office wall.

Yet, despite the two decades and several fortunes he spent in research and development, Pritikin never achieved the kind of stable resistance he was looking for. And his dreams of the perfect resistor proved to be more a trial by fire–causing him frustration, lost income, and a lengthy lawsuit– than an electronic rainbow.

In 1949 Nathan hired Harold Weinstein, a student at Illinois Institute of Technology, on a part-time basis to help him work on the resistor. Ilene had been friendly with Weinstein's wife and had introduced Harold to Nathan. When Weinstein graduated from college the following year, Pritikin hired the young engineer full-time. Weinstein was supervised by Pritikin and carried out his instructions during the work on the resistor. In March 1951, Nathan asked Weinstein to write out an agreement assigning all future patent rights to Pritikin. Weinstein replied, "Certainly you trust me more than that." Pritikin unwisely dropped the issue.

By the end of 1951, an improved resistor had been created. It had not yet achieved the level of stability that he had hoped for, but it was an improvement over existing devices. By spring 1952, Pritikin was ready to consummate a deal with Allen-Bradley Company of Milwaukee, Wisconsin, for the sale of his rights to the resistor he had created.

Before the negotiations were finished, however, Weinstein walked off his job without notice and had a lawyer contact Allen-Bradley telling the company that Weinstein, not Pritikin, was the inventor of the resistor and that if they consummated a deal with Pritikin, Weinstein would sue. Allen-Bradley broke off negotiations with Pritikin, and Nathan took Weinstein to court.

The case took nearly two years to decide. The lengthy court battle was slowed by the presentation of several hundred pages of documents, most of which were provided by Pritikin to demonstrate that he was an established inventor and engineer. Pritikin was forced to provide such documentation because Weinstein claimed Pritikin had no formal education in engineering or electronics and that Pritikin had learned what he knew about these fields from Weinstein himself. Weinstein claimed Pritikin was incapable of coming up with the design of the resistor because he lacked the formal background necessary to understand the concepts involved.

As the case dragged on, slowed by many delays and seemingly endless testimony, Weinstein offered to settle with Pritikin. His demands were simple: A payment of $25,000 would keep him out of the resistor field for two years; $50,000 would keep him out for four years. Nathan could have sole proprietorship of the resistor during those years, and Weinstein would agree not to use or share Nathan's processes.

Nathan was already in debt after spending exorbitantly on research and development. As his legal fees mounted, his attorneys pressed him to accept the offer, afraid that if he didn't settle they would never be paid their legal fees. After receiving Weinstein's offer, Pritikin's lawyer sent his client a stinging letter:

> The time I have spent in this litigation, even at a reduced per diem which I have been charging you, now amounts to $15,000. You have not been able to meet our charges as they were billed and the prospects are that you will be less able to meet them in the future. Your status with your patent lawyers is equally bad. If proof were needed your present debt situation and your present income should be conclusive that you cannot take the risk of pursuing the litigation course where there is a possibility of settlement. . . . I am leaving here Thursday noon for Washington to be gone the balance of the week. The case is set to proceed before the Master [judge] on Monday, May 25. Sober reflection will surely convince you that only one answer is possible and that is that you must accept the offered settlement.

For Pritikin, the issue at hand was painfully clear. He knew that if he acquiesced to Weinstein and paid the settlement, it would be tantamount to an admission that Weinstein was the inventor of the resistor. Pritikin had risen to prominence in the electronics and engineering industry the hard way: without formal education and on the strength of his creativity. By letting Weinstein claim credit for the resistor, Nathan would be broadcasting to the industry that he had no real skills or understanding and that his accomplishments were really those of trained people he had hired.

On the other hand, his lawyer had made it abundantly clear that Pritikin's top priority should be paying his attorney's fees—not justice. The existing costs threatened to bankrupt him as it were, and pressing the matter would only deepen his debt. Pritikin's attorney provided no real hope of a quick resolution of the case. Settlement seemed to be the prudent course.

But prudence alone rarely was a determining factor in Pritikin's mind, especially when the issue at hand involved what he considered an injustice. When his attorney returned from Washington that Thursday morning in May 1954, Nathan's answer was waiting: he would pursue a judgment in court.

It is likely Nathan somehow managed to draw the money out of his company to pay his legal expenses, but in any event, he got his attorneys to stay on the case.

Two months later, Superior Court Judge Alfred J. Cilella ruled in Pritikin's favor. In his lengthy decision, Judge Cilella stated that Pritikin had invented the photo-resist method which was a fundamental part of the resistor production in 1942, when he produced the reticle for the Air Force. The judge wrote that Pritikin was a "self-educated technician and scientific researcher; that although he was graduated from high school and attended the University of Chicago for only 'short of two years,' he acquired an intensive knowledge of photography, electroplating, metal and glass etching, largely through personal unsupervised study. . . ." Pritikin, the judge wrote, was regarded by various manufacturers, including the Air Material Command, as a source of resistors, inductors, and commutators as early as February 1949. Finally, Judge Cilella ruled Pritikin was entitled to the ownership of his invention and that no claims by Weinstein could be made against it.

Pritikin went on to produce his resistors and continue to search for a better design, but it would not be the last time someone would try to undermine his credibility on the basis of his formal education, or the lack of it.

CHAPTER 3

California Dreaming

The years 1955 to 1957 marked a turning point in Nathan's life in ways he would never have guessed. His 40th birthday brought with it a period of introspection and intimations of change on the horizon. This period saw him make his first important steps toward the improvement of his health, and, paradoxically, the singular mistake that would ultimately bring about his death.

Despite the fact that he owned his own business and had made important contributions to his field, Nathan had not achieved the kind of success he had dreamed of and worked so hard for. The Pritikins lived in a large, seven-room apartment in the South Shore district in Chicago, a middle-class neighborhood with comfortable apartments and single-family homes. They had a live-in maid, who helped Ilene with the housekeeping and the children, and many of the luxuries that defined the American dream. But Pritikin wanted more. He longed for financial independence, more time to devote to his research projects and his family, and a release from the tensions and pressures he currently was facing.

For all his hard work and inventive genius, Pritikin's business was still struggling. The electronics and engineering industry was becoming more competitive, and he felt enormous pressure to come up with new ideas that would keep his products in demand. He went to work before 8:00 A.M. and didn't return home until well past 7:00 P.M. He was under continual pressure to have his products ready in time to meet production deadlines and satisfy his customers. Most weekends he worked at the factory, conducting experiments on new products or trying to improve old ones. He seemed to struggle on slippery ground.

"We lived between success and disaster," Ilene recalled. "We were constantly thinking that success was just ahead, and failure about to catch us from behind. As it turned out, neither thing happened. We just kept going, without failing or achieving the final success that Nathan was always dreaming of."

One of Pritikin's more important dreams at the time was to get out of Chicago. Ever since he was a boy, Pritikin had abhorred the Chicago winters. Each winter seemed to get more intensely cold, the wind more biting and bitter. Everything he did between October and March seemed more difficult, from starting the car to getting home from the office. And each successive winter seemed to get longer.

He also wanted to live in a healthier environment. He dreamed of living in a climate that provided clean air, plenty of sunshine, and natural beauty. He yearned to escape the city, with its unending concrete and long, dark shadows cast by looming buildings. Chicago was fast becoming a gloomy state of mind.

In addition to his own personal desires was the fact that he had a growing family. By 1955, Nathan and Ilene had four children: Jack, 14, Janet, 6, Robert, 4, and Ralph, 1. A year later they would have one more child, a boy they named Kenneth. Nathan wanted to find a more hospitable place to raise his family.

Nathan's brother, Albert, had moved to Bakersfield, California, in 1941, and the following year Nathan visited him. Nathan fell in love with California and told Albert and others that he thought he would move in a year or two.

When the winter of 1945 was setting in, Pritikin wrote a letter to the weather bureau in Washington, D.C., requesting a summary of the weather patterns in Honolulu, Los Angeles, Miami, San Diego, Phoenix, Hot Springs (Arkansas), Brownsville (Texas), Palm Springs (California), and Chicago, the last to be used as a means of comparison. He had finally decided on California by the time he married Ilene in 1947, and was telling friends and associates that a move to California was imminent.

He and Ilene made several trips to southern California in the early 1950s. They drove up and down the coast looking at communities where they thought they might settle. Nathan approached the question of where to relocate with his usual scientific scrutiny. He subscribed to government publications for climate and weather patterns for cities and towns from San Francisco to San Diego.

In November 1953, Pritikin wrote to Professor A. J. Haagen-Smit at the California Institute of Technology for information on the effects of smog on plant life and animals. Haagen-Smit sent Pritikin some information on smog in Los Angeles, but nothing on its effects on plants and animals. Instead, he referred Pritikin to Dr. Paul Kotin at the University of

Southern California. After posing the same question to Kotin, Pritikin received a short note from Kotin stating that studies attempting to answer these very questions were now being done, but that nothing was available on the subject as yet. Unsatisfied, Pritikin ruled out Los Angeles.

Eventually, he and Ilene decided on Santa Barbara, a small city which, in 1955, had a population of 50,300. Santa Barbara is located on the southern coast of California, nearly 100 miles north of Los Angeles. It is built on a jagged coastline that stretches west, so that the city is bordered to the south by the ocean, and to the north by the Santa Ynez mountain range. Characterized by its Spanish architecture, with its clay-tiled roofs and stucco façades, Santa Barbara is built on the foothills of the Santa Ynez and the shelf that runs to the sea. The climate is nearly ideal–the temperature ranges from a winter low of 45 degrees to a summer high in the 80s and low 90s. There are cool ocean breezes and little rain. Nathan and Ilene fell in love with the city.

Nathan worked furiously to gain the capital necessary to move his business to Santa Barbara. In the meantime, he spoke to key employees about going with him when the time came to move. Most agreed to relocate.

A Meeting that Changed a Life

While he prepared to make his move westward, Pritikin continued to follow the scientific literature linking diet to health. He was particularly interested in the work done by Dr. Lester Morrison, a Los Angeles physician and heart disease researcher. Like Pritikin, Morrison was impressed by the mortality rates among European civilians on restricted diets during World War II. In fact, Morrison was so intrigued by the phenomenon that he decided to conduct his own study to see if he could duplicate the results.

Morrison began his study in 1946 by placing 50 of his patients on a restricted diet that moderately limited the fat and cholesterol levels to that comparable to the European regimen. He took another 50 patients, all of whom were following a typical American diet that was high in fat and cholesterol, and placed them in the study as well. He then followed the mortality rates of both groups for the next 12 years. At the end of 8 years, only 24 percent (about 12 people) on the high-fat diet were still alive; 56 percent (about 24 people) on the restricted diet were still alive. (At the end of 12 years, all 50 patients on the high-fat diet were dead, while 38 percent, about 17 people, on the low-fat diet were still alive.)

As of 1955, Nathan had been following Morrison's study for nine years and was well aware of its results to that point. He also realized its implications. In the fall of that year, Pritikin called Morrison and asked if he could come to Los Angeles to meet Morrison and discuss his research. Pritikin was already planning a business trip to Los Angeles and wanted to know more about Morrison's work. Morrison was glad to oblige. The two agreed to meet on December 21, 1955.

The night before he was to meet Morrison, Pritikin sat in a Los Angeles hotel room, called room service, and ordered a hot fudge sundae. Pritikin loved ice cream and ate about a pint of it a day. Ever since he was a boy, ice cream had been his favorite dessert. For him, the creamy richness, loaded with fat and sugar, was the most satisfying treat. Lately, however, his enjoyment was being infringed upon by growing suspicions.

On the basis of the World War II experience and a number of small studies such as Morrison's, Pritikin had come to believe fat and cholesterol were the underlying causes of heart and artery diseases. The prevailing view among doctors and scientists was that aging and stress were the causes of heart disease and that diet had nothing to do with the origins of the illness. But Pritikin believed the prevailing view did not seem to have the support of the evidence.

Despite his growing doubts about the healthfulness of the American diet, Nathan had not yet changed his eating habits. The very thought of changing his diet was unpleasant for him. One of his most enjoyable pastimes was to go out with Ilene to a seafood or ethnic restaurant for a gourmet dinner. Among his favorite dishes were lobster Newburg, eggplant Parmesan, steak, and roast beef. He loved dairy products and used six pats of butter on his baked potato. He also had a compelling sweet tooth. Besides ice cream, he especially enjoyed pecan pie and baklava, a flaky Greek pastry. The thought of giving up such foods pained him. All the pleasures he associated with eating, with going out to restaurants, would suddenly be gone, he feared.

And yet, like a seasoned tracker, he continued to stalk the scientific evidence linking diet to health, connecting small bits of information, watching for corroborating evidence, contacting researchers like Morrison. The trail was strong. He knew he'd have to change sooner or later. The question was, when.

By all outward signs, Nathan was in excellent health. He had a thin, wiry build and youthful good looks. His alert, slightly slanted eyes were charged with energy: when happy, his eyes and wide smile seemed to explode with a childlike delight; when confronting an adversary or facing a serious issue, those eyes gave off a razor-sharp stare that penetrated confusion or pretension like a knife through the rind of a melon. Pritikin exuded strength, confidence, and health.

Still, as he spooned the creamy dessert into his mouth, Pritikin told himself this would be his last sundae. Ice cream had lost its innocence.

Pritikin and Morrison met the following day at Morrison's office on Wilshire Boulevard. They discussed the evidence linking diet to heart disease. Both men believed fat and cholesterol in foods raised blood cholesterol and caused plaque, or cholesterol deposits, to build up within the walls of the artery.

Cholesterol is a waxlike substance used in cell construction and metabolism and in the formation of hormones. Small amounts are necessary for healthy cell development. Beyond these small, healthy amounts, dietary cholesterol and fat raise blood cholesterol. Doctors measure blood cholesterol in milligrams (mg.) of cholesterol per deciliter (dl.) of blood, and blood cholesterol is often written as mg.%, to indicate the percentage of milligrams of cholesterol in a deciliter of blood.

In 1955, doctors routinely maintained that a cholesterol level of 300 mg.% was normal, and well within a safe range. At that time, the role of cholesterol in the etiology of heart disease was largely unknown.

There was very little evidence to determine what a safe cholesterol level was, but Morrison believed that a safe cholesterol level was 220 mg.%. His assessment was based on the World War II data and his own study. Anything above this range would be increasingly dangerous, he told Pritikin. Since the evidence was scant on this point, no one knew for sure how high one could go before the cholesterol level became hazardous.

It was during their discussion about cholesterol that Morrison asked Pritikin a fateful question: "What's your cholesterol level?" Pritikin didn't know; he had never had it checked.

"If you're going to study heart disease, you have to know your cholesterol level," Pritikin recalled Morrison telling him.

With Pritikin's acquiescence, Morrison instructed his nurse to take a blood sample from Pritikin and to have his cholesterol level analyzed. After the blood sample was taken, Morrison asked Pritikin if he'd like to have a stress test done. Nathan said yes.

A stress test reveals the relative strength of the heart as a person goes from a resting state to varying degrees of exercise. The test is done by attaching electrodes to the person's arms at the biceps, or on the chest in the area of the heart. The electrodes are attached to an electrocardiograph. Each beat of the heart sends a signal through the electrodes to the electrocardiograph, which translates the beats into a jagged line written on graph paper, called an electrocardiogram. If the heartbeat is normal, the jagged line will be consistent and steady; if there is the presence of heart disease, the beats will become irregular during exercise, which in turn will be reflected in the irregularities of the jagged line on the electrocardiogram.

In 1955, a routine stress test was performed by having a person step up and down on a two-step box for about a minute and a half. It was called the Master Two-Step method. Today, stress tests are done on treadmills which can control the rate of exercise from a slow walk to a fast run.

Nathan stepped up and down on the box rapidly with the electrodes attached to his chest, while the electrocardiograph monitored the activity of his heart. After the test was performed, he put his shirt back on while Morrison interpreted the graph results. Meanwhile, Pritikin's cholesterol level came back from Morrison's lab.

Morrison told Pritikin his cholesterol level was 280 mg.%, which Morrison said was in the "high normal" range. Pritikin's stress test was normal. Morrison suggested that Pritikin have his cholesterol level checked again in a few months. Shortly thereafter, the two parted, agreeing to stay in touch.

Despite Morrison's lack of alarm and Pritikin's apparently normal stress test, Nathan was convinced that his cholesterol level was clearly in the dangerous range and might be leading to a heart attack. He wondered again how much longer he could go on eating a high-fat diet before he suffered from serious health problems. On the flight back to Chicago, Pritikin considered his options. There were no diets in 1955 that claimed to prevent or treat heart disease. He guessed that he might try to duplicate the European regimen during World War II, but wondered if that might have deficiencies. What was the ideal diet for humans? Does such a thing exist? These questions intrigued him. If certain foods promote illness, than surely others must promote health.

By the time the flight landed in Chicago, however, Nathan's concerns for his health had given way to those for Glass Products. It was always harder going back to Chicago after being in California, especially in December. For the next year, he struggled to increase production, save money, and find a solution to the problems of the resistor. His business continued to thrive, and gradually he managed to accumulate the needed cash to make the move. The resistor's solution, however, evaded him.

Pritikin decided to postpone any decisions about his diet or his elevated cholesterol during 1956, but in the early part of 1957 he did make one health decision he would later regret more than any other. Since his mid-thirties, Pritikin had suffered from a condition known as pruritis ani, or anal itching, caused by an imbalance in the bacterial environment within his intestines. The condition arose after he was given antibiotics for a particularly intractable sore throat. Pritikin later theorized that the antibiotics, which indiscriminately destroy bacteria in the body, killed many friendly bacteria in his intestines. He believed this caused an imbalance in the intestinal environment, resulting in the spread of many unfriendly bacteria, which, among other things, caused the itching. (Antibiotics are recognized today as a threat to intestinal flora.)

Pritikin consulted his physician about the anal itching; his doctor prescribed a series of ointments and external preparations, none of which was effective in treating the problem. The doctor then prescribed small dosages of meprobamate, an antifungal drug taken orally, but this resulted in skin eruptions elsewhere on Pritikin's body. The doctor then advised Nathan to take a series of x-ray treatments to destroy the fungus. Pritikin was concerned the x-rays would be hitting a part of the body very sensitive to radiation. His doctor assured him, however, that the treatments were safe. After considering the advice, Pritikin reluctantly agreed to undergo the x-ray treatments.

According to his medical records and a letter from Pritikin's physician, Nathan received 88 radiation absorbed doses (rads) of unfiltered x-rays on January 12, 1957. He got the same dosage of x-rays on January 19 and an additional 44 rads with the same quality x-rays on February 16.

Two days later, a blood test revealed that he had an elevated white count. A year later, Pritikin would be informed he had monoclonal macroglobulinemia, a condition characterized by an elevated level of globulins, or aggregated proteins and white blood cells, that form clumps in the bloodstream. It is a blood disorder that in its later stages can become leukemia.

But that information would come later. By spring of 1957, Pritikin was finally ready to make his long-awaited migration west. And on June 2, 1957, Nathan, Ilene, the children, and Glass Products–complete with several hundred tons of equipment and about ten key employees–moved to Santa Barbara, California, to start a new life. And a revolution.

CHAPTER 4

A Diagnosis,
an Experiment,
a Cure

*M*oving from Chicago's deathly cold winters and endless sweep of gray to Santa Barbara's warm sunshine, ocean vistas, and low white buildings was, for Nathan, like coming out of a tomb to a new life. He loved being close to nature. The tall eucalyptus trees, stately palms, and wide variety of flower-bearing trees and bushes–all of which flourished beneath the imposing presence of the Santa Ynez mountain range–gave Santa Barbara a radiant, exotic glow. Meanwhile, the relentless lapping of the ocean against the city's beaches provided a constant reminder of the fierce and primal heartbeat of nature.

Nathan became acutely sensitive to the fragrance of flowers and the development of plants. Clouds and weather patterns intrigued him. He continued to work obsessively at his business, but there was a new desire to enjoy life. He and Ilene took tennis lessons and played regularly; he accompanied the family to parks and on picnics. He even bicycled ten miles back and forth to work each day. Meanwhile, he continued to follow the heart disease research and regularly corresponded with Morrison. The findings were intriguing.

Nathan had read that at the turn of the century Sir William Osler, a British researcher, had found atherosclerosis was far more prevalent among the English rich than the poor. Osler conjectured that the diet of the aristocracy might be causing the disease. The rich, he observed, ate an abundance of fatty foods, while the poor ate more grains and vegetables– foods low in fat and free of cholesterol.

In 1933, a Russian scientist named Anitschkow reported that when rabbits were fed eggs, meat, and milk, they developed atherosclerosis; however, when the rabbits ate vegetables, they didn't get the disease.

Anitschkow demonstrated it was the fat and cholesterol in the foods that caused the atherosclerosis in the rabbits.

Other animal studies showed that when animals are fed a high-fat, high-cholesterol diet, their blood cholesterol levels increase, but when their diets are changed to lower the fat and cholesterol content, their blood cholesterol levels also decrease.

Pritikin also watched with interest as the famed epidemiologist Ancel Keys began his seminal work of examining populations, their eating habits, and disease patterns.

In 1956, Dr. N. Kimura, a Japanese physician, compared the autopsy records of 10,000 Japanese killed during World War II with those of Americans killed during the same period. Kimura found the Japanese had a remarkable absence of atherosclerosis, while the Americans suffered a high degree of the illness. He effectively correlated the two different disease rates to the differing amounts of fat and cholesterol in the diets of the Japanese and Americans.

The fat content of the Japanese diet was about 10 to 15 percent of its total calories, while the fat content of the American diet comprised as much as 45 percent of its total calories–almost half! (A year later, Keys and Kimura would find that when Japanese migrated to the United States and adopted more American-like eating patterns, thus raising their fat and cholesterol intake, their rates of heart disease–and certain cancers–increased to that of Americans. In short, the Japanese had no genetic immunity from coronary disease; the evidence suggested their diets protected them from the illness.)

That the American diet might be causing illness was a revolutionary thought. For one thing, the American diet and food supply were revered throughout the world. America was the breadbasket, the country with the most successful agriculture system in history. The American diet was considered second to none. Indeed, scientists at the time believed that, aside from obesity, the only problems associated with diet–even in Third World countries–were those resulting from nutrient deficiencies: pellagra, caused by lack of niacin; beriberi, from a deficiency of thiamine; and blindness, from a lack of vitamin A.

In light of these problems, fortification of foods–adding nutrients that had been lost during processing–became more widespread.

Aside from the problems of nutrient deficiencies was the general problem of hunger in underdeveloped nations. (Hunger in the United States went largely unnoticed during the 1950s.) Images of bloated bellies and humans reduced to skin and bones prompted the birth of C.A.R.E. and U.S. grain shipments overseas. Americans came to think of themselves as the best-fed people on earth. Moreover, it was during the 1950s that Americans developed their love affair with protein, and particularly with red meat, a food that came to symbolize nutritional superiority as well as American affluence.

It was this concern for lack of nutrition and the overwhelming reverence for the American diet that led the United States Department of Agriculture to develop nutritional guidelines–the "Basic Four Food Groups"–in 1956. The Basic Four were meat, dairy foods, fruits and vegetables, and breads and cereals. The guidelines were an overnight success. They were easy to teach–no home economics course would be without them as an instructional tool–and the food industry loved them. The National Dairy Council instantly saw the profit-making potential of the Basic Four and cranked up an entire nutrition education campaign around them. The Dairy Council quickly became the leading source of nutrition information in the United States, touting the nutritional benefits of dairy foods.

By 1958, the healthfulness of the American diet was unquestioned by the vast majority of scientists, doctors, and laypeople because it provided an abundance of nutrition. And so it was almost heresy to think this diet might be causing widespread disease and even death. But that was the idea beginning to take hold among a small handful of scientists in the world. Pritikin was among the first to see such a possibility and to appreciate the early scientific studies.

Diagnosis: Heart Disease

In the autumn of 1957, Pritikin began to make small changes in his diet. He ate red meat only two or three times per week, reduced the amount of butter he ate, substituted skim milk for whole, ate less chicken, and eliminated all egg yolks–egg yolks being very high in cholesterol and fat. He also introduced whole grain breads and pastas to his diet and started to eat more vegetables and fish.

These dietary changes were small, by any standard. Pritikin's diet remained essentially the same as that of most Americans, with the exception of egg yolks, perhaps, and the substitution of whole grain flour products. At the outset of 1958 he was still eating all types of red meat, including beef, lamb, and pork; he continued to eat butter, though in smaller quantities. Pritikin wanted to make prudent changes gradually.

On February 11, 1958, he went to Sansum Medical Clinic in Santa Barbara for a thorough health examination and a stress test. He was examined by Dr. Dale Creek, an internist at Sansum. Although Creek was retained as Nathan's physician, he was assisted from time to time by Dr. Clayton H. Klakeg, also a physician at Sansum. According to the Sansum medical records, Creek noted Nathan's two primary health concerns at his initial visit as chronic pruritis ani and an "abnormal EKG."

The abnormal EKG Creek referred to was the electrocardiogram given Pritikin by Lester Morrison more than two years before, when Morrison said Pritikin's test was "within normal limits." Since that time, however, Nathan had taught himself to read EKGs and noticed a small abnormality in the EKG tracings Morrison had done for him. Pritikin had read the EKG as showing the early stages of heart disease and told Creek of his observations. He also told Creek he had made some changes in his diet that he hoped would help him avoid heart disease.

As a result of Pritikin's concerns, Creek performed a series of blood tests and an EKG. He also sent Pritikin to a Sansum dietitian to have his diet evaluated.

The Sansum dietitian recorded that Pritikin's breakfast typically consisted of citrus fruit and cooked oatmeal with nonfat milk; he sometimes ate waffles and hotcakes made from whole grain flour. He also drank a glass of skim milk and occasionally ate some whole wheat toast with jam. For lunch he often had fish salad or a meat dish. At dinner, he ate fish or meat, potato, cooked vegetables, salad, some fruit or sherbet for dessert, and another glass of skim milk. He frequently ate nuts as a snack. The dietitian noted he drank about a quart of milk per day, ate only small amounts of salt, never drank alcohol or caffeinated beverages, and took only small amounts of water.

Under the head "deficiencies," the dietitian wrote, "Eggs especially," and then several spaces to the right a question mark before the word "fluid." The dietitian also noted in her summary: "Rather strict low-fat diet." Pritikin had trouble figuring out what was so strict or particularly low in fat about his diet. After he was through with the evaluation, Pritikin was sent back to Creek, who had the results of Nathan's blood test and EKG.

His blood cholesterol was 210 mg.%–a significant drop in cholesterol since his previous test two years before by Morrison. Creek said that his cholesterol level was normal. But Pritikin was troubled by the Sansum record which stated that a "normal" cholesterol level was anything between 150 mg.% and 300 mg.%. Based on his reading of the literature, Pritikin believed a cholesterol level of 300 mg.% caused rampant atherosclerosis and was probably life-threatening.

The EKG revealed Pritikin did indeed have heart disease. The Sansum record stated: "Posterior wall coronary insufficiency," a form of heart disease characterized by a lack of blood getting to the back, or posterior, part of the heart. The likely reason for his heart condition, Pritikin realized, was that he had advancing atherosclerosis in one or more of the arteries leading to the heart. At least one of his coronary arteries was being blocked by plaque, or cholesterol deposits, reducing the amount of blood and oxygen getting to the heart muscle. His heart was suffocating.

As a result of the diagnosis, Creek and Klakeg prescribed a drug called Atropine, which affects the flow of blood to the heart by influencing the vagus nerve, located in the neck. His doctors hoped that the Atropine would increase the blood flow to the heart, thus overcoming the insufficiency.

Pritikin was ordered not to exert himself. He was told not to walk more than four or five blocks a day, to take naps during the afternoons, and to eliminate all strenuous exercise, including bicycle riding and tennis.

Pritikin reacted to the advice with disbelief. He told Creek and Klakeg he had no symptoms of illness. They reminded him heart disease was, after all, a silent killer which often showed no outward symptoms until one was struck down. If he did not follow the advice, they warned him, he might one day find himself face down on the sidewalk as a result of a heart attack.

Pritikin left Sansum Clinic that day afraid and dejected; he had just come to California, where a new life seemed to be opening up to him. Now he was being told that he had to behave as if he were 20 years older than he was. But more puzzling news awaited him.

Three days later, on February 15, Creek did a blood test on Pritikin known as an electrophoresis, which reveals the balance of proteins in the blood. These proteins consist of albumins and a variety of globulins, or aggregates of proteins. In healthy adults there are fewer globulins than albumins, the ratio being at least two albumins to every single globulin. An imbalance of proteins can indicate the presence of cancer, hepatitis, cirrhosis of the liver, and other serious disorders. A diagnosis is made on the basis of which protein is imbalanced and to what degree.

Pritikin's electrophoresis analysis showed there was a distinct imbalance in his proteins. Sansum Clinic's record reads: "There is a gamma component in the protein electrophoretic pattern," meaning his test showed an abnormally high level of gamma globulins, or a type of globulin that contains and sometimes secretes antibodies. This abnormally high level of globulins is sometimes called a "spike." Clearly, there was something wrong with Pritikin's blood, but there was too little information for his doctors to make a diagnosis as yet. Nevertheless, a high gamma globulin rate suggests the potential for multiple myeloma, leukemia, and other forms of cancer. Apart from the heart disease, he showed no other signs of illness; all his other tests were normal.

From 1958 on, Pritikin's electrophoresis tests would consistently show this spike. That year the abnormality was small and no treatment was suggested. His physicians wanted to have electrophoresis tests done periodically to monitor his blood condition. They would have to wait to see what changes took place, if any. Nothing more was made of the test. It was puzzling, but even Pritikin did not consider it important.

As for the heart disease, neither Creek nor Klakeg believed that

Nathan's condition was especially severe. His EKG did not demonstrate an especially acute coronary insufficiency, according to Klakeg's assessment. As long as he followed his doctors' advice, there didn't seem to be much to worry about. In fact, both physicians expressed more concern over Pritikin's attitude toward his disease than the illness itself.

In addition, Creek was concerned about Pritikin's diet and on March 5, 1958, noted in Pritikin's patient record that he cautioned Nathan about his low-fat diet. He was afraid Pritikin might be depriving himself of vital nutrients. Creek wrote in Pritikin's record: "Be temperate in all things–including temperance." A year later, Klakeg expressed concern over Pritikin's attitude. In a March 18, 1959, letter to Lester Morrison, Klakeg noted Pritikin's "rather marked overconcern with his heart status, and this is his primary problem."

These rather patronizing comments by Creek and Klakeg illustrate the vastly different attitudes toward heart disease and its treatment taken by Pritikin and his doctors. For Pritikin, the conventional approach failed to address the underlying cause of the illness. It merely restricted his movements and tinkered with his nervous system. Unless he changed his diet, he believed, the cholesterol would continue to accumulate in his blood and further clog his arteries. The problem would only get worse. In time, more medication and restrictions would be necessary, until his arteries became so closed from plaque that he suffered either a heart attack or a stroke. The conventional approach seemed to guarantee such an end.

Pritikin did his best to convert both Creek and Klakeg to his point of view; he explained the literature linking diet to cardiovascular disease, and sent them additional studies in support of his argument. And while they recognized Nathan was well read on all subjects dealing with heart disease, they chose to ignore his pleas. Instead, the approach they took to Pritikin's heart condition was directly in line with standard medical practice. Neither one suggested he adopt a low-fat, low-cholesterol diet. Pritikin's desire to change his diet as a treatment of his disease was his own personal preference, and while Creek cautioned him about possible nutritional deficiencies, both doctors seemed to go along with Pritikin's desire to change his eating habits. In fact, at that time there was little, if any, support within the medical profession for altering one's diet to treat heart disease. (The American Medical Association did not endorse the concept of eating less fat and cholesterol until 1972, and even then the AMA refused to suggest how much of a reduction in these foods Americans should observe.)

Pritikin took the Atropine and restricted his activities. He gave up his tennis games, stopped bicycling to work, and tried to take an occasional nap in the afternoons. He did his best not to exert himself. Meanwhile, the Atropine so strongly affected his nervous system that it caused his eyes to dilate and forced him to wear sunglasses throughout the three-month period he took the drug.

It wasn't long, however, before he rebelled. Everything in his background as an inventor and a pioneer in other scientific fields, as well as his understanding of health, insisted he find another approach to his problems. The only approach he could believe in was one that addressed the underlying cause, which he believed was diet.

But where should he begin? Pritikin shared Creek's concern for dietary deficiencies. Eggs, meat, and dairy products are all high in fat and cholesterol, but they are also rich in protein, iron, vitamin B, and calcium. How many foods could he reduce or eliminate before he began to lose needed nutrients?

And yet, he could not remain on the Atropine. His eyes had grown increasingly sensitive to light, causing headaches and irritation, and the sunglasses were uncomfortable. At the end of April 1958, he stopped taking the drug and decided to treat his disease with a more restricted diet.

He wanted to create a diet that would be low in fat and cholesterol but met all nutritional needs. For that he needed an expert.

In May, Nathan contacted a nutritionist at the University of California at Los Angeles (UCLA) for an appointment to discuss his diet. As he strode along the university's well-manicured lawns and into the hallowed halls of academe, Pritikin was confident he and the nutritionist could devise the perfect diet to treat his heart disease.

Once in the nutritionist's office, Pritikin explained his dilemma. He told the scientist he wanted to create a diet for himself he could follow without fear of malnutrition. He asked if he could hire a graduate student to help him do it. The nutritionist said it couldn't be done.

The nutritionist told him lowering cholesterol by diet was dangerous, because it required that one "cut out foods high in fat and cholesterol and these are the best foods the body can eat.

"You've got to have those foods," the nutritionist told him.

Pritikin responded by saying animal studies had shown that when foods high in fat and cholesterol are lowered in the diet, blood cholesterol drops, which he believed reduced the chances of suffering a heart attack. The nutritionist countered that the elimination of such foods would lead to malnutrition. Also, lowering blood cholesterol would have no effect on his heart disease, the nutritionist said. One's cholesterol level is determined by heredity and, although it could be modified by diet, such altering would be dangerous.

"We can't help you," the nutritionist told Pritikin. "It's too dangerous; you might kill yourself."

His request for a graduate student was denied.

Pritikin left UCLA with the strong impression that there was a great deal nutritionists didn't know about diet and health. More than half the people in the world eat a diet that is low in fat and cholesterol and adequate in all the essential nutrients. Pritikin wanted to eat the same way they did. He wondered what was so difficult about that.

Nathan decided that if UCLA would not help him, then he would do it on his own. He got books on blood chemistry and nutrition and found out the levels of nutrients thought to be necessary to maintain health. He then got Creek to give him an open note to have regular blood tests performed, and within weeks of his meeting with the UCLA nutritionist, Pritikin showed up at the Blanchard-Dickson Laboratories in Santa Barbara with a list of 25 blood tests he wanted performed. In addition to a complete blood count, he wanted his blood values checked for pyruvic acid, fibrinogen, vitamin A and carotene, protein, folic acid, iron and iron-binding capacity, total lipids, protein-bound iodine, creatine, uric acid, macroglobulin, calcium, vitamin B, erythrocyte sedimentation rate, sodium, carbon dioxide levels, magnesium, free thyroxine, and leucine aminopeptidase. He planned to have these tests done every month or so to monitor the effects of his new diet on his blood values.

Dr. John P. Blanchard, who ran the laboratory, didn't quite know what to make of Pritikin and his rather lengthy request. According to Pritikin, it took Blanchard nearly an hour to figure out he would need four or five ounces of blood to conduct all the tests Pritikin wanted done. He then sent Nathan to the lab technician to have his blood drawn.

Pritikin expected his blood to be drawn in a syringe, but the lab technician took out a transfusion needle, telling him, "We can't get that much blood from a syringe."

The technician attached a rubber hose to one end of the transfusion needle and inserted the hose into a bottle. He then injected the needle into Pritikin's vein in the arm. Nathan turned white watching his blood drip into the bottle.

Seeing "my blood coming out in such volume, I nearly fainted on the chair," Pritikin recalled.

The technician noticed Nathan becoming ill and reassured him: "Don't worry," he said, "as long as you're sitting down you can't hurt yourself."

A Personal Experiment with Diet

For the next ten years, Pritikin kept meticulous track of his health through blood tests and urinalysis. Beginning in May 1958, Pritikin accumulated all his medical records to date and recorded the information on sheets of notebook paper which he taped together side by side to form

11-inch by 15-inch sheets. He drew vertical lines over the horizontal lines already on the notebook paper to form a graph design. At the top of the graph columns, he wrote the date of the blood and urine tests; the dates on his records begin in 1955 (he recorded the blood test given him by Morrison) and run through the late 1950s, 1960s, and 1970s. On the far left-hand side of the sheets, at the top of the page, he wrote the word "blood" and then "O-Group" (Pritikin had O+ blood). In the left-hand margin, he listed all the elements in his blood that he regularly had tested–more than 50 blood constituents in all. Included in the list were his red blood cell count, white blood cells, hemoglobin, platelets, lactic acid, rouleaux formation, fibrinogen, fasting glucose, nonfasting glucose, sodium, potassium, chloride, carbon dioxide levels, vitamin A and carotene, vitamin B, folic acid, iron, iron-binding capacity, calcium, cholesterol, total lipids, triglycerides, uric acid, neutral fats, and many others.

His urine chart was equally detailed.

By June 1958, at the age of 43, Pritikin started to make daring changes in his diet. He ate little else but lentil beans for weeks; then he switched to brown rice for another week; then he added beef. For the most part, his diet was centered around whole grains, vegetables, and fruits, but he would change the proportions of these foods–increasing fruit for a time, or rice, or beans–or simply add beef or fish or poultry for a week. He'd check his blood values and eliminate the food he was experimenting with, or bring it back into balance with the rest of his diet. He tried to isolate the effects of each food on his blood chemistry and his overall health. He would carry on this diligent experimentation for the next decade.

Pritikin recorded such details as "eating 10 dates after dinner"; "start fruit at 1,000 calories 55 percent total intake." One of his notes, recorded on December 17, 1968, states, "three weeks on fruit at 55 to 60 percent of total calories, 1,000-1,200 calories fruit."

He studied his body's reaction to every change in diet he made. On January 29, 1969, he wrote: "22 days on dried fruit, 12 dates, 60 percent calories on dried fruit; calories 1,800, was thirsty last two weeks, constant dry taste in mouth."

His cholesterol level rose and fell with his dietary changes. He noted his cholesterol high of 280 mg.% in 1955. From there it dropped steadily to 102 mg.% on December 24, 1963, after he started legumes as his exclusive protein source. His cholesterol level shot back up to 158 mg.% after he eliminated brown rice and started to eat one meal of meat or fish per day. From there his cholesterol gradually declined to 118 mg.% after he discontinued meat and resumed his normal diet of grains, vegetables, fruit, and occasional servings of fish.

Over the years, Pritikin came to have such a thorough knowledge of his body that he would be able to pinpoint obscure aspects of his diet as the source of a given symptom. Later, he would also be able to do the same for patients and for doctors who wrote to him describing patient symptoms that seemed to have no cause.

Pritikin's thorough investigation of how food affected his body reveals his remarkable ability to look at himself objectively. He refused to turn away from unpleasant or even frightening information. Unlike the typical patient, who surrenders to his doctor's advice, Pritikin took a cool and systematic approach to his health. His thoroughness and high degree of objectivity enabled him to make rational assessments based on the raw data.

This is not to say he wasn't afraid–years later he would admit as much when he told audiences how he created his program–but his fear did not stop him from doing what he thought best. And given the choice, he felt much more confident in his own plan than in orthodox methods, which promised no cure and required him to take drugs and restrict his movements.

If Nathan was secure in his decision, Ilene was anything but. Ilene had grown accustomed to her husband's unconventional ideas, but this time she felt he was really stretching it. Why didn't he take his medicine and be done with it? The disease did not seem life-threatening; many of her friends had high blood pressure or some other form of coronary disease and they seemed content to follow their doctors' orders. There were times when Ilene wondered if Nathan was just being difficult.

"I thought, 'Who is he to challenge the medical world and go off in a very strange direction?' " Ilene recalled. It seemed to her that Nathan was being extreme and a little peculiar; she also felt uncomfortable with what she considered his basically antisocial behavior.

Besides, Nathan's change of diet left Ilene a little offended. She took pride in the meals she prepared. Ilene read the conventional cookbooks, spent a lot of time in the kitchen preparing hearty and gourmet dishes, and felt she was providing the best meals she could for her family. Now Nathan had turned away from the pot roasts, the beef stews, and the meat loaves and started to eat what he was calling a "peasant diet."

Ilene was perplexed. What had gotten into him?

As Nathan said to Dr. John McDougall, physician and author, in a videotaped interview in 1982: "My wife thought I needed a psychiatrist more than I did a medical doctor."

Nevertheless, Ilene went along with him, preparing his brown rice, vegetables, beans, and fish, or, when he was experimenting, making some specific food in the quantities he wanted. As his experimenting began to show results, however, her skepticism slowly dissipated.

"Nathan did what he had to do at all times," Ilene recalled. "He conducted his own life. He relied upon me for companionship, but he was very self-directed."

Pritikin did not enforce his views on his family, or anyone else for that matter. He believed people would change when they wanted to. He maintained this attitude especially toward his children, who looked at his change in eating habits with a combination of wonder and humor.

"We kind of accepted that he was right," recalled his son Ralph. "Dad would explain what he was doing in the most rational way so that even us kids could understand. Pretty soon, everyone in the house wanted to eat what Dad was eating."

By the summer of 1958, Pritikin had some strong scientific evidence for his dietary program. The Framingham Heart Study, which examined the risk factors in the onset of heart disease among residents of Framingham, Massachusetts, published data showing that the higher one's blood cholesterol level, the greater the risk of heart disease. The Framingham Study, an ongoing study begun in 1948, revealed that people with cholesterol levels of 256 mg.% and over were 15 times more likely to suffer a heart attack than those with cholesterol levels below 193 mg.%.

In that same year, Dr. J. B. Hannah, a physician who worked for a Northern Rhodesian mining company, reported that the Bantus, a race of people who populate southern Africa, experience virtually no heart disease. They subsist on a low-fat, low-cholesterol diet, eat mostly whole grains, vegetables, and fruits, and suffer none of the common degenerative diseases that plague the modern industrialized world. During Hannah's five-year study, in which he followed the death rates of both Bantus and whites being treated in Nkana Nune Hospital, not a single Bantu died of heart disease. Among the relatively small population of whites treated at the hospital, 23 Europeans died of heart disease during the same period. And despite their vegetarian diet, Hannah reported, the Bantus experienced no nutritional-deficiency diseases.

Dr. H. M. Whyte studied the aborigines in New Guinea, who also eat a diet low in fat and cholesterol, and discovered the same phenomenon: a remarkably low rate of heart disease. Whyte also discovered that as the New Guineans got older, their blood pressure decreased by about ten points. In the United States, blood pressure tends to increase with age, thus increasing the risk of heart attack and stroke.

As a result of these and other studies, Nathan became intensely interested in the lives of so-called "primitive" peoples. All over the world, populations existed largely on vegetarian diets, supplemented by small amounts of animal foods. They carried on their lives outside the influences of technology, including food processing. They ate a diet that had been handed down to them through the millennia, and their physical health seemed to reflect the benefits of their diets and lifestyles.

The native population that would later inspire Pritikin the most was clearly the Tarahumara Indians of central Mexico, a tribe of 50,000. Pritikin would point to them as the best example of what human physical stamina was capable of on a simple diet. The Tarahumara, who were studied in the 1970s, eat mostly corn, wild plants, squash, beans, and small amounts of fish and meat. Animal products are consumed more as a condiment than a staple. They are a farming people who enjoy playing a game similar to kickball, but their wooden ball is kicked for more than 100 miles without stopping. The pace is 6 to 7 miles per hour, and research has shown that the only reason a player drops out of the game is for leg cramps or the need to urinate. Otherwise they keep right on running. As Pritikin would write years later, the Tarahumara "lead us to conclude we have hardly scratched the surface of man's physical capability when in his healthy state."

The study of native populations made Pritikin question many of the fundamental ideas in nutrition. He wondered if the Recommended Dietary Allowances (RDAs), the U.S. standard for healthy levels of specific nutrients, weren't inflated. He also questioned the Western world's dependence upon meat, eggs, and dairy foods for essential nutrients such as calcium and protein.

The Bantus, for example, eat only about 350 mg. of calcium per day. The RDA for calcium in the United States is 800 mg. to 1000 mg. And yet, Bantu mothers bear and nurse an average of nine children and have no calcium deficiencies.

He discovered that traditional peoples around the world stop drinking milk after they are weaned, and yet they suffer from no calcium deficiencies. Where do they get their calcium? Pritikin would find from his studies of nutrition that many green vegetables, such as collard and mustard greens, are loaded with calcium. A cup of milk contains about 300 mg. of calcium, while a cup of cooked collard greens contains about 320 mg. of calcium; a cup of cooked mustard greens has about 280 mg. Fish also contains calcium, as well as other minerals.

A diet consisting of whole grains, vegetables, and fruits can contain all the necessary vitamins and minerals, Pritikin would learn, with the possible exception of B_{12}, which is also available in vegetables that are not well rinsed or peeled, such as carrots or potatoes. Vitamin B_{12} exists in common bacteria, which are present in fermented foods and foods that are not peeled or washed.

Animal foods, of course, are rich in B_{12}. The amount of B_{12} required is so minimal that it takes between five and ten years for a B_{12} deficiency to manifest, but Nathan regularly ate fish and, for the time being, experimented with lean meat, so he did not have to worry about lacking B₁₂.

Nathan concluded that the so-called primitives, such as the Bantus and New Guineans, don't suffer from nutrient deficiencies, because unrefined, natural foods contain adequate nutrition.

But what about protein? Surely a diet low in meat, eggs, and dairy products will be low, and possibly deficient, in protein.

When he researched the literature, he found just the opposite. The average American diet, consisting of foods from the Basic Four Food Groups, derives between 17 and 25 percent of its total calories from protein. He discovered, however, that studies done on men eating as little as 6 percent of their total calories in protein showed no protein deficiency. He also found that when humans consume more than 15 percent protein, their bodies began to lose minerals, especially calcium, iron, zinc, phosphorus, and magnesium.

Pritikin began to suspect that the typical American diet was not just excessive in fat and cholesterol, but also in protein and refined carbohydrates. The whole diet was off, he realized, causing myriad problems. And he had just scratched the surface.

That summer of 1958, Nathan's program had begun to show some good results. His cholesterol level had dropped to 160 mg.% and his blood values were consistently normal.

"It really was not that complicated," Pritikin would say years later about changing his diet. "After a couple of months, I realized I was no different than any of the animal studies. The same way animals drop their cholesterol level, so do humans. I never did run into deficiencies, or have any problems at all with getting adequate nutrition. I was just frightened unnecessarily."

Nathan continued to refine and adhere strictly to his diet for the next year. He had always been spry and energetic, but he found his energy levels consistently high and his endurance better than ever. He discovered that complex carbohydrates–or long sugar molecules found in whole grains, vegetables, and fruits–provide far better fuel for the body than simple sugars. The sugar or carbohydrates from whole grains, for example, burn slowly, providing the body with a long-term energy supply. Simple sugars, on the other hand, provide a quick burst of energy that is burned rapidly– much like pushing the gas pedal to the floor of one's car–resulting in a net loss of energy and a condition known as hypoglycemia.

He was aware of an increase in mental clarity and an overall feeling of well-being. Nathan was convinced that he was on the right track.

A year later, on August 29, 1959–Pritikin's 44th birthday–Creek ran a series of blood tests on Nathan and found his cholesterol level was 155 mg.%, his calcium was 10.5 mg.% (normal), and his hemoglobin was 14.7 grams (normal). After more than a year on his diet, these and other blood values were all well within healthy ranges and his cholesterol level was low.

He did no exercise at all during this period. He thought it best to avoid physical exertion until his EKG showed that his heart condition was improving, and by December 1959, he hoped his EKG would show exactly that.

Unfortunately, the test, done on December 21, 1959, at Sansum Medical Clinic, showed no real improvement in his coronary insufficiency. His EKG still showed the presence of heart disease.

Once again, Creek sent Pritikin to the Sansum dietitian to have his diet assessed. According to the Sansum record taken that day, Pritikin's diet typically was made up of the following:

Breakfast usually consisted of oatmeal or seven-grain cereal with skim milk; he also ate a whole citrus fruit–either an orange or a grapefruit–or a sliced melon five times per week; hot cakes made with whole grain flour once a week; smoked fish with whole grain cereal once a week, and a glass of fruit juice daily. (Eventually, Nathan stopped drinking fruit juice. He maintained the best way to eat fruit was to eat the whole fruit; this way, one got all the nutrition and fiber available from the food, which didn't happen from drinking just the juice.)

For lunch, he ate salmon or tuna fish sandwiches on whole grain bread; brown rice or corn or potato; cooked vegetables; salad greens with dressing; fruit juice, lemonade, or water; and fruit for dessert.

For dinner, Pritikin ate fish four times per week, often as a casserole; he also liked shellfish. Dinner also included potato or brown rice, cooked vegetables, salad, and some type of fruit dessert.

He ate what the dietitian called "moderate" amounts of salt, "small" amounts of oil (usually corn oil), four or more bananas a week, nuts daily, and drank "moderate" amounts of water. His practice was to drink only when he was thirsty.

Obviously, he had deviated considerably from the Basic Four.

At the bottom of the Sansum record, the dietitian noted Pritikin's deficiencies as "milk, egg, meat."

Nathan was disappointed by the latest stress test. What was he doing wrong? He questioned whether a cholesterol level of 155 mg.% was low enough to reverse his condition, and whether he had given his program enough time. How long did it take to reverse heart disease?

Despite the hours he spent wrestling with these questions, Pritikin remained convinced his approach was correct. Once again, he pored over his records and made adjustments in his diet. He eliminated all nuts and the occasional piece of meat he was eating. He ate only small amounts of lean fish and poultry, along with ample servings of whole grains, vegetables, beans, and fruit.

By early spring 1960, his cholesterol level had fallen to 120 mg.%. In

June, Pritikin was ready to try another electrocardiogram.

Nathan didn't know what to expect from this EKG–surely his own reading of his health was good, but the last EKG test offered no real reason for hope and so he went into the test with an attitude of acceptance. To his great satisfaction, the test was normal. The June 15 EKG test record states: "Definite improvement since the tracing of December 15, 1959 . . . Normal electrocardiogram."

Next, A Personal Exercise Program

Nathan was elated. He had already proven he could lower his cholesterol level by diet without suffering from deficiency diseases. Now he had shown that by lowering his cholesterol level and keeping it low for a period of two years, he had improved the health of his heart. As far as he knew, he was the only person to have consciously done this.

There was still a long way to go. The EKG was again done with only minimal exertion, indicating his heart was getting enough blood and oxygen as long as he did not perform any kind of extended exercise, such as running or calisthenics. Exercise would cause the heart to beat faster, requiring more blood to pass through the coronary arteries and to the heart. Nathan realized there must still be atherosclerosis in his coronary arteries that would limit the amount of blood flow to the heart, thus creating insufficiency. In short, he had made progress, but he wasn't fully cured yet.

It was time to broaden his approach, he decided. Pritikin's studies had led him into an area that was little understood: the effects of exercise on the circulatory system. He had discovered research showing that when dogs were forced to exercise, they grew new capillaries in their legs and chest to better nourish the cells. The more they were exercised, the more capillaries they developed. This intrigued Pritikin. Could the human body grow new circulation with exercise?

The study suggested to him that if he could develop an exercise program for himself, he might be able to grow new circulation in parts of his body that were not getting sufficient blood and oxygen, including the heart.

The study on dogs was done in Germany. Nathan had had his copy translated into English. He knew of no other study demonstrating that new circulation could be produced, except in the case of coronary care patients who had recently suffered a heart attack. These patients often grow new coronary veins and capillaries as the body rallied to keep itself alive. Pritikin wondered if there was other research that might indicate that exercise helped to develop new circulation. Once again, he needed an expert–or so he thought.

Creek recommended a well-known circulation expert at a large California university. Pritikin called the researcher, who, for purposes of this book, will be called Dr. Smith, and made an appointment with him to discuss the literature.

Shortly thereafter, the two met in Smith's impressive office. Graduate degrees and various board appointments hung on the doctor's wall. A floor-to-ceiling bookcase, each shelf filled with books, ran along a wall that was 15 feet long and 8 feet high. The man himself sat imperiously behind a large desk, with an air of impatience and authority that seemed to hurry Pritikin to the point.

Nathan explained why he had come. "I want to grow collaterals," he said. Collaterals are secondary or accessory blood vessels to the heart and other parts of the body.

Smith dismissed the idea as ridiculous. "You can't grow new capillaries," he told Pritikin. "You only have what you were born with."

Nathan held up his study and explained the results of the research.

"First of all, that's about dogs, not humans," said Smith. "And is this the only study you could find?" Pritikin said it was, but that he planned to keep looking.

"What about people who have a heart attack?" Pritikin reminded him. "They grow collaterals right there in the coronary care ward."

"That's the only exception," Smith stated. When the body is near death, it will grow new collaterals to keep itself alive.

Pritikin suggested that if dogs have been shown to grow new capillaries from exercise, perhaps it was possible for humans, too.

Growing impatient now, Smith pointed to his enormous wall-length bookcase and said: "That will tell you that you can't grow new capillaries."

Pritikin looked at the bookcase and at his study and was "very discouraged."

What the scientist was telling him, in essence, was that heart disease could not be cured. There were only two ways to get more blood to the heart: grow new blood vessels or reverse atherosclerosis–that is, clear the artery's pathway of plaque. Studies done on monkeys at the University of Iowa had shown atherosclerosis could be reversed in primates given a low-fat, low-cholesterol diet, but the same type of study had never been done on humans, and very few scientists believed reversal of atherosclerosis in humans was possible. If the experts were right, then Pritikin could not grow new circulation or reverse his atherosclerosis–and he could not improve the condition of his heart. Once again, he faced another brick wall.

He went home that day thinking that exercise was out of the question.

In the following weeks, he continued to read the literature on exercise and found two more animal studies demonstrating the growth of new blood vessels as a result of exercise. He considered his conversation with

Smith, and Smith's enormous bookcase; he considered the warnings of Creek and Klakeg not to exercise; and he thought about the animal studies. And then he decided to start exercising.

The first thing he did was to go back to Creek and ask permission to have electrocardiogram stress tests done at Cottage Hospital in Santa Barbara whenever he wanted them. He explained to Creek that he wanted to begin exercising, but needed to keep track of the effects of exercise on his heart. The only way he could do that was to have regular stress tests performed. It would take too long to have to set up appointments with Sansum Clinic, he said; he wanted the tests done quickly in order to monitor the condition of his heart accurately. He told Creek he had taught himself to read EKG tracings and would take responsibility if something happened.

Creek didn't like it. He had warned Pritikin at length about the dangers of stressing his heart; moreover, he didn't know if Pritikin was capable of reading EKG tracings. After considerable debate, the two went to Cottage Hospital, where Pritikin was given a stress test that he read accurately for Creek. Finally, Creek relented and gave Pritikin an open note to have regular stress tests performed.

Pritikin started his exercise program slowly and cautiously. He was afraid that the experts were right: if he overexerted himself, he would bring on a heart attack that could be fatal. So he decided to start with short distances. He began by walking the total of six blocks per day in three walks of two blocks each. After he arrived at his office in the morning, he'd walk a block or so and then return. He walked again at noon and once more in the evenings in his backyard. After he'd walk a block, he would stop and check his pulse. He'd count the number of beats per minute and check to see if the pulse was consistent.

Pritikin carried on this routine for a week, after which he took a stress test at Cottage Hospital that showed no deterioration of his heart. For the next two weeks, he increased his daily distances to eight blocks per day. He had another stress test that again showed that his coronary insufficiency was no worse. Three weeks later, he was up to a total of nine blocks, and once again his stress test showed his heart was no worse.

For the next month, he walked for about a quarter mile a day without stopping. He increased it to two quarter-mile walks per day for another month and had another stress test. The test showed that the abnormality in his heart was starting to disappear; his heart was getting more blood.

He was clearly making progress. He was tempted to increase his distances markedly but he refused to be hurried; he was still concerned about the consequences of pushing himself too hard. Nathan was prepared to take the slow and incremental approach. Patience and persistence would lead to the goal. Besides, there was still a knife poised at his heart.

Pritikin gradually worked his way up to walking a mile and a half per day at a moderate pace without stopping. In the meantime, he continued his study of the literature on both diet and exercise.

The research detailing the effects of exercise on the body, and particularly on the heart and circulatory system, was still in its infancy in the early 1960s, but the studies pointed in the same direction–at least as far as Pritikin was concerned.

In 1955, Dr. Claude Beck demonstrated that oxygen differentials within the heart are responsible for a great number of heart attacks. There are three coronary arteries providing blood and oxygen to the heart. The heart is oxygenated unevenly when one or two coronary arteries are blocked with plaque to a greater extent than the remaining artery or arteries, therefore creating a condition whereby part of the heart is suffocating while the other parts are getting sufficient oxygen. When this condition occurs, the electrical currents constantly moving through the heart and causing the heart to beat also become uneven. Uneven electrical currents can throw the heart muscle into a spasm, which causes uncoordinated beating to occur, or a type of heart attack called fibrillation. Beck noted the heart's condition is more dangerous when it is unevenly oxygenated than when the arteries are uniformly clogged.

This study showed why bursts of exercise in people who are not well conditioned often cause sudden death due to fibrillation of the heart.

(Years later, Pritikin was to sound the alarm to runners who ate diets high in fat and cholesterol. His book *Diet for Runners*, which was published in 1985, reported many cases of runners who were struck down with heart attacks because they ate a diet high in fat and cholesterol and then stressed the heart by running.)

Other studies showed that the condition of the heart can be improved by a program of gradual exercise.

In 1957, R. W. Eckstein compared the arteries of two groups of dogs; one group was exercised regularly and the other was allowed to rest. He found that dogs that were exercised grew new blood vessels to the heart at a much greater rate than those left to rest.

In 1958, Dr. Paul Dudley White, who was President Dwight Eisenhower's personal physician, surveyed 335 former athletes and found that none of those who maintained vigorous exercise had suffered heart attacks. (Research has since shown that exercise alone is not enough to fully protect a person from heart disease caused by atherosclerosis. Only a low-fat, low-cholesterol diet will do that, but exercise will help to maintain the health of the heart and forestall a heart attack.)

J. Tepperman reported in 1961 that rats made to run one mile per day for 36 days experienced a 27 percent growth in their coronary vascular system, or what is known as the coronary tree.

The following year, H. L. Taylor and his co-workers studied railroad workers and found that clerks who remain sedentary experience twice as many heart attacks as railroad switchmen, whose jobs are physically demanding.

These and other studies reinforced Pritikin's confidence in his program and kept him exercising despite the warnings of doom that came from his doctors.

By the fall of 1961, Pritikin took a stress test that was almost normal at Cottage Hospital. Now he knew he had nearly beaten his heart disease. He felt it was time to increase his exercise routine. Each day, after he completed his mile-and-a-half walk, he went into his backyard and ran 10 to 20 steps. As always, he walked and ran in long trousers and street shoes. After he ran the 20 steps, he'd check his pulse. All was well.

After a couple of weeks of running 20 steps in his backyard, he gradually increased his distances until he reached a quarter-mile run without stopping.

And then his knee gave way. He was running laps in his backyard when suddenly a searing pain stabbed through his knee, buckled it, and sent him to the ground. He got up limping, his knee in agony.

After a few days' rest, Pritikin went to an orthopedic surgeon in Santa Barbara, who examined the knee and asked if he had been playing football with his children. No, Nathan replied. He'd been running.

"Running?" the doctor asked. "You can't run; you're 46 years old. You'll wear out all the cartilage in your knees if you run. By the time you're 50, you'll need a cane to get around. If you want to exercise, you'll have to swim. People over 40 can't run."

Nathan did not enjoy swimming and, as a result, did not think he could bring himself to swim enough to produce secondary vessel growth.

"I can't grow any collateral circulation by swimming," Pritikin responded.

"Grow collaterals? What do you mean?" asked the doctor.

Pritikin looked at the physician, realized he didn't have a sympathetic ear, and changed the subject.

"Can't I change my shoes or my gait or something to make it possible to run?" he asked.

"No. People over 40 can't run."

The verdict sounded final and Pritikin was disappointed. He had just started to enjoy running. He guessed he'd have to go back to walking, but his dreams of ever attaining a high degree of fitness seemed to evaporate in the doctor's office.

Three weeks later, his knee was healed. On a warm fall evening, Pritikin walked out of his backyard and decided to have one more quick run while he had some conditioning.

Before he ran, he uncharacteristically kicked off his shoes. He ran a few laps. He felt no pain in his knee, so he ran a few more laps. And then he realized his problem was not his knee.

"At that point, I realized that you can't run in street shoes," Pritikin would recall years later.

There was no running craze in 1961, nor was there the sophisticated running shoe that would come more than a decade later. So Nathan designed his own running shoe and brought his design to a shoe manufacturer, who made sneakers with specifically designed soles Pritikin had ordered.

"I never had a knee problem again," recalled Pritikin.

From that point on, Pritikin was literally off and running. Along the winding roads of Santa Barbara, running in long trousers and his specially designed sneakers, Pritikin was indeed an anomaly, a man so much ahead of his time that those who drove by him as he jogged didn't know what to make of him. Motorists would often stop and ask if he needed help; was he fleeing from some danger? "No, I'm fine," he would tell them, and keep right on going.

His conditioning improved rapidly and the miles began to pile up–one mile a day this week, two the next, three a month later. And he loved it. Running put him in touch with the wondrous endurance, coordination, and utility of the human body. "Man was made to walk," he used to say, but running was for him a more exciting expression of what humans were capable of. Physical conditioning was more than a concept–it was a way of reaching a high state of being. He marveled at the incredible abilities of the human machine, every system infinitely complex yet subtly coordinated, doing a million tasks at once, and yet doing them together. To push this beautiful machine, to make it perform feats of endurance and grace that were beyond its previous limits, was for Pritikin an almost magical capacity of the human body. Properly nourished and conditioned, there was no telling what the body and mind could do. It was this mystery of human potential that Pritikin was in search of as much as anything else.

Prognosis: No More Heart Disease

The new program resulted in a remarkable improvement in his stress tests. Both his resting EKG and his Master Two-Step stress test no longer detected any trace of coronary insufficiency. There were only two explanations for his accomplishment: either he had grown new circulation that provided increased blood flow to the heart, thus overcoming his insufficiency, or he had reversed his atherosclerosis, clearing the artery's pathway of plaque. The latter possibility was far more astonishing than the former, and so Pritikin assumed the more conservative point of view: he maintained that he grew new circulation, since he could not prove he had reversed the atherosclerosis. Reversal had never been shown in humans. Nevertheless, he did in fact think reversal of atherosclerosis was possible, and even likely on a low fat and cholesterol diet, but he didn't know how long it would take to accomplish. For the time being, he was content to say he had reversed his condition by growing new circulation and to leave the larger question to further study.

Pritikin's recovery left him with a feeling of rebirth. By the spring of 1962, he was exercising daily, was in excellent physical condition, and was maintaining a diet based primarily on whole grains, vegetables, fruit, and small amounts of fish and poultry. Moreover, it was a diet he enjoyed eating.

Pritikin realized that his battle with heart disease was of far greater significance than one man's struggle against a life-threatening illness. More than one million people died of heart disease each year in the United States, and another 40 million suffered from it. Heart disease accounted for more than $40 billion in research and treatment, to say nothing of lost productivity and human suffering. Illnesses of the heart and arteries represented the single greatest plague humans had ever faced.

He saw the established methods of treating cardiovascular disease as utter failures. As long as the cause of the illness was not addressed, the disease would continue to spread unchecked until it destroyed the patient. More important was the fact that most cardiovascular disease could be prevented. People could eliminate the threat of the disease from their lives by making significant changes in diet. In addition, thousands of people with heart disease could be saved by adopting a low-fat, low-cholesterol diet, Pritikin believed.

When he considered the scope of the problem and the standard treatment of the disease, he realized that his method for treating himself had far-reaching importance. He wondered if he could somehow standardize his approach to make it simple to understand and easy to use. Before he could do that, he would have to know a lot more about the effects of his program on other aspects of health.

Beginning in late 1963, Pritikin intensified his study of nutrition and analyzed every food he ate for its nutritional content. On April 3, 1964, for example, he noted that he ate 2½ oranges, 150 grams of oats, and 8 ounces of lentils for breakfast. The oranges gave him 300 international units (I.U.) of vitamin A, 0.15 mg. of thiamine, 0.05 mg. of riboflavin, 0.3 mg. of niacin, and 80 mg. of vitamin C. The oats provided 1.0 mg. of thiamine, 0.2 mg. of riboflavin, and 1.5 mg. of niacin. The lentils contained 1.25 mg. of thiamine, 0.54 mg. of riboflavin, 5.0 mg. of niacin, 11 mg. of vitamin C, and 1,270 I.U. of vitamin A.

He carried on the same kind of analysis for lunch and dinner. He wanted to know the value of every food available. He calculated the total nutritional value of his diet and then compared it to the Recommended Dietary Allowances. Nathan found that his diet was equal or superior to the nutritional content the RDAs recommended.

As he would say over and over again in years to come, unprocessed foods–"food as grown" was the way he liked to put it–were far superior in nutritional content to refined foods, which lose vitamins, minerals, protein, and fiber during processing.

From 1964 to the early 1970s, Pritikin experimented with his diet to come up with a regimen that promoted optimal health. He started his search by trying to formulate a diet for himself, but that led him to the larger question of what might be the ideal diet for people. The basis of this belief was twofold: the scientific evidence supported the view that certain foods promoted health while others promoted illness; the second was simple logic. Like everything else in nature, humans had evolved over millions of years, constantly adapting to the environment, gaining new abilities, losing old ones. It stood to reason that the highly specialized body had grown accustomed to, and dependent upon, certain foods in the environment. At the same time, it would find certain other foods foreign and, if eaten in sufficient quantities, even poisonous. Pritikin liked to use the example of cyanide, which is present in minute quantities in apricots. Because the quantities are so small, the body can tolerate the cyanide without adverse side effects. Fat and cholesterol can also be eaten in small quantities, he maintained, but when these quantities are exceeded, they become toxic. Later, he would coin the word "lipotoxemia" to indicate the poisoning of the body from excessive fats and cholesterol.

Based on the scientific evidence and the practical experience of native populations, Pritikin believed grains, vegetables, and fruit were the central foods for humans. These were the foods nature had provided in abundance. Certain other low-fat animal foods, such as fish, lean meat, poultry, and skim milk, could also be consumed, but in far lower quantities.

The modern diet, which is rich in animal foods–including beef, pork, eggs, butter, cheese, and whole milk–as well as highly refined foods such as processed grains, simple sugars, and artificial ingredients, is an anomaly when looked at from the point of view of evolution. It is only in recent history that such foods have become available in these quantities–as in the case of beef–or available at all, as in the case of artificial colors, flavors, or preservatives.

He accepted that the body would eventually decline and die–these were as natural as birth, he said–but the life span of humans should be far longer than 60 to 70 years, he maintained. Given the right foods and sufficient exercise and rest, the body should survive 120 years, Pritikin believed.

By February 1966, Pritikin believed he was ready for the ultimate test: a stress test done on a treadmill. Treadmills had been developed during the 1960s to mechanically replicate varying degrees of stress on the heart and circulatory system. The person stepped up on a treadmill and walked or ran at the speed at which the treadmill moved. Meanwhile, an electrocardiogram monitored the beating of the heart. Stress tests done on treadmills are extremely accurate and sensitive to methods of determining the relative health of the heart.

The only treadmill readily available to Pritikin in 1966 was in the university laboratory of the very scientist who five years earlier had told Pritikin that he could not grow new circulation: Dr. Smith.

Early in February, Pritikin went back to Smith and asked him if he could have a stress test done on the scientist's treadmill. Smith agreed, but told Pritikin to bring along a cardiologist because Smith did not want to take responsibility if Pritikin dropped dead on his treadmill.

On February 16, 1966, Pritikin arrived at Smith's lab with a cardiologist and was ready to take his stress test. Years later, Nathan recalled the events of that day in detail, and not without touches of absurd comedy.

According to Pritikin, the treadmill he was about to get on was enormous: three feet by ten feet. "It looked like it tested cows," Nathan recalled.

"Are you going to run in long pants?" Smith asked Pritikin.

"I always run in long pants," Pritikin replied.

"It's different here," Dr. Smith said. "When you run outside, you get a breeze, but here you're standing still while you run; you won't have any breeze that you create. Only the treadmill moves."

He then gave Pritikin a pair of shorts to wear; Nathan put them on and then told the doctor and his nurse standing by that he was ready for the test.

"Not yet," said Smith. "We've got to take some preliminary tests."

"What tests?" Pritikin asked. "I just want to run on the treadmill."

"This is a scientific laboratory; we have to run some tests," said Smith.

The scientist then explained that Pritikin's temperature would have to be taken and he'd have to be weighed; both tests would be done before he got on the treadmill and again immediately after he got off it.

"You're going to gain some temperature and we have to see how many degrees you gain," Smith said.

Pritikin acquiesced and opened his mouth for the nurse. The nurse promptly told him "We don't take temperature that way. It's not accurate enough. Bend over."

"Well, for the sake of science," Nathan replied, and bent over. A few minutes later, the nurse told him that his temperature was 99.5 degrees. She explained the rectal temperature is one point higher than normal.

"Thank you. I'm very glad to know that," Pritikin said.

The nurse proceeded to weigh him. Then he was told to get on the treadmill.

This particular treadmill was a very sophisticated device. The electrodes that were attached to the body were wired to a radio transmitter that sent a signal to the electrocardiograph, which monitored the heart. There were no wires between Pritikin and the treadmill to restrict his movements. Moreover, this treadmill registered a two-inch tracing every second, meaning that the electrocardiogram paper traveled two inches every second and therefore was able to give very precise readings on every single beat of the heart. (Most treadmills today provide only one-inch tracings per minute.)

Pritikin was then asked what protocol he wanted to use. He explained that he wanted to run at 8½ miles per hour, or 1 mile in 7 minutes, and he wanted to run for 20 minutes, or approximately 3 miles. That's what he was accustomed to doing. He also asked that the EKG tape run continuously so that he had a record of every heartbeat. The scientist agreed and Pritikin stepped up on the treadmill.

The machine began to roll slowly and Pritikin went from a walking pace to a brisk run within minutes.

"I was very glad that they had me put shorts on," Pritikin recalled. "Even though you're running, you're standing still; there's no wind at all. The sweat came down me in such a fury that my socks were getting wet."

After 20 minutes the machine began to slow down and soon stopped. Sensing he had accomplished what the experts said was impossible, Pritikin was bursting with anticipation.

"I was very, very happy when the treadmill started to slow down. I can't tell you how happy I was that the treadmill started to slow down," said Nathan.

He got off the treadmill and was eager to see the EKG tracings. "I was trying to catch my breath when the nurse said, 'Bend over.' "

After taking his temperature again, the nurse told him his temperature had risen several degrees.

"Don't worry, it'll cool down later," Pritikin assured her. He was then weighed and told he had lost two pounds, which he facetiously promised to drink back.

Meanwhile, Smith was looking at the tracings from the electrocardio-gram, "just like a broker in a stock market office where the ticker tape is all over the floor," Pritikin recalled.

Pritikin asked him if he saw any sign of coronary insufficiency.

"Not yet," Smith said.

The two of them looked through the tape twice but could find no trace of coronary disease. The EKG noted that Pritikin's heartbeat had gotten up to 177 beats per minute and stayed there. Not a single beat revealed any hint of coronary insufficiency.

There were only two ways that Pritikin could have overcome his coronary insufficiency: either he reversed his atherosclerosis or he grew new circulation.

Pritikin looked at Smith and asked, "Why don't we find any coronary insufficiency? The only way that could happen is if I have more blood [going to the heart]." The question came at Smith like a long, threatening sword.

"Well, you must have more blood," the scientist said.

"Where do you think it came from?" Pritikin asked slyly, as if inching the sword closer to Smith. "Is it possible I could have developed collateral circulation?"

Smith grunted and said, "Well, it's possible."

CHAPTER 5

A Mystery Disease Surfaces

"*I* can't tell you how elated I was. I knew I no longer had coronary insufficiency and I was finished with my heart problem. From that point on, I knew I would try to convert everyone in the world to a new way of living."

Those were Pritikin's thoughts after he completed his treadmill test in Dr. Smith's laboratory. It was as if he had passed through a door that separated sickness and health. He no longer thought of his heart–that most central of organs–as diseased. On the contrary, his heart was stronger and more alive than it had been in 20 years. And so was Nathan. He was running three miles per day and eating food he enjoyed and knew to be life-sustaining.

Equally exhilarating was the fact that he had once again stumbled onto the frontier. Through study, and trial and error, Pritikin had developed a program to treat heart disease, the number one cause of death in the United States and most of the Western world. Forty million Americans suffer from illnesses of the heart and arteries; one million die each year of such illnesses. The cost of cardiovascular disease, in terms of treatment, research, and lost productivity, is a staggering $50 billion annually. Pritikin had found an answer to the most widespread illness in human history.

Moreover, his program caused none of the side effects of drugs and surgery, nor did it require a patient to become less active. Just the opposite–it increased activity and improved overall vitality and strength.

Pritikin realized, too, that under his guidance the average patient with coronary heart disease could restore his or her health a lot faster and more efficiently than he himself had. Pritikin would later say that what took him eight years of trial and error to accomplish could now be done in nine months. He would also show that within weeks of beginning the program, the average heart disease patient would begin to feel rejuvenated.

Pritikin's victory over heart disease was not without its shadow, however. His blood tests had continued to show a disturbing imbalance of proteins ever since his original electrophoresis test at Sansum Clinic in 1958. On June 30, 1960, Pritikin's blood tests report stated that his "serum protein electrophoresis reveals a fairly homogenous component in the 'M' zone." This meant that Nathan's gamma globulins were still elevated. His doctors diagnosed him as having "paraproteinemia," meaning that he had an abnormal protein in his blood in quantities not normally observed.

In February 1965, another blood test–an erythrocyte sedimentation rate (or sed rate, for short)–indicated that whatever the problem was with Pritikin's blood, it might well be spreading. The sed rate shows how quickly red blood cells (or erythrocytes) settle to the bottom of a test tube in one hour. Normally, red blood cells remain suspended in the blood by virtue of the electrical balance and the overall health of the plasma, red blood cells, and other factors. In a healthy man, no more than 15 millimeters (mm.) of red blood cells will settle to the bottom of a test tube in one hour; in a healthy woman, no more than 25 mm. Nathan's February 1965 sed rate was 44 mm., well above normal.

The sed rate is nonspecific, meaning that it tells a physician if there is some systemic problem such as infection or even cancer, but will not indicate what specifically might be wrong.

In September 1965, Nathan consulted Dr. David H. Solomon at UCLA, complaining of tenderness of his left breast. Solomon did a series of tests on Pritikin but could find nothing to indicate the origins of the breast tenderness. Solomon did find that Pritikin had a slightly elevated level of estrogens in his urine, but said this was "not really diagnostic of anything." Solomon suspected Pritikin might have come into contact with estrogens, but in his report to another physician who was also seeing Pritikin, Solomon wrote that he could find nothing in Pritikin's diet or environment that might be the cause of his breast tenderness, elevated sed rate, or paraproteinemia. Solomon noted darkly, however, that these symptoms might be "part of a generalized systemic illness of some kind as yet undiagnosed . . . . "

In 1966, Pritikin began to experiment with his diet again to see what effects it might have on his elevated sed rate, gamma globulins, and other blood values. His records show that on April 21, 1966, he eliminated brown rice and added one meal of fish or red meat daily. Would a more traditional American diet improve his blood condition? he seemed to be asking. However, after increasing animal foods for five months, his blood condition showed no improvement and even seemed to worsen.

On September 26, 1966, Pritikin consulted hemotologist Dr. Jack W. Shields, a Santa Barbara physician, who recorded his findings in a letter to Nathan dated October 20, 1966. After noting that Pritikin had been "keeping rather extensive records on all [his] blood chemistry," Shields wrote that Pritikin's sed rate was now at 50 mm., up 6 mm. since his blood tests a year before. Shields also discovered an increase in the white blood cells in the bone marrow. He wrote: "There is a mild nonspecific increase in normal lymphocytes in the marrow, estimated approximately 25 percent of total cells. This is more than we see in most people normally, but is not great enough to be considered of any diagnostic significance at the present time."

Pritikin's gamma globulins were also slightly elevated since he had begun the meat-centered diet. His cholesterol level was also up, from 119 mg.% in April to 158 mg.% in August, and then back down to 144 mg.% in September when he began to go off the meat.

After his examination with Shields, Pritikin went back to his standard diet of whole grains, vegetables, beans, fruit, and fish.

Fifty and Feeling Younger

Though Pritikin's tests revealed the presence of some type of abnormality in his blood values and his white cell count in his bone marrow, doctors could not as yet diagnose his condition.

Indeed, references to Pritikin's striking good health turn up again and again in his physicians' reports. Wrote Shields: "It is my final impression, first of all, that you continue in excellent general health. We note that you have a persistently elevated sedimentation rate, a mild but questionably significant increase in Gamma M globulin . . . We note that there is a slight marrow lymphocytosis, but feel that this is of no diagnostic significance and can make very little of it at the present time.

"I really had no specific recommendations to make for your continued program except that we check you periodically with respect to these abnormalities and evaluating their situation . . . "

Pritikin himself could make nothing of his blood values. He was 50 years old in 1965, but he looked ten years younger. His hair showed no signs of gray. His skin was tight and supple, with little or no wrinkling. He was thin and wiry, but did not appear frail. His eyes radiated with the vitality he truly possessed.

Those who worked for Nathan at his engineering firm remembered him as a man who rarely *walked* to his given destination; he *ran* everywhere. He was exceedingly nimble; his body possessed a certain grace and agility that gave him the appearance of being light, flexible, and highly charged. He moved quickly when he moved; he seemed completely at rest when he stopped. He liked to take off his shoes once he entered his house and shuffle quickly to his front door to let someone in, or whenever he had to go from one end of the house to the other. At his office, and later at his Longevity Center, Nathan would race up and down a flight of stairs as if he were dancing. He was so light of foot that these movements were unobtrusive.

And yet, his blood condition persisted and gradually worsened. Two years later, on September 12, 1968, Shields performed the same thorough examination on Pritikin again and discovered an elevated level of macroglobulins in his blood. Like gamma globulins, macroglobulins are aggregated proteins, but of much greater size and weight. When they appear in the blood in abnormal quantities, they suggest the potential for a number of diseases, including disorders of the immune system and leukemia.

The normal level of macroglobulins in men ranges from 0.07 grams to 0.35 grams. Pritikin's macroglobulin rate was 0.7 grams, or twice the amount considered as the upper limit of normal.

Nevertheless, his other tests were normal and Shields stated that "your general health continues excellent."

For the next eight years, Nathan would monitor his blood values with the same results: elevated sed rate, gamma globulins, and macroglobulins. These blood values remained stable, though he did experience periodic and inexplicable bouts of mild anemia. Pritikin's hemoglobin during the late 1960s usually hovered at about 13 grams, about 1 gram below normal. Through the 1970s, it would drop to 10 grams and stay there. He suffered none of the typical side effects of anemia, however, such as lethargy or fatigue. He remained highly charged and extremely active. Doctors maintain that a person can live for decades with these blood values and never manifest any sign of a life-threatening illness. It was for this reason that his physicians took a wait-and-see position with his blood abnormalities.

For his part, Pritikin believed that he would just have to live with the abnormalities, though they puzzled him and he continued to have regular blood tests to see if any changes took place.

The importance of these signs in Pritikin's mind paled before the overwhelming significance of his program to treat heart disease. As he said, he wanted to "convert everyone in the world to a new way of living."

And now, he would set out to do just that.

CHAPTER 6

All Goals Turn to Health

By 1966, Pritikin's passionate study of health, nutrition, and medicine had completely overtaken him.

That year, Nathan withdrew from full-time work at his engineering firm. The long struggles to keep his business competitive had finally paid off in a series of expansions, increased sales, and a new plant. In 1960 Pritikin renamed the company Intellux and, in 1964, moved the business from its old and dusty warehouse in Santa Barbara to a brand new plant, which Pritikin had built and beautifully landscaped in neighboring Goleta. There, he employed 130 people and continued to provide high-quality electrical devices to large corporations and the U.S. Government, with annual sales of nearly $2 million. In 1966, he gave the daily operation of the company over to management and turned his attention to his study of health. He had no idea as yet where such knowledge would lead him, but his passion for the subject left him no alternative but to follow what he was now calling his new "avocation."

Telling the world about his program was not going to be easy, however.

Shortly after his treadmill test, Pritikin attended a party at which he overheard a man telling some friends that he had just been diagnosed as having coronary insufficiency. He was having chest pain, the man said, and his doctors had placed him on medication.

Later, Nathan buttonholed the man and asked him if he wanted to cure his coronary insufficiency.

"Sure," the man replied. "Are you a doctor?"

"No," said Pritikin.

"Are you a Ph.D.?" the man asked.

"No."

"Then don't bother me," the man said, irritated that Pritikin would presume upon him. "I've got a doctor and he's taking care of me."

The experience was so surprising to Pritikin that it came as a minor awakening. "I realized that my advice really wasn't wanted because I had no credibility," he recalled. That someone would reject his ideas on the basis of his formal education, or the lack of it, was remarkable to Pritikin. Being so accustomed himself to examining data and appraising it on its merits, it had not occurred to him that people would take information on health only from a health professional.

Pritikin would find, however, that many more would listen than would turn away.

From the Ordinary to the Extraordinary: Pritikin Success Stories

For the next ten years, Pritikin would privately advise the sick by telephone or in his study. He began giving advice to relatives, friends, and friends-of-friends, but soon the number of people he saw grew. He counseled people with a wide variety of illnesses, often consulting with a client's physician about the advice he was giving. He provided all advice for free.

Most of Pritikin's clients suffered from forms of heart disease, such as coronary insufficiency, angina, or high blood pressure. Others had adult-onset diabetes–which often accompanies coronary disease–and still others suffered from gout, kidney stones and gallstones, arthritis, and claudication (a disease characterized by severe leg pain, caused by poor circulation).

In addition to people with these illnesses, Pritikin counseled many people with bizarre or inscrutable illnesses that would not yield to standard medical treatments. His records show that he saw a woman who had been vomiting almost every night for the previous three years. Another woman, who all her life had enjoyed being in the sun, was suddenly unable to tolerate the sun for more than ten minutes without terrible headaches and a pain that traveled down her nose to her front teeth. A man from Oxnard, California, just south of Santa Barbara, came to Pritikin complaining of perpetual drowsiness. The most routine tasks, such as shaving in the morning, required a herculean effort and forced him to lie down after he was finished.

For those with most forms of heart disease, gout, adult-onset diabetes, and claudication, Pritikin's advice seemed to work miracles. One of Nathan's patients at the time was Eula Weaver, an 81-year-old woman who Pritikin later turned into a minor celebrity by presenting her case history before lay and professional audiences all across the country.

A spirited and determined woman, Mrs. Weaver was suffering from heart disease, severe angina pain, hypertension, arthritis, and claudication. She couldn't walk more than 100 feet without angina and leg pain. Mrs. Weaver had already been hospitalized once after suffering a heart attack. She had to wear gloves in the summertime because poor circulation left her hands permanently cold. When Eula Weaver hobbled into Nathan's study, she didn't know what to expect or to hope for. She had seen many doctors already and had taken every conceivable medication, without success. Pritikin recommended a dramatic change in diet to one consisting entirely of whole grains, fresh vegetables, and fruits. He also advised her on how to prepare the food. After she had been on the diet for a time, he counseled her to begin taking short walks. She followed his instructions to the letter. A year later, she was off all medication and was jogging daily. At 85, Mrs. Weaver entered the Senior Olympics and won two awards for the 800 and 1,500 meter races. She competed six consecutive years and won 12 awards in all.

Even with offbeat diseases, Pritikin often experienced remarkable success. For the Oxnard man suffering from continual exhaustion, Pritikin's methods succeeded where others had failed. After following Nathan's advice for a month, the man wrote the following letter to Pritikin:

> Over a month ago, I spoke to you on the telephone concerning my continuous drowsiness. Perhaps it may be of interest to you to know what has happened since I last spoke to you . . .
>
> Last September, I started becoming drowsy throughout the whole day. I would literally fall asleep on the job and was working at an efficiency of less than 50 percent. I also became very weak. Walking up one flight of stairs would exhaust me, as would just standing up. The few minutes of standing up required for shaving so exhausted me I would have to rest immediately after shaving.
>
> One Los Angeles physician told me I had narcolepsy [an illness characterized by the uncontrollable need for sleep] and prescribed Ritalin. A Los Angeles neurosurgeon prescribed Dexedrine [an amphetamine]. My EEG [electroencephalogram] was similar to that of a person having convulsions. Another Los Angeles physician told me I had Addison's disease [pernicious anemia] and prescribed Decadron, then Dilantin. None of these medications did any good. The third Los Angeles physician then stated that I was losing vitamins and minerals by hemorrhaging into the colon. He suggested removal of the colon.
>
> When I first spoke to you, I mentioned that I always had two eggs for breakfast accompanied by cheese, margarine, white bread, and pastry. In general, I ate a lot of cookies, cakes, and sweets. You said that such a diet was raising the fat level in my blood to such an extent that my brain was being

deprived of sufficient oxygen, causing the drowsiness. You recommended that I switch to a diet of romaine lettuce, oatmeal, brown rice, and fresh fruit. I tried this diet on Saturday and Sunday. I did not switch over to this new diet gradually but went into it suddenly. The result was that by Monday morning I had substantial cramps, diarrhea, and was extremely weak.

I felt so poorly that I went to an Oxnard physician. He told me I was anemic and had only half the amount of blood in my body as I should have. He prescribed Stuart's therapeutic vitamins, iron sulfate, and a low residue diet. Within a few days the cramps and diarrhea disappeared but the extreme drowsiness remained. When I spoke to you a second time, you said I should have switched over to the diet you recommended gradually.

I then studied the diet you sent me, and stopped eating the following: eggs, margarine, sweets, anything made with eggs, milk, and shortening, peanut butter, jelly. I switched to sourdough bread and pita bread and pea soup. In addition, I take daily vigorous 20-minute walks, as you recommended. *The result has been that the drowsiness has completely disappeared!* [letter writer's emphasis] In addition, my strength is returning and I even feel energetic.

I shall always be grateful to you for pointing out which foods were making me drowsy. Now that the drowsiness is gone, I am able to work efficiently again and feel like a completely new person. . . .

It was during the late 1960s, when Pritikin was advising people regularly on their health, that he began to develop a keen eye for telltale signs of illness by observing a person's face, eyes, and manner. Years later, he would tell Ilene he couldn't look at anyone anymore without privately assessing their health.

In December 1969, Nathan's son Robert and his friend Dick Brotherton, both 18 at the time, walked into the Pritikin home. Nathan was perched on a stool at the kitchen counter engaged in his daily routine of eating lunch while reading a medical journal. When the two young men entered the room, Pritikin was surprised to see Brotherton wearing eyeglasses.

"What's wrong?" Nathan asked Brotherton. He had never seen him wearing glasses before.

"The doctor tells me I need glasses," Brotherton said.

Pritikin had an eye chart hanging on the wall in his library. He escorted Brotherton into the library, told him where to stand, and then asked him to read the chart. Nathan examined the lenses of Brotherton's glasses as the young man read the chart.

"The doctor tells me I'm farsighted," Brotherton said after he finished reading the chart.

"That's ridiculous," said Pritikin. "Your eyes test perfectly, better than normal."

After a few minutes of questioning, Pritikin then proceeded to tell Brotherton how the eye focuses. He told Brotherton that all he needed to do was exercise his eyes to restore his vision. At that point, Pritikin gave what came to be known as his patented command before he gave his advice: "Here's what you do," said Pritikin.

He told Brotherton to read for as long as he could each day. When his eyes were tired, he should rest them. When his eyes felt fully rested, he should resume reading until his eyes were tired again, at which point he should stop reading. He should read for at least one extended period each day.

The second exercise Pritikin gave Brotherton was to lie in bed and trace the dimensions of the ceiling with his eyes. "Make squares with your eyes," Pritikin said. "Do this for five minutes, twice a day–once in the morning and again at night before bed." Do it for a month, and your eyes will be fully recovered, Nathan told him. In the meantime, don't bother wearing your glasses; they'll only make your eyes weaker, he said.

Dick Brotherton laughed. He had just been given a whirlwind tour of the workings of his own eyes.

"What do I do with my glasses?" he asked.

Nathan was already walking toward his study. "Keep them as a souvenir," Pritikin replied.

In a month, Brotherton's vision was fully restored, and he never wore glasses again.

One woman Nathan counseled for years struggled with multiple sclerosis.

Laura Ornstein was 51 when she met Nathan at a dinner party in Santa Barbara in August 1970. Mrs. Ornstein had been suffering from multiple sclerosis for nearly ten years by then, and she had recently reached a low point in her degeneration process. Just before meeting Nathan, she was having great difficulty walking more than 100 feet. At the end of her workday at New York's Nassau County Social Services, Mrs. Ornstein could barely walk to her car in the parking lot behind her office building without the aid of a friend who helped her keep her balance.

She came to California that August to visit her sister, Eddye, and then met Nathan. In his forthright and confident way, Pritikin asked Mrs. Ornstein if she would like to stop the progression of her disease. She said she would. "Then come to my house tomorrow and I'll give you a program to help you," he told her.

Laura Ornstein and her husband Bob arrived early the next day at Nathan's front door. He escorted them into his study where he already had an enormous pile of scientific literature laid out on his desk. The Ornsteins and Nathan talked for five hours, during which time Pritikin convinced them that the fat and salt content of Mrs. Ornstein's diet was contributing to the degenerative process of her illness. He explained the disease in detail and then used metaphors to make it understandable. Pritikin said that the nervous system is like wires with insulation around them. Mrs. Ornstein's nervous system, he said, had the insulation removed in places, where it was creating short circuits, thus impeding the flow of energy along the nerve. This created her problems in walking and keeping her balance.

Pritikin maintained that fat, cholesterol, and salt were contributing to the illness. He felt if Laura Ornstein were to stop eating these foods, her condition would improve. Mrs. Ornstein recalled that he never said the illness would be cured, but that the degeneration process could be halted and that her condition would even improve–to what extent, he didn't know.

He outlined his low-fat, low-cholesterol diet for them; he told her specifically to avoid animal protein, nuts, eggs, butter, and any other foods containing fat. She must eat grains, vegetables, and limited amounts of fruit. He also said that she must begin walking. "Walk as far as you can until you can't walk anymore," Pritikin told her. "Then rest, and then walk back home." He told her she would have to walk every day in order to see progress.

"Laura, you'll find that your progress will be two steps forward and one step back. But you'll see gradual improvement and your disease won't get worse."

Pritikin's advice was in stark contrast to the recommendations of her physicians, who told her there was no cure or treatment for multiple sclerosis and the only thing she could do was rest. Exercise of any kind exacerbated the illness and hurried the degeneration process, her doctors said. This, Mrs. Ornstein had discovered, was the standard approach to the illness in 1970.

Despite the revolutionary approach Pritikin was advocating, Laura Ornstein believed him. She went home to New York, and immediately went on the diet, following it to the letter. Meanwhile, she started walking each day and gradually her condition did indeed improve.

"In 1970, I had noticed that my right eye had begun to drift outward and I had spells where I would stumble," she recalled. "After I was on the diet for a few months, I could walk by myself. I didn't need assistance. Pretty soon I could walk a quarter mile and then a half mile."

Mrs. Ornstein saw other improvements, as well. "I felt like I had lots more energy, unlimited energy, really." Her eye stopped drifting and her gaze became straight and true.

For several months, Laura Ornstein called Pritikin weekly; afterward, she telephoned him once a month for several years. She regularly sent her blood records to him and he provided all his counsel for free.

After a couple of years, Pritikin set up an appointment for Mrs. Ornstein to see Dr. Roy Swank at the University of Oregon Medical School. Swank pioneered the use of a low-fat, low-cholesterol diet and exercise in the treatment of multiple sclerosis. His dietary program, however, was not as low in fat and cholesterol as Pritikin's. Like Pritikin, Swank was a maverick who seemed to be breaking all the established rules of medical treatment of multiple sclerosis. Mrs. Ornstein saw Swank, who evaluated her and kept her on the low-fat, low-cholesterol diet. He also encouraged her to exercise.

In 1978, after Pritikin had opened his Longevity Center, Laura and Bob Ornstein visited Nathan at his home. Pritikin had several physicians visiting him on the day the Ornsteins arrived. Nathan greeted the Ornsteins warmly and then invited Laura Ornstein to tell the doctors her case history. After she concluded, Pritikin asked her to walk across his living room for the doctors. The living room was large–just over 30 feet long. She got up from her chair and walked perfectly across the room and then back again. Pritikin beamed.

"He was so proud of me, but not as much as I was of myself," Mrs. Ornstein recalled.

From that low point she reached in August of 1970, Laura Ornstein steadily improved until she reached a plateau at which she was self-sufficient and able to walk alone about a half mile at a stretch.

"I think I could walk farther if I pushed myself and I think my condition would further improve," she said in 1986, "but I never felt the need to push myself after I got better on the diet."

In the early 1980's the Multiple Sclerosis Society began to recognize that a low-fat, low-cholesterol diet was effective for many patients in slowing the degeneration process and, for some, even producing an improvement of their condition.

Pritikin saw hundreds of patients from 1966 to 1976. It was during these years that he developed his approach to illness and his own motivational techniques.

Pritikin asked his clients to keep records of what they ate over the course of a day, and sometimes a week, after they adopted his program. Common daily menus included oats and oranges for breakfast; romaine lettuce, a variety of green vegetables, and whole wheat bread or a whole grain–such as brown rice–for lunch; brown rice, potato, carrots, green vegetables, and sourdough bread for dinner; fruit for dessert. Pritikin also allowed people to eat hoop cheese, a skim-milk cheese exceedingly low in fat and cholesterol. Other animal foods he suggested, if desired, were a variety of fish, including halibut, flounder, cod, snapper, seabass, and others; the white meat of chicken or turkey, without the skin, and small amounts of lean red meat, usually no more than three ounces (if a person desired red meat).

Pritikin placed a great deal of emphasis on blood tests. Very often he had his clients send him their blood records, blood pressure readings, and stress test results, if such tests had been performed. Though he considered all the data available from blood tests, he saw blood cholesterol level as the key indicator. It gave him insights into how sick a person was, and what the person might have been eating over a period of time. As dietary fat and cholesterol increases, so too does the cholesterol level in the blood. Increased dietary fat and cholesterol give rise to a whole host of illnesses, including heart disease, adult-onset (or type II) diabetes, and certain cancers. Conversely, the reduction of fat and cholesterol can prevent these illnesses and, in the case of heart disease and diabetes, often reverse them.

Pritikin counseled most of his patients for only brief periods of time. Once a person adopted his diet and exercise program, he or she usually experienced rapid results and no longer needed Nathan's guidance.

There were people, however, who could not follow Pritikin's advice. A physician who had retired to Santa Barbara whom Nathan counseled for two years appears to have had great difficulty staying on the program. According to Pritikin's records, Nathan first saw the man in November 1967, when his cholesterol level was 360 mg.%. By January 1968, after being on the diet just two months, the doctor's cholesterol level was down to 250 mg.%, a drop of more than a third. However, he was unable to make substantial progress following the initial drop; his cholesterol level climbed back up to 260 mg.% by November of that year, went back down to 224 mg.% in April 1969, but rose to 253 mg.% by December 1969. Pritikin saw the doctor regularly and counseled him to do his best to stay on the program, but he couldn't. In early 1970 the physician died of a heart attack.

It was not in Pritikin's nature to cajole or pressure a client to make changes. He responded to the specific complaint at the time, gave his advice, and let the person do whatever he or she wanted to do afterward. If the client wanted to come back to him for more advice, Nathan was happy to give it. He never turned anyone away, even if the client clearly had failed to follow the advice. Pritikin was prepared to go right on advising the person as long as the person wanted such advice.

Patience Born from Caring Detachment

The root of Pritikin's patience was his detachment from people. Without being critical or jaded, Pritikin didn't become personally attached to what other people did. He maintained that the actions of others had only a minor influence on events that were important to him. Anything that was important to him was his responsibility, Pritikin believed. He also felt people would naturally adopt a more healthful diet if they were properly educated on diet's effects on health. It was simply a matter of putting out the information, and letting nature take its course.

He maintained, too, that his actions spoke louder than his words. "Be an example," he once told his son Ralph, when asked how he got people to change their behavior patterns. "Never lecture."

These characteristics combined to give Pritikin a rather neutral outlook on people. There were only a handful of people in his life for whom he had strong feelings. As his son Robert said, "People used to come up to me and ask me what my father thought of them and I would say, 'He really likes you,' or 'He respects what you are doing,' but the truth of the matter was that my dad didn't think much about people or what they were doing. He loved humanity, but he didn't get close to many people."

Nathan's detachment gave him a kind of humorous perspective on life. When confronted with anything but a life-threatening issue, he would often make a pun out of the problem. His daughter Janet recalls that she would very often have to ask him to be serious when she came to him with a problem. At that point, he would become rational, serious, and focused, but he would have to be convinced first that the problem warranted that kind of attention.

Nathan's son Ken recalls the time his father worked for months on an experiment at his electronics business. When the experiment was about to finally reach fruition, the whole effort broke down in a series of disasters. Ken had been working with his father on the project and felt dejected about the failure. Nathan's reaction, on the other hand, was rational and light. He very calmly explained what to do next and then made a joke about the ongoing problems they were facing. Ken asked him how he could have such an attitude in the face of such frustrating difficulties.

"My father's reaction was that he had been through so many situations that were much darker than what we were going through at the time and that he didn't think the matter was so grave."

There was one other characteristic that seemed to give him enormous patience when it came to advising people: he loved counseling others. As Ilene recalled, "Nathan loved to help people, and he loved teaching. He enjoyed being the person with the answers. He would describe to the person his or her condition in very simple, understandable terms, and after he had finished talking he would love it when the person sat back in wonder and said, 'Really?'."

Even when telephone calls from people he was counseling threatened to upset the harmony of his household, he refused to limit the amount of time he gave to others.

Very often Pritikin would get calls just when the family was about to sit down to dinner. He would drop everything and take the call, which would often run 30 minutes or more. Ilene often pressed him to limit the time he spent on the telephone, at the dinner hour especially, but he absolutely refused to cut anyone short.

A Remarkable Mind for Remarkable Detail

When it came to his study of health and anatomy, Pritikin's intellectual curiosity knew no bounds. Everything about the human body fascinated him–the heart, vessels, blood, bones, individual organs. Even the finger-nails excited his curiosity. He wondered why he had ridges in his nails, when most other people did not. He read the available literature on fingernails as if the subject would reveal some great secret. He didn't seem to come up with anything, but he continued to puzzle over his ridges.

He made a great study of the teeth and gums. Page after page of his notes reveal he went from a very basic understanding to a sophisticated knowledge of the structure and biology of the teeth and gums. Two pages of his notes are dedicated to the names of the teeth and the "definitions of positions": "cervical–neck of tooth; corneal–exposed above the gingiva; mesial–toward the midline (center); proximal–surface that is next to the adjacent tooth . . . " and so on. Nathan studied the book *Oral Histology and Embryology,* by Orban, with fervor. In notes written in tiny, detailed, and highly legible handwriting, Pritikin recorded every fact in the book he regarded as important.

A sampling of Pritikin's notes reveals the respect he had for Orban's highly technical treatise.

> P. 55–Enamel is the hardest calcified tissue in the body. . . . Max thick-ness is .100 inches over molars. Composed of 96 percent inorganic, 4 percent organic. . . . Enamel is composed of rods (.0001 diameter) cemented together with a cementing interprismatic substance. . . . P.114–Dentin is considered a tissue. Dental lymph circulates in the dentin. Originates in pulp, goes through the dentin and returns to pulp. . . .

Pritikin made more than 100 such notes on the biology of the teeth and gums. Most of these notes are highly technical; they are punctuated by graphs and drawings Pritikin made to better illustrate and understand the workings of the teeth and gums. He studied the teeth on molecular and macroscopic levels. After reading his notes one might be led to think that he was considering going into dentistry. But he had no such interest. Pritikin was merely studying this subject in the same way he studied every subject: with a passion for thoroughness and an insatiable hunger for knowledge.

He joined this hunger with a remarkable memory. Part of his method for retaining information was to write it out himself, as he did with Orban's book. Once he had written it down, it remained with him indefinitely. But even without writing the points he wanted to retain, he possessed the capacity to recall scientific studies and obscure details years after he had first encountered them.

As his son Robert got older, he also became interested in science and would tell his father about the literature he had been studying at the time.

"He would correct me on studies I had just got done reading, studies he hadn't read for ten years," Robert recalled.

The Foundation Is Laid for a Health Revolution

In 1970, Nathan was invited to join a small group of local scientists and laypeople who wished to advance the study of aging: how and why humans get old and die. The group held regular meetings and soon became incorporated as the Longevity Foundation (no relationship to the Longevity Center that Pritikin would eventually create).

Pritikin had little interest in what he considered the less pressing issue of how and why people get old. While the Longevity Foundation focused most of its attention on the search for biochemical methods of extending life, Pritikin emphasized the need for making the most of the natural capacities humans already possessed. Nathan stressed that people get old prematurely because of their diets and sedentary lifestyles. Fat and cholesterol, he said, burden the body and cause it to fall victim to degenerative diseases that otherwise would not occur in the human organism. He maintained that life is actually cut short by the typical diets of the Western world. Human life, he said, would last naturally to 100 and beyond if the body were fed the proper foods and exercised regularly.

One of the members of the Longevity Foundation, mathematician Jon Leonard, took an interest in Nathan's ideas. When Pritikin introduced Leonard to the great library of research he had accumulated, Leonard suggested that they write a book together under the aegis of the Longevity Foundation. Pritikin agreed. In the early part of 1971, Leonard began laying the groundwork for the writing of what would become the bestseller, *Live Longer Now.* Leonard was assisted by J. L. Hofer, also a member of the Longevity Foundation. To help Leonard understand the studies and put them in proper perspective, Pritikin began to write a summary based upon his compilation of the research. He assimilated all the relevant medical literature that he had collected over the previous 25 years–a body of information that by this time filled two rooms of his house–and began to write a technical treatise on diet's relationship to the leading killer diseases.

Pritikin's writings were originally meant to help organize and interpret the studies so that Leonard could put them into a readable text for the layperson. However, the task soon began to obsess him. Hidden away in the quietest room in his house–his bedroom–and seated in a comfortable armchair, Nathan worked day and night, assembling and interpreting the studies, writing and rewriting his finely honed analysis, like an attorney marshaling the evidence for an intricate case. His innumerable studies were arranged on the floor all about him, organized in piles. All the studying he had done during the previous 2½ decades, all the knowledge he had accumulated to that point, was suddenly given voice. Each day Ilene would type his notes, and together they would edit his material until it satisfied them both.

Within two years, he produced three volumes that would become the foundation for his approach to virtually every degenerative disease facing the modern world. These three volumes would be the basis for all his lectures at the Longevity Centers and his many presentations that were yet to come before lay and professional audiences around the country. The ideas presented here would change the lives of thousands–including his own.

The range of illnesses he addressed in these three books is astonishing: heart disease (including atherosclerosis, angina, and high blood pressure), adult-onset diabetes, the common cancers (including lung, colon, breast, and prostate), gout, arthritis, kidney stones and gallstones, and many illnesses affecting hearing and sight, including glaucoma.

These illnesses, Pritikin strongly maintained, had their origins in the diets that are typical in Western industrialized nations, such as the United States. Pritikin even suspected that sickle cell anemia and multiple sclerosis might have a dietary component, and discussed this in his writing.

Pritikin's documentation was exhaustive. The heart disease book contains 207 technical references; diabetes, 206; cancer, 91; arthritis, 65; gallstones, 28; sight and glaucoma, 79; hearing, 10; exercise, 47; and dietary recommendations, 58. The medical literature Pritikin based his arguments on originally appeared in many of the most prestigious medical journals in the world. Some of the publications he cites most frequently include the *Journal of the American Medical Association, New England Journal of Medicine, American Journal of Clinical Nutrition, Archives in Pathology, Lancet, Annals of Internal Medicine*, and many others. The fact that all of Pritikin's points are supported by existing medical literature already published underscores a point he made for more than a decade, namely, that all the scientific evidence needed to make clear and definitive conclusions about the origins of degenerative diseases and their treatments had already been done. All one had to do was to see the common threads that ran through the existing research and assemble them into a coherent whole. At that point, Pritikin said, the conclusions would become obvious. This is what he had done. As he wrote in the introduction to the three volumes:

> Can valid insights be drawn second-hand by one who merely surveys
> the research of others? That this can be done–at times with brilliant and

revolutionary results, is beautifully illustrated by the work of two eminent biologists, Watson and Crick, who collected and analysed data from work entirely done by other investigators, then came up with their revolutionary interpretation of the structure of DNA, which gave birth to molecular biology; there was no first-hand observation or research involved.

He addressed each illness according to a fairly standardized structure. He began by discussing the disease in general, and the human and animal data linking it to diet as a causal factor. He then plunged into the biological mechanisms for the disease–how certain constituents in the diet affect the body on a cellular level, thus giving rise to the illness. He showed how the disease could be prevented and, in many cases, how it could be reversed by making changes in the diet.

Pritikin then critiqued the standard therapies used against the illness, including both drugs and surgery. In the case of pharmaceuticals, he analysed each drug commonly prescribed, how it worked, and what its side effects were. He also assessed surgical procedures–including bypass surgery and heart transplant–as well as coronary care units, their procedures and the drugs used in the treatment of acute coronary cases.

Pritikin's exhaustive analysis takes the reader through the disease process (which often starts in infancy, as in the case of cardiovascular disease) and shows that in each case the principal causes are dietary–not fatalistic heredity or the wear of aging.

In the introduction to the three-volume set, Pritikin stated:

The civilized world is confronted with a giant paradox: as the benefits of modern technology and advanced medicine become more readily available to the inhabitants of these developed nations, life expectancy drops. The immense hospital complexes, the increasing number of care centers, the sophisticated and expensive diagnostic equipment, the huge and costly research programs designed to develop drug cures and to ferret out the causes of the disease fatalities which cut down so many even before they have lived their promised three score and ten years, and often in the very prime of their lives–all of this is to no avail. The various degenerative diseases–atherosclerosis, including coronary heart disease, hypertension, diabetes, cancer, glaucoma and arthritis–proceed relentlessly to claim many millions of victims. If not fatal, these diseases may be severely crippling, but millions suffer quick and unsuspected deaths, and millions more suffer slow agony, uncertainty and equally untimely deaths.

Definitive solutions have been provided by modern medicine for many of the health problems that have plagued mankind historically–most of the infectious diseases, maternal and infant mortality in childbirth, surgical repairs necessitated by injuries or congenital defects, etc.; but the cause or causes of degenerative diseases remain largely a mystery from the standpoint of most–lay and professional alike.

In the absence of accepted definitive views concerning the cause(s) of the common degenerative diseases, speculation abounds. These are among the widely held views: 1. The degenerative diseases are mainly a natural consequence of aging and there is no way by which these processes can be prevented; 2. Heredity is a major factor in many of these conditions–such as coronary heart disease and diabetes–and again, one accepts the consequences fatalistically; 3. Many of these diseases are associated with emotional factors, such as tension of modern life and strained family relationships; 4. There is much discussion that autoimmune etiologies are the factor in arthritic diseases, and so on.

Adherents to these views regard the degenerative diseases as being largely outside of our control so far as prevention is concerned and look to drugs and surgery as the primary resources for therapy. The lack of success of this approach is reflected in the growing degenerative disease epidemic and the mortality rates for these diseases.

A large and convincing body of scientific evidence, the subject of the chapters that follow, points in another direction entirely. The weight of this evidence indicates that the common degenerative diseases are largely due to nutritional factors, and do not require explanation in terms of such concepts as heredity, inevitability of aging, stress, etc. While acknowledged by only a small segment of the medical profession presently, recognition of the validity of the evidence upon which this viewpoint rests is gaining momentum.

The evidence demonstrates that the cure for many of the degenerative diseases also has a nutritional basis: as the offending dietary factors are removed from the food regime, the symptoms of many of the degenerative diseases regress, often completely.

Pritikin's hypothesis was simple: common foods in the diets of Westerners–especially in the United States–are eaten in excess, causing a wide range of illnesses and premature death. The most dangerous constituents in today's diets are fat and cholesterol, found most commonly in red meat, dairy products, and eggs. He created the word "lipotoxemia" to describe the poisoning of the body by the overconsumption of fats and cholesterol. He likened the consumption of fat and cholesterol to that of cyanide, which is found in very small amounts in lima beans. As long as humans consume only minute quantities of cyanide, the poison has no adverse effects. However, when the quantity of cyanide consumed exceeds a certain level, it becomes highly toxic. Fat and cholesterol are safe when eaten in very small amounts, he said, but extremely harmful when taken in larger quantities.

In addition, most people eat an overabundance of protein, refined grains, salt, and sugar. These also contribute to the degenerative process, though they are usually less toxic than fat and cholesterol. The standard American diet, rich in all these harmful constituents, poisons the body and causes a variety of diseases, including heart disease, cancer, diabetes, gout, kidney stones and gallstones, arthritis, and others.

Interestingly, Pritikin believed these seemingly diverse illnesses were in fact only one single disease, manifesting itself in a variety of symptom-states, which we have come to call heart disease, cancer, diabetes, and by some other names. In any case, they all spring from the same origin: a diet high in fat, cholesterol, refined foods, salt, and sugar. He showed that a change in diet would not only prevent these diseases, but–for millions of people–would cure them.

Pritikin realized that these were revolutionary ideas and expected many scientists to react with incredulity. As he further stated in the introduction of his three volumes:

> Such a postulation linking diet and the scourge of degenerative diseases may seem far-fetched, until one reflects upon some basic biological facts. All animals, man included, have a diet that emerged from the long-term experience of the species in nature over many thousands of years. Now, man no longer eats foods his body was designed to eat, but has created a synthetic diet–the penalty of which is to endure the adverse effects of short-term experience. The more man's diet departs from foods to which he is biologically suited, the more the adverse effects.

Though Pritikin would come to know firsthand just how startling were his ideas to the vast majority of researchers, there were enough public statements by spokesmen of the medical profession by 1972 to anticipate accurately the scientific community's reaction to his diet-health hypothesis.

That same year, Dr. Philip White, head of the American Medical Association's Department of Foods and Nutrition, stated, "There is no assurance that a casual change in diet will be of any benefit, and little assurance that a significant change will be, either."

Dr. Donald S. Fredrickson, who would later become director of the National Institutes of Health (arguably the most powerful scientific position in the United States), said in 1972: "I admit here to a bias of one long preoccupied with genetically determined hyperlipidemia (elevated cholesterol level) . . . The problem in the majority of the 'most susceptible' is not to be solved by general dietary advice."

Dr. E. C. Naber, at Ohio State University, echoed the concerns many researchers had for dietary lowering of fat and cholesterol, a concern Pritikin had personally dealt with in 1957, namely the possible loss of important nutrients present in the typical American diet. Naber said, "It is too early to tell how large a part cholesterol plays in heart disease and drastic attempts to avoid foods high in it are probably harmful."

These men were among the leaders of the scientific community who would set public policy and who would form the intellectual and political resistance to Nathan Pritikin–and others–who would try to change the eating habits of Americans.

As he would prove over the next 14 years, Pritikin was undaunted in the face of such powerful opponents. He believed in his message and his ability to convey it to scientists and laypeople alike. More importantly, he maintained the firm conviction that once people applied these ideas, the effectiveness of his diet would be persuasive enough.

As he further wrote in his introduction:

> The message of this book is this: one need not fall prey to the degenerative diseases. Coronary heart disease, diabetes, arthritis, glaucoma, hypertension, gout, angina, and some cancers are all entirely avoidable. There is a price to pay for health: this is a return to simpler foods and a more active existence. If you are not prepared to pay this price, the reading of this book will not benefit you; if you are, the evidence assembled in the chapters of this book will convince you that you will be rewarded with the good health and long life which nature intended for you as your return for your investment.

The completion of his three-volume set on diet's relationship to degenerative diseases was, for Pritikin, a major achievement. After searching the scientific literature for 25 years, he was aware of no other text that provided such a comprehensive analysis. While individual researchers in the fields of cardiovascular disease or diabetes or cancer had seen the importance of diet within their own specific fields, no one–to Pritikin's knowledge–had scientifically documented diet's relationship to all the common degenerative diseases.

With Pritikin's analysis in hand and his guidance readily available, Jon Leonard moved quickly through *Live Longer Now.* Leonard and Pritikin hoped for a wide audience for their groundbreaking book. Meantime, Pritikin wrote to a number of leading scientists in the fields of cardiovascular disease and diabetes asking them to review *Live Longer Now* prior to publication, but after seeing the manuscript each scientist declined Pritikin's request. Grosset and Dunlap, a New York publisher, accepted the manuscript in the spring of 1973 and scheduled it for publication the following year.

Pritikin's unique analysis was finally going public.

CHAPTER 7

The Turning Point—
Pritikin Goes Public

*I*n the fall of 1973, Nathan received an invitation from a friend to attend a medical meeting in Los Angeles. The friend was a medical doctor. He knew Nathan well and was aware of his longstanding interest in health and nutrition.

During their drive from Santa Barbara, Nathan noticed that his friend had brought with him a large bag containing his lunch. Pritikin thought little of it since the medical meeting would probably allow for a lunch break. They arrived at the meeting, took their seats, and started to listen to the first speaker. The lecturer had just completed his opening remarks when Pritikin's friend removed a large basket of chicken legs from his lunch bag and started eating them.

Surprised and amused, Pritikin turned to his friend and said, "You obviously like chicken legs."

"I hate chicken legs," the friend replied.

"But you've got at least ten chicken legs in that basket," Pritikin said.

"That's because I've got hypoglycemia," the friend answered. "I have to eat chicken legs."

"Don't tell me you're on that high-protein diet," Pritikin said.

"Of course I'm on a high-protein diet; that's the only diet there is for hypoglycemia. I've had it for ten years," said the friend.

"And you'll have it for the rest of your life if you continue to eat that diet," Pritikin replied.

The doctor insisted his diet was the only answer to his problem, which he said was acute. He told Pritikin he suffered from fatigue, nausea, and dizziness caused by the hypoglycemia, and that it had affected his medical practice. The fatigue forced him to nap at noon each day and to limit the number of patients he scheduled. He feared if he did not eat this high-protein diet, which he detested, he might have to further reduce his practice.

Pritikin asked him to try a different diet that would reduce the amount of protein he had been eating, but sharply increase the amount of complex carbohydrates, which Pritikin said would give him more energy.

The friend became annoyed with Nathan's persistence. "Look, I got my diet from a doctor who has been treating this type of problem for 25 years. I'm not going to change now."

It took Pritikin two months to convince his friend to go through the pertinent medical literature that Pritikin had been collecting. Together they went over hundreds of studies. Finally, in the winter of 1973, the doctor agreed to start Pritikin's dietary program.

Ten days later, he called Pritikin on the telephone and announced that he felt much better. He said that he no longer felt the need to nap in the afternoon. He had plenty of energy and felt wonderful.

"You're cured," Pritikin pronounced joyfully. "Go out and play tennis."

The Big Breakthrough

Pritikin's friend would not let the experience drop, however. He wanted Nathan to talk to the doctor who prescribed the high-protein diet for him in the first place. The friend said he would set up an appointment with his physician, Dr. Wilbur Currier, who lived in Pasadena, California, so that Nathan could share his ideas with him.

Shortly thereafter, Currier called Pritikin and asked him how he scientifically justified giving a high-carbohydrate diet to a person with a blood sugar problem.

Nathan told Currier of some of the studies supporting such a diet in the treatment of hypoglycemia, as well as adult-onset diabetes. Currier was unconvinced but he agreed to see Nathan; he asked Pritikin to bring some of the medical literature that supported his ideas.

Pritikin was nervous about seeing Currier. "No one had ever cross-examined me who was a physician," he later confessed. And he had every intention of showing up well armed. Pritikin gathered more than 100 scientific studies investigating the relationship between diet and health with an emphasis on sugar metabolism, and drove to Pasadena to see Currier. The two met at Currier's club. Nathan expected to talk to Currier for about 45 minutes. They talked for six hours without stopping. Currier was so impressed by Nathan and his ideas that he told him he was going to change his entire practice to include Pritikin's dietary recommendations.

Currier wanted Nathan to come to his office in Pasadena and act as his consultant. There Pritikin would see patients with Currier and advise the doctor on the dietary information each patient should receive. Pritikin agreed.

A few days later, Nathan joined Currier at his office. Pritikin asked the doctor what he should do. The first thing Pritikin should do, Currier told him, was to put on a white coat. He then told Pritikin his plan. Nathan would join Currier in his examining room while the doctor saw patients. After listening to each patient's problem, Nathan and Currier would step outside the office, at which time Pritikin would tell Currier what kind of nutritional advice he should give the particular patient. The two would then go back into the office and Currier would prescribe the diet. Nathan, amused and incredulous, agreed.

The plan worked fine, according to Pritikin, and after a couple of days of this, Currier had the system down and Nathan left Pasadena.

A few months later, in January 1974, *Live Longer Now* was published and Jon Leonard traveled around the country to promote the book. Leading newspapers and magazines wrote mostly lukewarm reviews of the book. However, sales were brisk and eventually it would reach the *New York Times* paperback bestseller's list.

That same month, Nathan received a call from Currier, who invited him to speak at an upcoming medical conference arranged by physicians belonging to the International Academy of Preventive Medicine. Currier was an officer of the medical society and would be elected president at the conference. The meeting was to take place in March in Miami Beach, Florida.

Pritikin was wary. How many people would attend the meeting? he asked. And who would make up the audience, laypeople or physicians or both?

Currier told him that there would be several hundred health professionals in the audience, the majority of whom would be medical doctors, and that doctors and Ph.D.'s would be the speakers.

"Who will you have that has no credentials, like myself?" Pritikin asked.

"You'll be the only one," Currier said, "But we need to shake them up a little bit."

With great trepidation, Pritikin agreed to do it. He had never appeared before a medical audience and he was understandably nervous.

Meanwhile, *Live Longer Now* was stirring up more interest. A few days after Currier called him, Nathan got another call from a physicians' group called the American Academy of Medical Preventics. They, too, wanted Pritikin to give a talk at their medical meeting, which was taking place in Miami Beach the same week Currier's group was meeting there. Once again, Pritikin agreed.

For the next two months, Nathan and Ilene worked tirelessly on Nathan's talks. As she would do for many of his speeches, Ilene edited and typed the two talks nearly a dozen times. Nathan compiled hundreds of studies supporting his basic points and rehearsed the speeches in front of Ilene over and over again. These two speeches would change both of their lives forever.

While he was in the electronics and engineering business, Nathan's and Ilene's lives did not routinely intertwine. He was there when Ilene and family members needed him, but it was usually upon request. He devoted long hours and many weekends to his businesses and his study of the medical literature. Ilene raised the children, while Nathan concentrated on his work.

However, with their five children well on their way to adulthood, Ilene now unstintingly turned her attention to Nathan and his work. The speeches he was about to give would mark a turning point in their lives. From that time on, their worlds would join. Ilene and Nathan were no longer separated by the responsibilities of their mutually exclusive roles as parent and scientist-businessman. His dream to reshape the world according to his own vision now became hers. In the years ahead, Ilene would become his editor, consultant, and confidante. In the early days of the Longevity Center, she would organize the kitchens, create menus and meal plans, and generally oversee the quality of the meals they were offering. Though the emphasis was always on Nathan and his ideas, Ilene helped to tailor his talks to make them more appealing, literate, and understandable to the layperson.

Their abilities seemed to complement one another perfectly. While Nathan possessed a brilliant mind and a creative genius, he nevertheless was a poor judge of character. People often did things that surprised or baffled him. He was a person directed toward the masses. He had an enormous capacity to inspire and lead people in the direction he wanted them to go, but it was never his forte to understand individual human behavior. These were Ilene's strengths. Ilene had a penchant for under-standing people—what they wanted and needed. She was shrewd yet retiring, always avoiding the limelight that he traveled in but keeping an eye on how he was presenting himself, and what others were up to. While Nathan's writing tended to be blunt and pointed, Ilene possessed an ear for a well-turned phrase and the qualities of a diplomat. She made Nathan's broadsides more palpable and, at times, perhaps more palatable to his audience.

Finding a place in his world gave her great satisfaction and fulfillment. As she would say years later, "I was never happier than when I worked with

Nathan in preparing the material with which he would do battle with the medical world. I worked with his notes, polishing them into a form that I thought would do justice to his point of view."

Medical World Takes Notice

When they finally arrived in Miami Beach for the March 21 conference, Nathan and Ilene had two suitcases with them: one very large case weighing 80 pounds that contained Nathan's references, and another, smaller case containing their clothes. After they arrived at their hotel, Nathan arranged his references in order "so that I could immediately get to them in case anyone challenged me on any point," he recalled. He wanted to be prepared for the worst. How would the doctors react to his talk? he wondered. Would they attack him outright, or politely question where on earth he had gotten this crazy idea.

The conference began the following day. As expected, about 300 physicians and scientists gathered in the large auditorium to listen to the speakers.

When his turn to speak arrived, Pritikin mounted the dais and put his speech on the lectern. He wasted no time in getting to the point.

"It is a privilege for me to address your organization," he began. "When Dr. Currier extended the invitation to speak to you, I was impressed with his unusual open-mindedness for two reasons: One, I am not a member of your profession and two, the views I wish to present run counter to the high-protein, low-carbohydrate approach, a dietary practice that many of you have been emphasizing.

"A large aspect of your concern has been the nutritional deficiencies. My views deal with the danger of nutritional excesses–that is, with excess intake of fats, simple carbohydrates and cholesterol. It is my thesis that the high fat content of Western diets is the primary cause of most of the degenerative diseases rife in most of the developed nations in the world. Simple carbohydrates and cholesterol are potent secondary factors in this worldwide crisis."

It was a theme he would reiterate in talk after talk for the rest of his life.

When he finally finished his speech, he nervously awaited the doctors' response.

Nothing happened. Pritikin asked for questions. Not a single question came. The silence was loud.

"I had never seen such glum looks on so many faces before," Nathan recalled. "I could see that they were not taking seriously what I said. It didn't look like anyone was even listening to me. I could see I was not wanted."

Disheartened and let down, Nathan descended from the dais and told

Currier that he felt he should leave right away. The conference was scheduled for another two days, but Nathan didn't feel there was any reason for him to remain.

"Don't go just yet," Currier said. "You're scheduled to give a workshop." Workshops were informal meetings with small groups of doctors who would ask questions and discuss a particular topic. Pritikin didn't believe there would be enough interest in his ideas for anyone to attend his workshop, but he agreed to stay.

The next day, he reported to the small room where his workshop was to be given and was shocked to find it packed with physicians. All the seats were taken and still more doctors stood up along the walls. There were more than 50 people present and it was standing room only.

Nathan opened the door, saw the crowd and closed it immediately. He hurried to the secretary and told her that she had given him the wrong room.

"I'm supposed to give a workshop," he said. "Half a dozen people around a small table."

The secretary looked puzzled. "There are only two workshops scheduled for this hour–yours and someone else's, and that's your room," said the secretary.

Disbelieving, Pritikin walked back to the room and stood in front of his waiting audience. Not sure what to do, he asked for questions. About 20 people raised their hands and the questions began coming.

"And then I realized what was wrong the day before. The kind of nutrition I was talking about was so different from anything they had ever heard that they didn't know what to ask me. And now the questions came out like a torrent."

The following day, he gave his talk to the American Academy of Medical Preventics at the Deauville Hotel in Miami Beach. After his talk, a group of enthusiastic doctors gathered around him. Many of the physicians wondered if guidelines for a dietary therapy such as the one Pritikin had described were available. The program Pritikin had described would be helpful for many of their patients, the physicians said, and even for themselves and their families.

Sensing an opportunity, Nathan responded on the spot by suggesting that he and the physicians combine forces to conduct a large study. Pritikin proposed that they pool their patients and use his low-fat, low-cholesterol diet on those suffering from heart disease and adult-onset diabetes.

Many of the physicians liked the idea, and Nathan collected business cards. He told them he'd be back in touch.

Pritikin had been a hit. While he had maintained for years that his ideas were fresh and worthy of attention, this was the first time he had put them out publicly before a medical audience that could just as easily have pulverized them if they were without foundation. Just the opposite happened. He not only managed to educate and inspire his listeners, but he drew them to him. Now he had his first chance at doing a credible study that could bring his program wider attention.

First Study Launch: Trial and Error

When he returned to Santa Barbara, he obtained mailing lists from both groups he had addressed and sent his proposal to the physicians to do a large-scale experiment that would study the effects of a low-fat, low-cholesterol diet on adults with coronary heart disease, angina, hypertension, claudication, and adult-onset diabetes. His idea was to have the doctors prescribe the diets to their patients, monitor their responses, take blood samples, and send the blood to Bio-Science Laboratories in Los Angeles. Bio-Science had agreed to furnish reports on all the patients and keep track of patient records.

Pritikin was flooded with physician inquiries and requests for more information. Nathan and Ilene responded to the requests by sending an information kit that contained a 20-page manual for physicians, including 92 references of studies that provided the scientific basis for the dietary program; an 18-page Patient's Manual with an explanation of the diet; a table of foods to use and to avoid; a sample menu for a day and some basic recipes; a monthly dietary diary to be kept by patients; some exercise instructions; and several case histories of people who had high blood pressure, angina, and adult-onset diabetes, and who had been treated successfully on the program.

Pritikin had hoped to interest leading scientists to participate as advisory board members; however, despite his efforts, he was unable to enlist the help of any of the ranking researchers he contacted. Nathan single-handedly supervised the study and kept the records, with help from Ilene. He called the project the Low Fat and Cholesterol Study, or LFC for short.

The study officially got under way in May 1974, when a handful of physicians started placing patients on the program and following their responses. Eventually, 21 doctors from many different parts of the country and nearly 1,000 patients participated in the LFC study, which would run for one year, to June 1975. The study would cost Nathan and Ilene more than $25,000, much of which went to typesetting, printing, and mailing the manuals and other materials.

The project got a major boost when the *Journal of the American Medical Association* (JAMA) published an announcement in its September 2, 1974, issue for the study, which Nathan had sent. JAMA printed a picture of Eula Weaver running in her jogging clothes, along with a description of her condition before and after she adopted the low-fat, low-cholesterol diet. The JAMA article stated that interested doctors could write to Pritikin for study kits that included a complete manual for doctors and patients.

Thanks in large part to the JAMA publicity, Pritikin got hundreds of requests for more information from such diverse places as the assistant White House physician in Washington, D.C.; the medical director of the Medical Services Division of the City of Los Angeles, who considered placing a group of police officers and fire fighters on the diet; and the North American Reassurance Company, a large insurance company that recognized the potential benefits to policyholders. None of these high-ranking business and government officials participated in the study, however.

In fact, Nathan ran into insuperable problems, the most important of which came out of a general lack of understanding of his program. It was so radically different from orthodox medical therapies and typical American eating habits that, under the conditions of the study, misconceptions and poor implementation by physicians and patients seemed inevitable. People didn't know how to make the food and doctors didn't know how to treat patients with the program.

As the White House physician put it in a letter to Nathan:

> Thank you very much for sending me the material on the LFC Study. It looked very interesting, and I think the concept may prove valid. Unfortunately, the patient population that I deal with is composed primarily of "workaholics" who frequently do not eat regularly, let alone have the opportunity for a fifteen-minute walk after each meal.

Pritikin understood the doctor's position, even though it was based on the altogether erroneous perception that people who work long hours do not have time to eat well and exercise. Nathan himself was a workaholic, a man of incredible productivity; however, he also found time to eat a healthy diet and exercise regularly.

More importantly, it was Nathan's position that a program of sound diet and regular exercise actually enhances productivity, since it reduces sick time, increases energy, and promotes mental clarity. He saw the typical American diet as antithetical to productivity, because it reduces energy levels and leads to sickness, disability, and premature death. From the standpoint of productivity, a diet made up of whole grains, fresh vegetables, fruit, and restricted amounts of low-fat, low-cholesterol animal foods was the diet of choice. Pritikin also maintained that once a person became used to the new way of eating, he or she would spend no more time preparing the food and consuming it than they would if they were eating a typical American diet. And in the long run, it was time well spent.

The biggest problem the study faced, however, was the relative lack of nutrition knowledge physicians possessed. Using diet to prevent or treat disease was as foreign to many as the lunar surface.

Up to the early 1980s, doctors were given little nutrition education in medical school. While they were taught about various dietary components, such as vitamins and minerals, their nutritional education focused primarily on deficiency diseases. Pritikin's approach was based on the consequences of consuming too much of certain foods, not too little.

Breakdowns in communication and confidence between doctors and their patients occurred regularly. Physicians were often unsure of what effects the diet would have on those who had just begun the program, nor did they know how and when to reduce their patients' medications as the symptoms abated on the diet.

In truth, Pritikin possessed a rare knowledge. Very few people had experimented with diet in the manner that he had, and fewer still knew how to treat illness using diet alone. Physicians had to stay in constant touch with Nathan in order to understand what their patients were going through on his diet. Pritikin's correspondence with doctors participating in the LFC study not only reveals his vast knowledge of nutrition and medicine, but also his confidence in his methods.

To a physician in Blooming Glen, Pennsylvania, Pritikin wrote on October 27, 1974:

> Enclosed is your data form for patient 32-002M71 and the ECG tracing. After four weeks on the LFC diet, his [the patient's] blood pressure could return to normal without the Hydrodiuril [hypertensive medication]. Try taking him off the hydrochlorothiazide since it is raising his uric acid level. 7.5 mg.% is too high and if he is off the drug, uric acid will drop below 6 mg.% and his arthritis should improve enough so that Indocin [medication for arthritis] may not be required.
>
> At a level of 6 mg.%, Tylenol in small dosages can keep him comfortable.

On November 24, 1974, he wrote to a doctor in Gainesville, Georgia, who requested his guidance:

> You may consider the LFC regimen for pregnant women. It is almost a guarantee for prevention of toxemia, as well as to arrest and reverse diabetes during pregnancy. It is quite effective in lowering the hyperlipidemia associated with the third trimester of pregnancy, and will keep the newborns' blood levels in proper range.

To a physician in Bellevue, Washington, on September 15, 1974, he wrote:

> Enclosed is data form [patient] 42-007M57. He reports blurred vision, headache, and postural dizziness. These all could be caused by the niacin.

Suggest deleting niacin for a three-week trial to note if symptoms disappear. He will not require a vasodilator on the LFC diet.

Patient 42-004M46 has a drastic rise in triglycerides which has raised the cholesterol and uric acid levels. He should be closely questioned as to his daily food intake. Either a high quantity of fruit or simple carbohydrates in the form of honey, sugar, etc. can have this effect. Let him write down everything he eats for 2-4 days; then mail it to me . . . The triglyceride rise could be due to a recent infection or fever. Has he had a recent illness? Keep me advised on him.

Pritikin also wrote letters to patients directly and published a newsletter entitled "LFC Study Progress Report: News about the Low-Fat, Low-Cholesterol Study," to keep physicians informed and to inspire them to stay with the program. He did everything in his power to keep up the compliance of both the physicans and the patients.

But to little avail. Patient compliance was discouraging–a mere 5 percent. By March of 1975 Pritikin tried to round up the results of his LFC study by circulating a questionnaire among the study's physicians to ascertain the effects of the diet on their patients.

There was some good news, however. For those who managed to change their eating habits and stick to the program, the results were very good, the physicians reported. Many patients were indeed able to reverse serious diseases, and those physicians who used the program were able to wean patients from drug therapies.

Pritikin was not at all discouraged by the results of his study. He remained confident of the essential efficacy of his approach, and was buoyed by the results of those who were able to follow the program. Moreover, he had learned a great deal in carrying out the study. Now, more than ever before, he realized that patients needed closer supervision if they were to stick to the program. They needed to understand fully why they should eat this way, and how to prepare the new diet. He began to consider other ways of applying his approach, ways that would allow for closer monitoring of patients so that the program would have the best chance at treating serious diseases.

It wouldn't be long before an opportunity to do just that would present itself.

CHAPTER 8

A Breakthrough for Diabetics

*O*ne of the leading medical scientists in the United States would one day say that Nathan Pritikin's role in changing medicine was similar to that of the little boy in the story "The Emperor's New Clothes," in which a young boy dares to say what no one else will: the emperor is wearing no clothes.

While the majority of scientists and doctors were going along with conventional thinking, Pritikin had the insight and the courage to spread a revolutionary approach to disease. And then he went on to prove he was right. Nothing in Pritikin's health career better exemplified his pioneer thinking than his approach to diabetes.

Diabetes is the third leading cause of death in the United States and much of the Western world. It is an illness characterized by the body's inability to convert sugar in the bloodstream to fuel. Without fuel, cells die.

There are two types of diabetes. Type I, or juvenile diabetes, is characterized by a failure of the pancreas to produce insulin and often occurs early in life. In type II, or adult-onset diabetes, the pancreas is able to produce insulin but the insulin is unable to convert blood sugar to fuel for cells.

Nine to ten million Americans suffer from type II, or adult-onset, diabetes. One to two million suffer from juvenile diabetes.

Both forms of diabetes cause a wide variety of other illnesses, including blindness, gangrene, palsy, and hearing loss. They are also associated with a higher-than-average rate of heart attacks and strokes. Even those who take oral drugs or insulin are at high risk of contracting all these illnesses.

In 1974, when Nathan set out to change medicine's approach to diabetes, the American Diabetes Association (ADA) was advocating a diet high in fat and protein and low in carbohydrates as part of the diabetic's treatment. The specific dietary recommendations in 1974 were 40 percent of calories from fat, 20 percent from protein, and 40 percent from carbohydrates. (Those recommendations didn't change until 1979.)

The rationale behind this diet was that if diabetics could not metabolize sugar, then all carbohydrates–both refined and complex–had to be limited. The most important goals of the diet were to control calories (obesity increases the severity of the disease) and limit sugars.

In addition to diet, physicians prescribed oral drugs, such as Orinase, Diabinese, or Tolinase, which stimulate release of insulin from the pancreas, the organ that produces insulin.

Finally, insulin was also administered to both type I and type II diabetics who did not respond adequately to diet or drugs.

The diet recommended by ADA, Pritikin argued, actually was increasing the incidence of the disease or making it worse among those who already suffered from it.

Pritikin made a radical distinction in the type of carbohydrates consumed by diabetics. He agreed diabetics should avoid simple carbohydrates, such as table sugar, but maintained that the vast majority of the diabetic diet should consist of complex carbohydrates, from grains and vegetables. This diet could reverse type II diabetes and restore health, he believed. In most cases, drugs–which have severe side effects–or insulin were not necessary.

Although diet could not reverse juvenile diabetes, Nathan maintained it could prevent many of the other illnesses normally associated with the disease, such as heart disease, blindness, and gangrene.

Nathan also encouraged diabetics to walk daily. He said it could improve circulation and metabolism and control weight and appetite.

Once again, Pritikin had unearthed the research to support his thesis.

He had found numerous studies done at the early part of the twentieth century demonstrating that a high-fat diet was actually the cause of diabetes. The researchers had found that when healthy people are placed on a high-fat diet, they can be made diabetic. On the other hand, diabetics who eat a diet low in fat–and high in complex carbohydrates–can actually reverse the disease.

The key question was, how could he get doctors and scientists to look at this evidence and test the hypothesis. The leading researchers and experts in the field believed exactly the opposite of what Pritikin was saying.

He considered various ways of publicizing the diet and the research he had collected, but realized the scientific establishment was unlikely to be convinced by a layman. No, he would have to find another way to prove his program worked.

The best way to convince the scientific world, Pritikin believed, was to have an eminently respected scientist test Nathan's diet as a treatment for diabetes. Done by the right investigator, such a study would draw a great deal of attention from the scientific and medical communities, and could perhaps change the way diabetes is treated.

In the early spring of 1974, Nathan wrote letters to researchers at many leading institutions, including Stanford University, the University of Washington, Sansum Clinic in Santa Barbara, and the City of Hope research center in Duarte, California. He represented himself as a member of the Longevity Foundation and a scientist interested in diabetes research. In several cases, he sent the scientists his volume on diabetes (from his three-volume work), which documented the cause of most diabetes as a high-fat diet. Pritikin was so determined that a study be done that he offered to help raise the money needed to do the research. Scientists at Stanford were interested in his ideas, but said they would need $30,000 to fund the research. Pritikin set out to find the money.

One of the first places he contacted was the philanthropic offshoot of the McDonald's hamburger empire, the Kroc Foundation. The Kroc Foundation was founded by Ray Kroc, a diabetic who also created the McDonald's hamburger, and it was run by his brother, Dr. Robert L. Kroc, a biochemist. The Foundation was interested in new drugs or surgical procedures for diabetes, but Pritikin pursued the matter because he was hopeful he could obtain the funding from them and he saw a certain justice in having some of the McDonald's fortune go toward finding a dietary cure for an illness he believed its own food was helping to create. Following an exchange of numerous letters, Pritikin and Robert Kroc engaged in a lively telephone discussion on the subject of diabetes. After the two had talked for a while, Kroc finally asked Pritikin whether he was an M.D. or a Ph.D. Nathan answered that he was neither; he added that he had no degree at all. With that, the conversation came to an abrupt halt, Pritikin recalled years later.

One philanthropist was interested in Pritikin's ideas. That man was Richard Berk, a trustee at the David and Minnie Berk Foundation in New York. The Berk Foundation funded health-related research and had a particular interest in finding a cure for diabetes. Pritikin sent Berk a number of studies supporting his ideas, as well as his speech to the International Academy of Metabology, given in March 1974 in Miami Beach. In May 1974, Berk wrote to Pritikin in bewilderment:

> Your address to the International Academy of Metabology indicates that scientists have done similar studies for many years. What has happened that these theories are not known and are contradicted by almost every major diet being recommended today. . . . I am thoroughly confused, so please

bear with me. Too many diets, so many different suggestions, and now your approach which is new, at least as far as I am concerned.

Pritikin responded by saying that for 50 years doctors and scientists have labored under the mistaken notion that diabetes was caused by a defective pancreas. This led to endless research and therapies that never addressed the real problem: fat in the bloodstream rendered the body's insulin inert, thus making it impossible for insulin to make blood sugar available to cells. A high-fat diet was causing the onset of adult diabetes, Pritikin stated. He pointed out that recent research had shown the average diabetic actually produces more insulin than a nondiabetic. These studies showed that the problem with diabetes is not so much the pancreas as the effectiveness of the insulin.

During these 50 years, studies had shown repeatedly that the drugs used for diabetes do not prevent the ravages of the disease, and, in addition, often have severe side effects. The most exhaustive study performed in the United States examining the side effects of diabetes medication, the University Group Diabetes Program, concluded that even with the use of the drugs, diabetics have 250 percent more death from heart attacks, as well as other serious disorders.

As Pritikin provided more studies, the Berk Foundation became more enamored of his ideas, and even suggested that the foundation might support a study examining his hypothesis if he could get one going.

In the meantime, Stanford scientists told Pritikin that they were no longer interested in doing the kind of study he had in mind. Pritikin would have to look elsewhere.

In May 1974, Pritikin telephoned Dr. James W. Anderson, chief of Endocrine-Metabolic Section at the University of Kentucky Medical School. Anderson was an internationally recognized researcher in the field of diabetes. He had studied the effects of simple sugars (or simple carbohydrates) on diabetes and found that when simple sugar makes up as much as 80 percent of the total calories in the diet, many diabetics actually need less medication, such as oral drugs and insulin. On a diet of 80 percent sugar, the level of fat in the diet is reduced to 10 to 15 percent of total calories–a very low level. Pritikin had been saying for years that it wasn't sugar that was the main cause of diabetes, but fat, a conclusion Anderson's research seemed to support.

Anderson's work had actually contradicted the long-held belief that carbohydrates were harmful to diabetics.

In his telephone conversation with Anderson, Pritikin suggested that Anderson do a study using Pritikin's diet as a treatment for diabetes. Anderson liked the idea.

A Bittersweet Success

On May 13, 1974, Pritikin wrote Anderson a letter and included a protocol, or a description of the study he had in mind. The letter reviewed the results of early studies showing that a high-carbohydrate, low-fat diet reversed adult-onset diabetes.

Pritikin then described the study he wanted done. A number of diabetics who were using oral drugs or insulin should be placed on the ADA diet for one week and monitored to see what effects the diet had on their blood sugar levels. After the week was over, two-thirds of these same patients should be placed on the "experimental" or Pritikin diet for one year to see what effects this diet had on the diabetic condition. He described the experimental diet as "foods in their original state, and approximately 12 percent protein, 10 percent fat, and 78 percent slowly absorbed carbohydrates. No simple, quickly absorbed carbohydrates [such as table sugar, or sucrose, which Anderson had used before] will be used and cholesterol would be limited to 100 mg. per day."

Pritikin stated that the patients "should be housed in a controlled environment, preferably a metabolic ward."

He also suggested that all subjects should take three 20-minute walks per day, one after each meal.

On June 6, 1974, Anderson wrote back to Pritikin, "I am very interested in participating in a study such as the one you have outlined and would very much like to do some detailed studies on hospitalized patients."

Anderson concluded his letter by saying, "I think it would be extremely beneficial for me if you could come through Lexington and we could discuss this in greater detail."

On June 24, Pritikin wrote back to Anderson telling him that he could be in Lexington sometime in the early part of July. The two finally met on July 2, 1974. They discussed their prospective efforts together, and the research up to that point. Pritikin shared with Anderson his book on diabetes, which outlined all of Nathan's ideas on the relationship between diet and adult-onset diabetes.

On July 10, Anderson wrote back to Pritikin telling him he would need $10,000 to do the study. The money would go toward paying the salary of a Ph.D. in nutrition for one year.

Anderson also included a revised protocol, which was essentially the same as Pritikin's earlier version submitted to Anderson in May. Anderson described the experimental diet as a "high-carbohydrate diet" that will "contain 75 percent of calories as carbohydrate and will exclude sucrose and simple sugars in as far as possible. This diet will largely consist of starches and other polysaccharides. The protein content will be 15 percent of calories and the fat content 10 percent of calories. The cholesterol content will be restricted to 100 mg. per day."

This was essentially the same diet Pritikin had suggested to Anderson originally.

On July 20, Pritikin wrote back to Anderson that the "experimental design is fine" and that he hoped "to have funds for you in six to eight weeks." Pritikin had been writing to the Berk Foundation and was now hoping it would support Anderson's research with a grant for $10,000.

Berk responded positively to Pritikin's overtures, and in September the Berk Foundation gave Anderson $10,000 as a result of Pritikin's lobbying on his behalf. In his letter of thanks to Richard Berk, Anderson wrote, "I greatly appreciate the $10,000 which the David and Minnie Berk Foundation has contributed to my research in diabetes. As Nathan Pritikin and I have indicated to you, we think this is a very important area of research in diabetes and one which will have an important impact on the treatment of many diabetics in the future." He concluded that he would keep Berk informed. At the bottom of the carbon copy of the letter, which he sent to Pritikin, Anderson wrote in longhand, "Thanks again, Nathan. Jim."

Nathan was effusive in his gratitude to Berk. In a letter to Berk dated October 1, 1974, Pritikin wrote, "Needless to say, your grant is appreciated more than I can express in words. It represents the first funds I have ever obtained for health causes."

The study Anderson was about to undertake was the realization of a dream for Pritikin. His ideas were finally being taken seriously and, if the study results turned out as he thought they would, his hypothesis would be proven true.

Anderson wanted to begin the study in January 1975. On October 23, 1974, Pritikin provided Anderson with meal plans and suggestions for the research.

"Enclosed are three copies of the proposed diet," Pritikin wrote. "I decided to make it cholesterol-free to improve the blood lipids in the fastest possible time. The lower the lipids [blood fats], the more efficient the insulin should be." He recommended that people in the study take walks and then noted that "special precautions to avoid any infection problems–respiratory, etc.–should be made. Patient[s] should have adequate sleep every night. Care of the feet, due to blisters or other problems caused by walking, etc., must be closely watched. If a toe becomes infected or if the patient contracts any infection that will generate a fever, the increased insulin requirement will negate the experimental results, at least for several weeks until the pre-infection status returns."

The study finally got under way. Thirteen diabetic men were followed for one year. All of them were on oral drugs or insulin: five were on drugs and eight required daily injections of insulin.

Pritikin's expertise in all areas of diet, nutrition, and health were offered to Anderson without restraint. His only interest was in seeing that nothing interfered with the study's results. He regularly discussed various fine points of nutrition and metabolism with Anderson throughout 1975, when the study was conducted. Anderson reciprocated by keeping Pritikin well informed about the progress of the study and thanking him in his letters for his help.

Within weeks of beginning the "experimental" or Pritikin diet, all the men showed improvement in their condition. All the men on oral drugs were able to stop taking the drugs, and four of the eight men on insulin were able to stop taking the insulin entirely. Eventually, a fifth man on daily injections of insulin could reduce his insulin by nearly half.

The study showed that the high-carbohydrate, low-fat diet was clearly the treatment of choice for diabetics on oral drugs, and for some on insulin.

Anderson was scheduled to give a talk in Japan on August 7, 1975, where he planned to report the preliminary results of the study. Pritikin apparently asked Anderson specifically to give him (Pritikin) credit for originating the diet and helping with the study.

On August 5, Nathan wrote Dr. Melvin L. Weidman, a physician who headed the Kirsten Foundation, located in Manhasset, New York, which had also become interested in Pritikin's ideas. Pritikin's letter states that, "Anderson's whole approach now is to use our diet, confirm our results, and explore what makes the diet work. I phoned him and he promised me that from now on he will credit my name as the originator of the new diet, and will start with his Japan talk."

Anderson did make a passing reference to Pritikin in his Japan talk, saying that the diet Anderson used in his study was "similar to the one used by Nathan Pritikin and his associates. . . . " No mention was made of Pritikin's participation in the study, however, or that he helped raise the money to conduct the research. In fact, this would be the last public reference he would make to Pritikin.

Privately, however, in correspondence with Pritikin, Anderson was giving Pritikin credit for the dietary regimen used in the study. On October 30, 1975, Anderson wrote to Pritikin to give him the latest progress report on the study and seemed to congratulate him by saying, "When these patients were switched to a 75 percent carbohydrate diet similar to that which you advocate which contained large amounts of starch and generous amounts of dietary fiber, each one showed improvement. In each instance the plasma glucose value dropped to under 100 mg.% and we were able to discontinue all insulin or oral agent therapy."

Anderson's study was published in the *American Journal of Clinical Nutrition* in August 1976. In it he expressed his thanks to the Berk Foundation for its financial support, but made no mention of Pritikin. He did mail Nathan a copy of his paper in advance with the words "Nathan, Best regards, Jim" written on it.

The results of Anderson's study showed that the Pritikin diet significantly improved the health of the diabetics. On the ADA diet, the 13 men in the study all needed some type of medication to treat their diabetes. On the diet suggested by Pritikin, 9 of the men were weaned of drugs or insulin entirely, and a tenth had his insulin requirement cut in half.

"Official" New Diet Reflects Pritikin Program

Anderson went on to use the high-carbohydrate, low-fat diet in numerous studies after his 1975 collaboration with Pritikin. The research had a major impact on the scientific community, and was instrumental in changing the dietary recommendations of the American Diabetes Association. The 1979 guidelines by the ADA urged diabetics to eat up to 60 percent of their calories from carbohydrates and as little as 20 percent from fat. It was the first time the ADA changed its dietary recommendations in 50 years. Anderson served on the ADA committee that changed the guidelines.

Pritikin was gratified that the study and Anderson's subsequent work had had such a powerful influence on the scientific community. There was no doubt that, as a result of the research, thousands of diabetics who followed the ADA's advice had been helped. However, Pritikin was hurt by Anderson's failure to mention any association with him.

Years later, Anderson maintained that he had intended to do such a study before Pritikin contacted him and that Pritikin's contribution was minimal to insignificant. He insisted that Pritikin had little to do with the research and that Nathan exaggerated his role in the study. In short, Pritikin didn't deserve to be mentioned, Anderson felt. He did admit Pritikin was a controversial figure and that it was not politically wise to associate with him, especially after Pritikin opened the Longevity Center in 1976. Anderson also acknowledged it was Nathan who raised the money to do the study, without which the research could not have been done—at least not then.

Anderson later modified the diet somewhat to include 70 percent of its calories in complex carbohydrates, 9 percent fat, and about 21 percent protein. He renamed this diet the HFC Diet, or high-fiber, high-carbohydrate diet. He also emphasized the role of fiber in the diet, which distinguished it from Pritikin's emphasis on complex carbohydrates and fat. However, when asked by a reporter in 1980 which of the constituents in the diet played the major roles in the treatment of diabetes, Anderson stated the fiber plays "a minor role: the major influence here is probably increased complex carbohydrate and limited fat. The diet used 9 percent fat and 70 percent carbohydrate, the HFC diet."

Anderson continued to pursue Pritikin for financial support of his research, and Pritikin managed to provide Anderson with another $10,000 for other studies. Anderson did agree to serve on Pritikin's Board of Advisors after Nathan had opened the Longevity Center in January 1976, but resigned nine months later for "personal and other reasons." Anderson never mentioned his collaboration with Pritikin in his public writings or talks.

It would not be until 1981 that Pritikin expressed his desire to be given some credit for his role in the landmark research on the low-fat, high-complex carbohydrate diet. In a letter dated April 27, 1981, Pritikin wrote to Anderson saying:

> While I was in London a few days ago, I met with the publishers of [Dr.] Denis Burkitt's book, Martin Dunitz. Mr. Dunitz told me he was publishing a book for you on diabetes. I know that you have hesitated over the past years to mention any association with me in any of your medical articles, since you felt it would not be appropriate.
>
> Your book for the layman, as opposed to a scientific article, would not inhibit you from recounting my role in your starting the use of the high-fiber, high-carbohydrate diet. A paragraph or two would probably cover my contribution. I understand from Mr. Dunitz that the book will be typeset in the next period of weeks. Although I have not discussed this with him, it would be an opportunity to include mention of our collaboration if you wish to do so.

Anderson chose not to mention Pritikin in his book.

CHAPTER 9

Innovator, Inventor, Businessman

*T*hough health and nutrition were Pritikin's avocations and, in fact, the fields he loved the most, it was the electronics industry that was the source of his income.

By 1974, Pritikin owned a controlling interest in five corporations. These included: Nalene Industries (named by joining the "Na" from Nathan and "lene" from Ilene), a company that made high-precision dies and die-stamped metal parts; Renco Corporation, which made a type of optical encoder, a device Nathan designed that gave commands to automated machines and computers, telling them what to do and when to do it; Penex Corporation, a company that produced retractable, porous-tipped pens that was still in the research and development stages; Epod Engineering, which made measuring instruments; and finally, his flagship company, Photronics.

Photronics was Pritikin's last of a series of businesses in the electronic and engineering fields that evolved from Glass Products, which he started in Chicago in 1948 and moved to Santa Barbara in 1957. Pritikin changed the name of Glass Products to Intellux in 1960 and finally moved the company to Goleta, the neighboring suburb, in 1964. He sold Intellux to Harvey Radio in 1967 and retired that year to oversee his other business interests and concentrate on his study of health and nutrition. In 1972, he "wandered" back into the electronics industry, as he put it, and formed Photronics, which picked up where Intellux had left off.

Photronics produced electronic devices and printed circuits, including the circuit boards in hand-held calculators and the memory banks for computers. In 1975, Photronics employed nearly 150 people, had $4 million in gross sales, and had a $2 million annual payroll.

Meanwhile, Nathan had his fingers in half a dozen other enterprises, including real estate, production of liquid crystals (which are used in making numerals appear on watch faces and other digital displays), and several inventions then under development at the same time.

By 1975, he had 19 U.S. patents and 24 foreign patents. Among his inventions were: a new method for making inlaid circuits that were flush with their insulation base (patented in 1954); a new method for making printed circuits (patented in 1955); an improved electrical resistor and the technology for producing them inexpensively (1958), which was followed by several other improved versions, all of which were patented through the 1960s; thin films that were used as electrical conductors and the technology to produce them (1964); a new process for embedding circuits in insulated bases, making them resistant to heat and moisture, and protecting them from shock; and better inlaid circuits and methods for producing them (1965). Other inventions followed which were variations on these same themes.

Pritikin was widely respected throughout the electronics industry as one of the leaders in his field. In September 1977, when he was to speak to the Western Electronic Manufacturers Association in Santa Barbara, Nathan–then 62–was heralded in premeeting publicity as "an extremely innovative talent in the electronic technologies."

Pritikin was anything but a typically successful businessman, however. He came to work most days on a bicycle. He replaced his sports jacket with a lab coat once he got inside the building, and everyone in the place called him by his first name.

His dress was always understated. Even after he started the Longevity Center and became a nationally known figure, he dressed in modest suits and sports jackets. He rarely wore a tie. His clothes were bought off the rack and occasionally seemed a little too big for his slender frame. Because of a foot injury that he had suffered as a child, he often wore sandals, which gave his feet greater comfort.

Pritikin looked more like a university professor than a hard-driving businessman. His utilitarian approach to clothing and simple diet caused many of Pritikin's associates to see him as monkish and even ascetic. This was enhanced by the fact that his personality tended to be serious and completely without artifice. He was so totally focused on whatever he was doing that even at home the main topic of conversation with Ilene would invariably be his latest project.

Though he was simple in his style of living, he was downright reckless when it came to pouring money into his inventions.

For Nathan, money allowed him creative freedom and therefore was essential to his happiness. His ideas were the things he prized the most, and he needed money to bring them to fruition. "If it [an invention or a business venture] was something Nathan was interested in–even when it was an idea that others had given up on–he didn't see it as a risk," recalled his attorney, Howard Parke. "He had great faith in his ability to make his ideas work."

Strictly speaking, Pritikin had little interest in business for its own sake; he saw business as the playground for his ideas, the matrix from which his creativity flowed.

Despite all his successes, many people regarded Pritikin as a poor businessman, and indeed, his priorities were such that profits and the security of his businesses were secondary to finding ways to capitalize on his latest invention. No one knows how many fortunes he poured into his search for the ideal resistor, a project that spanned more than 20 years and never achieved the success he had hoped it would.

He was forever in the laboratory carrying out experiments or in his office devising new ones. Pritikin's attitude was always that his current invention would be his ticket to great success. His crowning achievement was always just over the next hill. As a result, Nathan financed his ideas with the attitude that each one would bring the long-sought payoff he had dreamed of. But as Ilene said, "We never achieved the ultimate success Nathan was always hoping for, nor did we fall victim to the disaster that seemed to threaten so often."

(A few times they came close. In fact, five years later, in 1979, Pritikin's personal fortune and his entire health empire would be threatened at its roots when he was forced into personal bankruptcy.)

Yet, despite the vicissitudes of his businesses and personal health, Pritikin remained remarkably composed, which always seemed to amaze his family. One of the ways he dealt with stress was to walk the trails of his five-acre estate.

In 1960, Nathan had a large, five-bedroom home built in Montecito, a beautiful, wooded section of Santa Barbara. The house, which he helped design, was built on the side of a gradual rise. The sides of the house facing south and west were constructed almost entirely of glass, allowing the sun–which shines nine days out of ten in Santa Barbara–to pour in throughout the daylight hours. Ilene decorated the house with contemporary and Oriental art from India, China, and Japan.

The land was densely populated by California live oaks and a wide variety of flowers and bushes. Nathan had ferns planted along the trails, which he had meticulously maintained. In many places, the paths were covered by a carpet of moss. They wound through the garden beneath the towering oaks, over a ravine, and through various thickets.

Nathan seemed to lose himself here. He'd walk along these paths, inspecting and admiring new life. There was such a balance between well-ordered plants and wild shrubbery that it created the illusion of being removed from Santa Barbara, from civilization itself. It was wild and alive and he loved it.

Sometimes while he walked the trails one of his children would accompany him to discuss their lives or ask about his. As they walked and talked, Nathan's attention would occasionally, and quite suddenly, be diverted by a small flower or the growth of a young plant.

"He had a way of tuning into nature," recalled his daughter, Janet, who often accompanied her father on these walks. "He would suddenly become very aware of a flower or a plant. If it were a flower, he would close his eyes, take a whiff of it and sigh, as if he had experienced a bit of ecstasy, and then he would move on. He could block out everything when he walked his trails. He was happy and you could see it. Afterward, his mind would be moving a mile a minute again."

Once his walks were over, he was back on the job, seemingly rejuvenated and even playful.

"Throughout his business life, my father was faced with countless predicaments any of which could easily be called a crisis," said Janet. "There was never a time I can recall when Dad seemed unduly anxious, let alone frenzied or hysterical, about a work crisis. In fact, sometimes even if I knew there were problems, he would still be whistling, joking, or smiling, or perhaps commenting on a wonderful aroma in the kitchen or fragrance of the flowers outside. And I don't think it was necessarily a matter of 'putting on a happy face' for the rest of us; I truly believe he was able to separate the dismal state of his business from life itself and what he valued most–family, nature, small pleasures."

Pritikin was the kind of father who bore his burdens silently and cheerfully in front of his family. He rarely shared his difficulties with his children, and when he did, his purpose was to reassure them. He shielded the family from the problems of his world and let the children tend to their own lives.

Two of Nathan's sons, Robert and Ralph, saw their father's attitudes toward life in terms of the sport they both loved, which was surfing.

Ever since Robert and Ralph had been in their early teens, they thought nothing of getting up at 4:00 A.M. if the surf was "up." By 5:00 A.M., they would be in the ocean and perched on their boards, waiting eagerly for the water to rise up and carry them landward.

Surfing is all balance and instinct, a willingness to let go and gamble when everything rational is telling you to hold back or hold on. For those who can put fear aside, and let instinct and balance guide them inside a canopy of salt water and glittering sunlight–inside the very cup of the wave–well, any surfer will tell you there is no experience like "being tubed."

Secretly, Robert and Ralph referred to their father as the greatest surfer, despite the fact that Nathan had never been on a surfboard–indeed, never got into the ocean. To Robert and Ralph, Nathan lived all of life like a surfer, always heading for the dangerous waters, always ready to gamble everything on the prospect that his next project–his next wave–would carry him all the way to a remote shore that only he could see.

Nathan, Ralph, and Robert shared an insider's joke about surfing, because–on its surface–it represented everything that was outside of Nathan's world. Nathan had taken the work ethic to its outer limits, while surfers–who view life as something to be enjoyed, rather than labored over–were trying to turn the good life into an art form.

Eventually, the words "the surf's up" took on a generic meaning in the Pritikin household, a shorthand way of saying that something good and propitious hung in the balance or was about to happen. "The surf's down" meant the opposite: difficulties, trouble on the horizon. It would be this very metaphor that Nathan would use to tell Ralph that his life was coming to an end.

An Unusual Boss

When he wasn't dreaming up new ideas in the electronics field, and working slavishly to implement them, Pritikin was in his office reading medical journals. He estimated that a third of all his time at Glass Products, Intellux, and Photronics was spent reading the scientific literature on nutrition, health, and medicine.

His employees were well aware of his passion for health and nutrition. In the February 1975 issue of *The Readout*, the Photronics employees' monthly newsletter, Nathan's longstanding interest in health and the Long Beach Study were the subject of an article:

> Ever notice how Nathan Pritikin bounces around the plant as though he was made of India rubber? Ask him what keeps him feeling so fit and you're likely to get a 15-minute lecture on the evils of fat and cholesterol in our diet and the need to get adequate exercise in the maintenance of good health and warding off diseases of aging, like heart trouble and diabetes.
>
> Last year, his ideas found their way into print in a book published by Grosset and Dunlap called *Live Longer Now.*

Those who worked with him and knew him well uniformly stated that Pritikin was a genius when it came to finding creative solutions to technical problems. He was also a workaholic. He arrived at the plant early in the morning and stayed, on the average, until 7:00 P.M.

Conversely, he was disproportionately lacking in management skills. In fact, he hated to manage people, and instead hired others to oversee his operations while he focused his attention and most of his business profits on research and development. People who worked for Nathan at Glass Products, Intellux, and Photronics state that he was extremely mild-mannered and hated confrontation. He refused to discipline or fire anyone, no matter what an employee's work habits. His brother Albert, who worked for Nathan for more than 25 years, recalls that even when a group of employees had gathered to gossip during working hours, Nathan would leave them to their scuttlebutt until they decided themselves to go back to work. If he had a question for an employee who happened to be socializing on company time, he would interrupt with a sincere, "Excuse me." Pritikin's secretary at Glass Products, Gloria Harms, recalled the way Nathan handled a female employee who had a longstanding problem with alcohol, which caused her to call in sick frequently. Whenever the woman telephoned Nathan's secretary to say she wouldn't be coming to work that day, Pritikin would tell his secretary to call the woman back every 15 minutes until she agreed to come to work. The woman would inevitably relent and come to the office. Pritikin said nothing about the episodes, according to Ms. Harms.

Gloria Harms remembers the day when one of Nathan's employees was in trouble with a creditor who threatened legal action against the man. Pritikin telephoned the creditor and asked him if he would drop the charges if Pritikin paid the debt. Pritikin then got his employee to agree that he would pay Pritikin back in monthly installments from his salary. Ms. Harms recalled, however, that Pritikin took one installment payment out of the employee's salary and forgave the rest of the debt.

When it came to managing people, Pritikin's only tool was time. He never threatened or cajoled. He simply endured; he waited the human problems out. According to his secretary, his standard answer to anyone who complained about another employee's work habits was: "He needs time" or "She needs time." He believed that most human character flaws that got in the way of work would eventually go away, or the person would decide on his or her own to leave the company. His stock reply to anyone who asked him how a particular business problem would turn out was simply, "We'll know in 90 days." Meanwhile, he turned his attention to the technical aspects of his business and let the personality problems take care of themselves.

This attitude sprang in part from his inherent lack of confidence in handling relationships, and particularly personality conflicts. Instead of trying to correct such situations, he responded with tolerance and compassion, choosing to say nothing and wait.

His refusal to confront people openly got him into endless trouble with business partners, however. His attorney, Howard Parke, said that Nathan would participate in important business conversations seemingly in a state of complete agreement with his partners. After the conversation was over, however, Pritikin would go off and do just what he wanted. Some of his business partners said Pritikin at times was difficult to pin down, becoming remote or elusive.

Ted Barash, a marketing expert and the man given credit for making Weight Watchers a success, went into business with Pritikin to form the Pritikin Better Health Program, which sought to provide weekend seminars on the Pritikin program around the country. Barash and Pritikin negotiated for months before Nathan was willing to sign a contract giving Barash the rights to begin marketing the program. Barash recalled how Pritikin postponed numerous meetings with attorneys and principal participants for months on end, costing Barash and Pritikin many thousands of dollars in legal fees and lost time.

"Nathan was a genius," Barash recalled. "He deserves enormous credit. But like all geniuses, he had major deficiencies." Clearly, the greatest of these was in business. According to Barash, Nathan would sign papers he should not have and, at crucial times, change his mind in midstream, holding up a project or turning it in a new direction.

Parke maintained that the chief source of conflict between Pritikin and his business partners was the fact that Nathan tended to be soft-spoken and indirect, and as a result people often "heard what they wanted to hear." Frequently, however, the source of the trouble with business partners or associates was Pritikin's unwillingness to state his aims plainly.

He could also be stubborn. Even when he deliberately brought in experts to advise him, said Parke, he often did exactly the opposite of what he was advised to do.

Compassionate and tolerant with weakness, often a poor judge of character, a genius inventor who cared little for business, remote with peers, and aggressive with antagonists–Nathan Pritikin possessed a complex character with remarkable paradoxes. To most of the people in his life, Pritikin represented the embodiment of paternal solicitude, offering jobs, money, and better health. With partners in business he often became guarded and elusive, seeking always to maintain his independence and control over his business affairs. When it came to dealing with adversaries and powerful institutions, Pritikin's mild manner took the offensive. The warrior side of his nature emerged and he would fight endlessly for what he believed was right.

In August 1974, Nathan turned 59. He didn't know it then, but his greatest battles still lay ahead.

CHAPTER **10**

Heart Health
and the Pritikin Program

On January 5, 1975, Pritikin stood in the living room of a small two-bedroom house in Long Beach, California, looking at 13 severely ill men. All 13 were on complete disability from the Veterans Administration; some were not very far from death.

They ranged in age from 50 to 70. As a group, they suffered from heart disease, angina pain, high blood pressure, cerebral ischemia (lack of blood to the brain, often caused by atherosclerosis), diabetes, arthritis, gout, congestive heart failure, elevated cholesterol levels, elevated triglyceride levels, and xanthomas (nodules of flesh that appear on the body caused by fatty deposits in the skin). Most of the men couldn't walk a block without severe chest and leg pain from insufficient circulation.

The group ranged in educational levels from a couple of college graduates to one man who had left school after the third grade. Their occupations before going on complete disability were equally varied. One of the men in that living room, Alex Berger, who in 1975 was 62, had retired from the U.S. Army with the rank of full colonel. Another, Sam Freedman, 68, was a retired journalist. Most of the men, however, had worked as manual laborers–sheetmetal workers, gardeners, and shipyard workers. Several had had long periods of unemployment. One man had made a fortune, lost it, and had spent several years living in flophouses and YMCAs.

"It was a real cross section of society," Alex Berger recalled in 1986. "Some of the guys were really beaten up by life."

They were not an inspiring lot, but to Pritikin these men were a dream come true.

Nathan was about to place these 13 men–plus 6 more who would

113

follow the program at home–on his program, and then follow their progress for six months. The men would receive no treatment except Pritikin's diet and exercise regimen. The exercise would consist entirely of two to three 15-minute walks per day. The men would increase the distance they walked as their condition improved.

The men would also be encouraged to stop smoking cigarettes and drinking alcohol for the duration of the study.

At the conclusion of the six-month study, the health of Pritikin's group would be compared to another group of 19 men who received the standard medical care for heart disease, claudication, and diabetes. This second group, called a control group, would also be encouraged to walk daily and to stop smoking and drinking. They would consume a standard American diet, made up of 20 percent protein, 40 percent fat, and 40 percent carbohydrate.

Nathan saw it as a chance to prove once and for all that his diet was more effective in the treatment of these diseases than orthodox medicine. If the results were what he hoped, it would be a landmark study.

Still, by the looks of things–especially in the expressions of doubt on the faces of the men who now looked back at him–it was not going to be an easy task. But then, few things in this study had been easy so far.

A Study Begins in Long Beach

The project had started because of a fortuitous coincidence. Five months earlier, in August 1974, Dr. John Kern had happened across a tape recording of Pritikin's memorable talk to the annual meeting of the American Academy of Medical Preventics, which had taken place the previous March in Miami Beach. The conference officials had recorded the talks given by the speakers and made them available by mail order to doctors around the country. Kern, chief of General Medicine at the VA Hospital in Long Beach, California, was intrigued by Pritikin's thesis that diet could prevent and even reverse many degenerative diseases, including atherosclerosis.

Kern had been studying the effects of chelation–an experimental therapy based on the hypothesis that certain drugs can eliminate plaque from the arteries–and vitamin and mineral therapy on atherosclerosis. After hearing Pritikin's talk, however, Kern became excited by the possibility of using diet as a means of treating heart disease. He telephoned Pritikin and the two met later that month.

At their meeting, Kern suggested he and Pritikin collaborate on a study testing the effectiveness of diet as a treatment for heart disease. The plan was simple: two groups of men with proven coronary heart disease would be studied. One group would get Pritikin's diet and exercise program, while the other got conventional medical treatment. After a period of six months, both groups would be compared to see what effects, if any, the Pritikin program had had on the experimental group, as compared to the standard therapy group.

The Veterans Administration would provide the patients for both groups and all the necessary medical tests, including blood and EKG stress tests and angiograms, Kern said. An angiogram is a test done to ascertain the degree of atherosclerosis clogging the arteries and where the blockages are located. The test is done by injecting radioactive dye into the bloodstream; the dye collects in the arteries throughout the body. X-rays are then able to reveal the extent to which atherosclerosis has accumulated in the arteries. The test can reveal the condition of main arteries throughout the body, including the femoral arteries in the legs and the coronary arteries of the heart. (There is some risk to the patient. Angiograms have been responsible for bringing on heart attacks and a small percentage of patients have died from the test.)

Kern said the VA would provide before-and-after angiograms; that is, each patient would receive an angiogram at the outset of the study and another at the conclusion of the project, to see what changes took place in the arteries of both groups.

Another measurement for the patient progress, Pritikin and Kern decided, would be claudication, an illness of the circulatory system.

Claudication is often caused by atherosclerosis blocking the arteries at the periphery of the body. The lack of circulation results in pain in the limbs, and especially in the legs when walking. People with severe claudication cannot walk more than a short distance before they suffer from acute pain in the legs and are forced to stop walking. Claudication would serve as a good test disease, because it was easy to gauge whether a functional improvement had been made on the program simply by measuring the distance the men could walk at the outset of the study and comparing it to how far they could walk at the conclusion of the study.

Pritikin and Kern wanted the men in both groups to be well-matched, meaning that each man in Pritikin's group should have a counterpart in the control group with a similar illness at a similar stage of development. Ideally, a man in the experimental group with a 50 percent closure of the femoral (thigh) artery should be compared with a man in the control group with approximately the same degree of closure in the same artery. This would provide a clear comparison between the two therapies applied in the study.

Pritikin realized from the start that he would need help administering and supervising his program. He needed someone to ensure that the men ate the proper diet, took daily walks, and maintained the program. He also needed help sifting through the more than 800 relevant patient records at the VA Hospital to find at least 20 well-matched pairs. There was only one person who had the necessary expertise and time available to help him, and that person was his son Robert.

Born on August 29, the same day as his father, Robert Pritikin was about to turn 23 years old in the summer of 1974. Like his father, Robert was fascinated by science. His degree in biology and his familiarity with the scientific literature on diet and health made him a natural protégé to Nathan. But Robert was now in Bali, Indonesia, on a surfing holiday, with no immediate plans of returning.

Initially, Nathan wanted Robert to come home to become a traveling fellow for the Kirsten Foundation, a New York-based philanthropic institute that was interested in Nathan's ideas regarding diet's relationship to diabetes. But now Nathan needed Robert's help to conduct what Nathan was calling his "Long Beach Study." Since the Kirsten Foundation was interested in finding a cure for diabetes, and since the Long Beach Study would examine the effects of diet on diabetics, Pritikin proposed to the Kirsten Foundation that it pay Robert's salary while Robert supervised the study. The foundation director, Dr. Melvin Weidman, agreed.

Knowing how much this study meant to his father, Robert readily acquiesced to come home from paradise.

New Life for the Severely Ill

Together, Robert and Nathan found 38 VA patients to participate in the study, and divided them into two groups of 19 each. Nathan had blood tests performed at the VA Hospital on each of the patients and now turned to the VA for angiograms. That's when things began to get difficult.

The VA now refused to administer the angiograms. VA Hospital director, Dr. Wilbert S. Aranow, prevented the angiograms because several VA patients had recently died while the tests were being administered. Aranow was now cutting back on all such tests.

But there was another problem: Kern and Pritikin hadn't gone through formal channels for VA approval of their study, and although Kern could provide certain tests and facilities on his own authority, he couldn't deliver the angiograms himself. Nathan asked VA officials how long it would take to get VA approval for the study–which would guarantee the tests–but the answer was daunting: the process could take up to two years.

"All my patients will be dead by then," Pritikin told the VA officials. That didn't seem to impress them much, however.

Nathan suggested that he would pay for the angiograms himself and asked how much each test cost. The answer was $1,200; with 38 men in his study, that would come to more than $45,000–too much for Pritikin to fork over himself.

Pritikin refused to give up. He told Robert, "Don't worry. Give me a few days and I'll have the whole thing put back together." As usual, his perserverance paid off.

After being refused assistance by local health institutions, Pritikin got Loma Linda University–a Seventh-day Adventist hospital in Riverside, California–to perform the angiograms. Loma Linda advocated a vegetarian diet and saw Pritikin's study as a chance to test the effectiveness of such a program on serious illnesses. Pritikin had his angiograms.

But now he had another problem: where to conduct the study. He wanted to use the VA personnel and kitchens, but dismissed the idea when he found that the available kitchens were only equipped to feed the thousands of people who were inpatients at the VA complex. "The smallest pot they had was four feet long," Pritikin recalled. Remarkably, the VA had no small test kitchen in their entire facility.

Nathan and Robert worked out an elaborate neighborhood scheme in which the men would be divided into small groups and take turns eating at one another's homes. The logistics of that plan proved untenable, however, and Nathan ultimately decided to rent a house where he would install Robert as the supervisor and cook.

That house was located at 2020 Kallin Avenue in Long Beach, near the VA Hospital. The plan was for Robert to spend the weekdays with the men, from Sunday night to Friday afternoon. Nathan and Ilene would arrive Friday afternoon and relieve Robert, who could then take the weekend off. Robert would see that the men got their meals (he cooked the food or reheated meals already prepared by Ilene) and supervise the exercise of the men during the week. Robert kept all the records on the men, coordinated the tests at the VA, and answered questions about the program whenever they arose.

Even with Robert's salary being provided by the Kirsten Foundation, the study was still going to be expensive. Feeding 19 men for six months plus renting a house in Long Beach came to well over $20,000.

Nathan's attempts to raise the money through 50 private health foundations were quickly denied. He wasn't a medical doctor or a Ph.D. or affiliated with a university. The National Institutes of Health informed him that it would take nine months before the bureaucracy could render a decision on his grant request. Once again, the "damn-the-torpedoes" streak emerged in him; there was nothing else to say but "full speed ahead." He wanted this study done, and if that meant picking up the costs, so be it.

Nathan did get some help, however. Since the study was designed to show the health benefits from eating a low-fat, low-cholesterol diet, several food companies solicited by Pritikin provided quantities of whole grains, breads, rice cakes, crackers, canned tomato products, nonfat milk and hoop cheese, fruit, and herbal teas. Among these companies were Erewhon, Fisher Mills, El Molino, the Hol Grain division of Gold Grain, Chiquita Brands, Hunt's Foods, Pure Gold, Knudsen Dairy, and Celestial Seasonings.

Pritikin responded to each company with ebullient gratitude.

> The success of the program was greatly helped by your contribution to the study. You may not have been aware but we had no outside funding to feed the men, and without contributions such as yours the study might not have been possible.
>
> It should be pointed out that food was offered to us that we refused because it did not meet our nutritional standards. Your product, of course, did, and it is our pleasure to let the scientific world know that.

Pritikin did turn away a large apple distributor who offered Pritikin a free supply of apples for the duration of the study, because the apples were covered with a wax polish that Nathan suspected might be unhealthful. He checked with the Johnson Wax Company in Racine, Wisconsin, where the wax for apples was made, and found that the apple wax had a strong chemical resemblance to wax used to shine cars. He decided to pass on the apples.

As a final measure of support, Nathan enlisted his nephew, Dr. Stephen Kaye, a medical doctor, to assist in providing regular medical checkups for the men.

By January 5, 1975, everything was in place: the men were present; Kern and Kaye were standing by, ready to keep track of their patients; Robert was ready; the food was available, and Nathan was chafing at the bit to get started. He had 19 sick people to treat and to transform.

That day, the study began.

Because most of them had nowhere else to go, the men began showing up at the house at 6:30 in the morning. Robert would be up only a few minutes by then and preparing breakfast. One by one, they would appear in the kitchen, sit down, and start talking to him.

"We had guys who were in their seventies, so our group had representatives from World War I, World War II, and the Korean War." For six months, Robert listened patiently to every kind of war story imaginable. He heard the seemingly never-ending account that ran from Verdun to Normandy to the freezing cold along the 38th Parallel. For many of these men, their best years were behind them, and they relived them endlessly, from breakfast till dinner and then through the evening snack.

Breakfast usually consisted of cracked whole wheat or rolled oats, sliced banana, and skim milk. Both grain cereals got heaping tablespoons of bran flakes sprinkled on them. The meal was accompanied by a cup of herb tea.

After breakfast, Robert sent the men off on their walks. There was a park nearby and the house was situated in a pleasant neighborhood. At the outset of the study, most of the men could barely walk a few blocks without severe claudication pain. Soon they would return, complaining of leg pain and wanting their morning snack, which consisted of a piece of fruit–an orange or half a grapefruit, usually. After their snack, the men walked again. Like the former soldiers that they were, they marched reluctantly after Robert's coaxing. Nearly crippled with leg cramps, they quickly returned, most of them wondering how in heaven's name they had ever got themselves involved in such madness.

Lunch was at noon. It usually consisted of a variety of greens, soups, whole grains, and bread, and was finished off with one of several herb teas. Specifically, the Pritikins provided a green salad, usually made up of romaine lettuce and other vegetables; one of several soups, including vegetable, minestrone, lentil, split pea, bean, and potato; a variety of grains, including brown rice and bulgur wheat; occasionally some nonfat hoop cheese served on a sandwich made with whole wheat bread.

After lunch, the men took another walk. At 3:00 P.M., they returned for soup.

Dinner was served at 5:00 P.M. A typical dinner consisted of a salad, beans, whole grains, and an herb tea. Ilene and her assistant Esther Taylor, who worked for the Pritikins and would eventually become the first chef at the Longevity Center, converted a number of ethnic dishes into Pritikin-style meals. They made enchiladas, tostadas, lasagne, and falafel, using a variety of beans, whole grain products, and vegetables.

The men were scheduled to leave at 6:00 P.M. and return home. Robert provided them with a snack for later at night, which usually consisted of rice crackers and a piece of fruit. Again, many of them hung around until Robert chased them out around 8:00.

At the outset of the study, the men complained regularly about the food and often poked fun at it. They had spent their lives eating everything imaginable and now suddenly they were eating "birdseed." Grains and beans were peasant food–not American. Cries went out for emergency hamburgers and french fries. Smokers drifted off into the bushes in the park to sneak a few puffs. Few gave up beer and alcohol initially. For the most part, though, compliance among the 13 men who came to the house each day was excellent. They ate the food they were given and took their walks, even though they didn't know what to expect, if anything.

As the weeks went by, Robert settled in to his job. He prepared the meals, did the cleaning, sent the men on their walks, and kept track of their progress. He answered their questions on how the diet would help them as a therapy against their various illnesses and kept them focused on what they were trying to accomplish. He scheduled their appointments for their physical examinations and blood tests at the VA and made sure they got there by driving most of them to the hospital. He was study coordinator, big brother, father confessor, analyst, chief cook, and maid rolled into one.

He worked hard at keeping morale up, but the culture shock of the program caused tensions to build. Personality conflicts began to develop.

As Alex Berger pointed out, the men were from a wide variety of backgrounds and education levels. There were natural antagonisms. Coming to the same house every day for meals brought them into close contact with one another; for some of the men, that meant being in the company of people they didn't care for, and in a couple of cases actually despised. Like caged animals, they tolerated each other until eventually the grumblings turned to outright conflict.

As Nathan would recall years later, "Two of the men, in their sixties—one with congestive heart failure and the other with serious angina—got into a fistfight." The two were pounding each other when suddenly they were both struck, simultaneously, by severe angina, a stabbing pain through the heart. They threw their arms around each other—not in hostility anymore but in fear—and held onto one another for dear life, afraid to let go lest they fall down dead. "They were so gasping for breath," Pritikin recalled, that Robert "could hardly get them apart." The other men stood around them in shock, watching helplessly as the two combatants gasped for life.

With considerable effort, Robert managed to fight his way between the two and separate them. Their chests heaved furiously. For several tense moments, no one knew what would happen next. But soon the tension passed. The two men started to breathe easier. Everyone began to relax.

But the fight awakened the men to the seriousness of their conditions. Their very lives hung by a few tenuous threads. Many were suddenly forced to decide whether this program was simply a social obligation, to be carried out as if it were a troublesome break from the routine, or a serious attempt at getting well.

One of the men involved in the fight decided to leave the study. Two months later, he was dead of a heart attack. An autopsy revealed that he had died of fibrillation (heart spasm), more than likely caused by his return to smoking and a high-fat diet after leaving the study. (Remarkably, the autopsy and a subsequent angiogram showed some regression of the man's atherosclerosis in the femoral arteries. The results of the angiogram later performed at Loma Linda University would be disputed by National Heart, Lung and Blood Institute as inconclusive, however.)

The men who tried to maintain the program at home demonstrated poor compliance, and most left the study.

In the end, 12 men stayed with the program. They had nowhere else to go and little to support them on the way. There were three square meals waiting at 2020 Kallin Street every day, an assortment of snacks, and Robert's company. Besides, the food was growing on them. The 12 remaining men did indeed give up their standard ways of eating, as well as smoking and alcohol. They adhered strictly to the diet and exercise program.

Every weekend, Nathan and Ilene would arrive with bags of produce and large containers of frozen soups and dinner entrees that Robert would heat during the week. Robert would then leave for the weekend. Ilene prepared the meals on Friday night, Saturday, and Sunday while Nathan saw each man privately to discuss his progress on the program.

"When Nathan arrived," Berger recalled, "he would go over each person's file in depth with them, covering every aspect of the program and any symptoms he might be experiencing. He was totally dedicated to every person in the study."

When Nathan saw each man, he ferreted out every little detail about the man's health, his personal problems, his complaints about the program or his general condition. As always, Pritikin was totally focused on the person in front of him, giving the impression that no one else mattered but this man. One by one, they left Pritikin, convinced that better days and greater health were at hand. All they had to do was stick to the program and keep walking and they would see results. Later, he gave them the facts relating diet to health and the information was powerful in itself.

"He knew the information so well that you believed him," Berger recalled. "He convinced you that you were getting a new lease on life."

By the simple strength of his personality, Pritikin gained each man's implicit confidence. He also inspired them.

"By Friday, everyone was ready to quit, kill themselves, or go back to drinking, smoking, and high-fat foods, but by Sunday they were enthusiastic and ready to go back at it," said Berger.

At night, Pritikin would give a lecture on diet's relationship to health and the benefits of exercise. In his lectures, he showed the men in simple yet graphic terms just what was happening to their bodies on his diet and exercise program. In his step-by-step approach, Pritikin showed the men how their former diets had caused their illnesses, and how their current eating and exercise habits were restoring their health. Pritikin in effect convinced each one of these men that he was indeed fortunate to be a part of this program.

The participants responded with respect not only for the program but for the man who had created it.

"The men were like little children around my father," Robert said. "They were on their best behavior. They had the sense that to act rude or disruptive in front of him would be the worst kind of embarrassment."

Still, there were problems Pritikin could do nothing about. Most had to do with the VA. Despite Kern's participation, Pritikin's study got an extremely low priority at the laboratories at the VA. Pritikin's patients were the last people to get blood and other tests performed, and, if the analysis was to be done late on a Friday, the vials of drawn blood would often mysteriously disappear. Pritikin was forced to have his men come back time and again to have the same test performed in order to ensure accurate record keeping of their blood values. Getting the laboratory technicians to run treadmill stress tests got to be so difficult that Kern took to doing the tests on the weekends. He ran the tests himself to avoid the resistance he and Nathan were getting from the VA.

Meanwhile, neighbors began to complain about the strange men gathering every day in front of the house at 2020 Kallin Street. When the neighbors found out that Pritikin was running a clinic in the house, they threw a collective fit. They had the Long Beach Housing Authority send cease-and-desist orders to Pritikin. Housing authority officers began showing up weekly with summonses ordering Robert to close down the house immediately. Robert responded by telling the officers that they would have to take him to court to get him out of the house. It would be at least six months before the case could be heard.

"By that time, we'll be out of here," Robert told the evictors. "So why don't you save everyone the headaches and legal expenses and leave us alone." Logic didn't seem to impress them. Cease-and-desist orders continued to arrive.

Eventually, Nathan went to the housing authority and tried to convince the Long Beach officials of the importance of his study to the good of the world. He tried to work the same magic on them that he did on his men, but to no avail. Finally, he fell in with Robert and threatened to get his lawyers involved. Ultimately, the Long Beach authorities saw the wisdom of leaving the Pritikins alone, as long as they vacated the premises by late June.

As the turmoil settled down, the program was able to return to its uninterrupted healthy routine, and by February, it was showing some results.

"In a month, most of the men were off their medication," Berger recalled. "People started to feel better, and gradually we started to see miracles right in front of our eyes."

Pritikin wrote enthusiastically to a doctor in the early part of the study about the results so far. In his letter, he states the "results [of the Long Beach Study] to date are phenomenal. The controls are unchanged, but of the [Pritikin] diet group: the 9 hypertensives [9 men who had high blood pressure at the outset of the study] are normal without drugs; the [adult-onset] diabetics are off all their drugs, including two diabetics who had been on insulin from 10 to 15 years; severe arthritis has disappeared; walking capacity has increased from blocks to miles; blood levels of cholesterol and triglycerides have dropped 30 to 70 percent."

On February 24, Pritikin wrote to Dr. Weidman, director of the Kirsten Foundation, with a progress report on the diabetics in the study.

> Both W.K. and C.Q. [two men in the study] have advanced atherosclerosis and have had arterial reconstruction work done. Their angiograms show considerable arterial stenosis and occlusion. W.K. couldn't walk 200 feet without holding onto a fence or other support. His balance was poor and endurance zero. Now he walks 5 miles every day. C.Q. had claudication problems not as bad as W.K.'s and has increased his walking capacity to 8 to 10 miles per day.
>
> Another diabetic, E.B., on Orinase [an oral drug for diabetes] has now normalized, and still another, J.K., who had been spilling [sugar through the urine] for a year and a half (2 hour postprandial 311 mg.%) is now spill-free.

Robert kept records on the men, but Sam Freedman, the journalist, kept an extensive daily journal of his experience in the study.

When he entered the study, Freedman noted that at 63 years of age, he was five feet, four inches tall and weighed 162 pounds. He could only walk three blocks before his severe angina and claudication pain forced him to stop exerting himself. In addition to the heart disease and angina, Freedman had high blood pressure, kidney and urinary problems, and was overweight. He was taking nitroglycerin tablets to keep his heart pumping during angina attacks; Aldomet, a medication for high blood pressure; Ismelin, for high blood pressure specifically caused by atherosclerosis blocking blood flow through the kidneys; and Hydrochlor, a diuretic to assist the function of the kidneys and bladder.

On January 20, Freedman noted in his journal after taking a short walk: "chest pain, severe, 15 minutes duration; aborted with one tab nitroglycerin." He also wrote that he had calf pain in his left leg caused by the claudication. On January 27, after another walk, "anginal paroxysm, painful and paralyzing, extreme left pulmonary area. . . . Aborted by 1.015 gr. nitroglycerin."

On February 1, however, he wrote: "No regression. Left leg stronger."

On February 3: "Left leg feels better on walking today. . . . Notable that I was able to walk 21 blocks. Have just returned and leg feels good."

On February 6: " . . . Off all medication at this time. Effect of termination awaited in next blood pressure reading."

On February 8, he wrote: " . . . Feeling of well-being. Slight lessening of nocturia [frequent urination at night]."

On February 9: "Improved renal function. Parabolic arc of urine has resumed normality, with full and stronger flow. Nocturia has lessened. Termination of diuretic [drug] last week shows no ill effect now."

Two days later, Freedman wrote: "The food regimen here has resulted in an improved gastrointestinal condition, with elimination all that can be desired. There is diminishing flatulence. Sleep has also improved, ending some insomnia in the early A.M. hours. There is now no doubt that a saltless dietary, simple nonfat, and walking can do wonders for the body. The blood pressure, no longer under Aldomet, Ismelin . . . is well within normal limits. Diastolic consistently holds at 80 to 74 and systolic, on February 10 test, 155. *Now on no medication* [emphasis Freedman's]."

On February 19, Freedman noted that his blood pressure test was 138 over 65, another large drop in just seven days.

On March 20, he recorded his weight at 130 pounds, a loss of 34 pounds in less than three months.

On May 3, Freedman marveled at his ever-improving kidney condition. "Now I rise once a night, whereas formerly it was 3 or 4 times. Could this mean that the kidney ischemia which obviously exists [his angiogram indicated advanced atherosclerosis in the kidneys] has lessened?"

On May 14, just three weeks before the study was to end, Freedman made a summary entry in his journal.

> Seldom, if ever, suffer from fatigue, now that diet is so beneficial and frequent; also marked decrease in weight from 164 lbs . . . to 126 today . . . . Seldom, if ever, feel hunger on this dietary. Find simplest foods satisfying and do not have any vague cravings for indefinable food elements. This I believe is significant, indicating complete nutritive value of dietary used in this regimen. The ample salads, twice a day (at least once a day) provide the vitamins and minerals amply needed to fuel the system. I attribute this as the main factor for lack of fatigue and nervousness. No medications have been found necessary since mid-February. There has been no recurrence of angina pectoris, which formerly was frequent, occurring at rest, and at night in bed. There has been no edema, and kidney function has improved. Elimination has been normal . . . . Avoiding all fats, sugars, white bread, salt, alcohol . . . and tobacco. Drinking water and nonfat milk. No preservatives in food.
>
> The complete cessation of substernal pain episodes may be highly significant as to cause. Probably the remarkably lowered cholesterol is the primary factor.

When he concluded the study, Freedman was walking more than 5 miles per day. Berger, who could walk as many as 3 miles in a day at the outset of the study, finished the six-month program walking 15 miles a day.

As each man began to see the benefits of the program, morale and enthusiasm made quantum leaps.

Diabetics were off oral drugs and insulin; hypertensives were off medication with normal blood pressures; all the men with angina experienced complete cessation of the painful attacks; the men with arthritis no longer needed medication for pain.

Heart Disease: "It's Gone!"

One day in February 1975, a stranger showed up at the doorstep of the 2020 Kallin Street house looking for Nathan. The man's name was Leon Perlsweig and he had just been told that he needed bypass surgery if he was going to continue living much longer.

Perlsweig was a 54-year-old Los Angeles attorney. Silver-haired and handsome, the five-foot, six-inch Perlsweig could barely walk a block without suffering from severe angina pain caused by the exertion. In January, 1975, the pain was getting worse. The cool Los Angeles nights caused his blood vessels to constrict, further reducing the amount of oxygen to his heart and bringing on the angina. Perlsweig had been taking nitroglycerin tablets for his angina and now he was taking the pills more frequently–and more fearfully.

The time had come to do something. Perlsweig went to the UCLA medical center for an examination, where doctors performed an electrocardiogram, a treadmill stress test, and an angiogram on him. Then they gave him the shocking diagnosis. One of his coronary arteries was nearly 100 percent occluded, another was 89 percent closed, and a third was 79 percent blocked. His doctor informed him that he would need triple bypass surgery in order to go on living.

Perlsweig spent the next two weeks considering the surgery. One afternoon that month, he read an article in the *National Enquirer* about Eula Weaver and her remarkable experience using the Pritikin program. The article detailed Mrs. Weaver's long history of heart disease and other illnesses, as well as her full recovery and her success in the Senior Olympics. Perlsweig called Mrs. Weaver and engaged her in a lengthy conversation about her health and the Pritikin program. After talking to Mrs. Weaver, Perlsweig was convinced that the program was indeed responsible for her recovery. The next call he made was to Nathan. The two agreed to meet at the Long Beach house.

After talking to Pritikin, Perlsweig was skeptical. His doctors had informed him that he needed bypass surgery to survive, but Pritikin was saying that a simple diet and exercise program was all that was needed. Could Pritikin be right? he wondered.

Perlsweig went to Kern for more information about the results Pritikin was having with his Long Beach patients. Kern explained that he was looking at chelation and vitamin therapy, as well as comparing Pritikin's ideas with a control group. Perlsweig asked him which of the therapies seemed to be having the best results.

Kern "hemmed and hawed," Perlsweig recalled. "He told me it was too early to tell which therapy was having the best results. But as a lawyer, I'm pretty good at using my cross-examination technique to pin a person down and get him to tell me the truth. And so, after telling him that I realize it's too early to get final results, and that we must be cautious, I asked, 'Up till now, who has the best results, Pritikin's group or the other therapies?' And he told me that Pritikin's group had far and away the best results."

Perlsweig considered his options. "Pritikin wasn't asking me to do something that was so radical, like have bypass surgery." He started the diet.

Perlsweig ate the whole grains and vegetables Pritikin had prescribed. He avoided all meat, dairy products, eggs, and refined grains and took walks each day. Periodically, he checked with Nathan on his condition.

"He was quite thorough and very patient," Perlsweig said of his meetings with Nathan. "And he really gave of himself. I offered to pay him several times, but he refused." It wasn't long before Perlsweig began to feel the effects of the program.

"I knew in 30 days that I was getting better," he said. The angina pain began to recede until it disappeared. His overall vitality improved dramatically. In two months, he lost 18 pounds, his weight dropping to an optimal 139. Perlsweig discontinued the nitroglycerin and other drugs he had been taking, and gradually increased the length and speed of his walks. Four months later, he went back to UCLA medical center for another EKG and a treadmill stress test.

Before his physician conducted the treadmill stress test, he told Perlsweig that there was no cure for his coronary disease. Once you have it, the doctor said, you have it for life. He didn't want Perlsweig to be disappointed when his tests showed no real change in his condition. Perlsweig got on the treadmill and started to walk . . . and walk . . . and walk. Perlsweig felt great. Meanwhile, his physician examined the EKG tracings and marvelled at Perlsweig's results. His physician could not find any trace of coronary insufficiency.

"While I was taking the test, my doctor, in a very undignified and unprofessional manner, kept on repeating the same words over and over again," Perlsweig recalled. "He kept on saying, 'It's gone, it's gone; it's not supposed to be gone, but it's gone.'"

After a year on the diet, Perlsweig was running nine miles per day. In 1987, he was still on the program and still running up to four miles per day.

Creeping Criticism

Not all of Pritikin's patients experienced such remarkable recoveries. On July 10, Nathan wrote to Weidman again, giving an update on the study's success rate with its diabetics. He told Weidman that two juvenile diabetics in the study had had relapses and had fallen back on insulin after being off the synthetic hormone for a short time. Pritikin would concede later that his diet would not cure juvenile diabetics, though he felt they could be helped and would need less insulin on the program. Still, a complete restoration of health would be impossible using just the diet and exercise program, he would later say. Pritikin's real success with diabetics came with those who suffered from adult-onset diabetes. People with this disease–both obese and lean adult-onsets–could be restored to what Pritikin termed "normal function," meaning complete freedom from oral drugs or insulin.

Despite his disappointment with juvenile diabetics, Pritikin's program did show some remarkable results and demonstrated–at least to Nathan–how powerful his diet and exercise program was for patients with heart disease, high blood pressure, angina, and for adult-onset diabetics.

In his write-up of the Long Beach Study, Pritikin reported that the control group made no significant changes in high blood pressure or diabetes. They did show a 448 percent improvement in walking distance, an impressive feat, given the high-fat diet they consumed. Pritikin attributed this improvement to the fine California weather, which permitted the men to walk in pleasant conditions for six months of the year.

The Long Beach experimental group showed a 6,000 percent increase in walking distance–the greatest improvement of walking distance in patients with claudication recorded anywhere in the scientific literature. Pritikin also reported remarkable improvement in patients with coexisting diseases. One hundred percent of all patients with angina were returned to normal and weaned of all drugs. The same success rate was achieved with all patients suffering from gout, arthritis, and elevated blood lipids– that is, cessation of symptoms and elimination of medication. Seventy-five percent of all the hypertensives were relieved of symptoms of high blood pressure and taken off all medication. One hypertensive patient who was weaned of his drugs had been on antihypertensive medication for 20 years.

Two of the men–including the man who died–showed some reversal of atherosclerosis in the femoral arteries, located in the thighs.

For the next several years, Pritikin would claim on the basis of his Long Beach Study results that his diet was reversing atherosclerosis. He would be widely criticized for this claim, since reversal had not been shown in the coronary arteries.

But his was not the only criticism leveled against Pritikin's study. Dr. Robert Levy, director of the National Heart, Lung and Blood Institute, would later point out that the study had never been approved by the VA; he would also criticize it because the control and experimental groups were never well matched. He questioned Pritikin's claim of reversal in two patients, stating that the angiographic studies were poorly done and inconclusive. Levy also criticized the study for not being "double-blind." A double-blind study is one in which neither the participating scientists nor the people being studied know which one is getting the special treatment–in this case a low-fat, low-cholesterol diet–and which one is not. This prevents either group from being prejudiced by expectations as to the outcome of the study. In the Long Beach Study, the men in the experimental group clearly knew they were getting Nathan's diet and exercise program, as did the researchers. Levy would later conclude in essence that the study was meaningless, regardless of the positive results. But Pritikin pointed out that it would have been impossible to conduct a double-blind study, and in any case prior knowledge of the diet could not account for such outstanding results.

It was true that the study never received VA approval. Pritikin conceded, too, that the control and experimental groups were poorly matched. Moreover, he had conducted the study under extremely difficult conditions, given the resistance from the VA, the Long Beach Housing Authority, the lack of money, and the need to get maximum results in a very short period of time. Reversal of heart disease in monkeys usually takes as long as 18 months to accomplish. There was no reason to believe Pritikin could accomplish the same feat–even under the best of conditions–in six months.

Nevertheless, the program had an incredible impact on the health of the men in Pritikin's group. In fact, the results were so good that, as John Kern would say years later, Pritikin could have been justified in simply calling the project a "pilot" study, rather than a "controlled double-blind." The study showed the impact of the Pritikin diet and exercise program on severely ill men. Although it was flawed from the point of view that it was not double-blind and yes, the angiographic studies may well have been difficult to interpret, the study nevertheless demonstrated that the program would restore severely ill men to health in a matter of months. That was no small accomplishment. Pritikin expected sincere scientists to be able to look past the study's flaws and see into the substance of the results. As would become eminently clear to Pritikin later, Levy and other scientists refused to do this. Indeed, the study's flaws would be used to dismiss not only its results, but also its basic premise: that diet could be useful in the treatment of heart disease and other serious illnesses.

Over the next decade, Levy and Pritikin would become bitter enemies. Their points of view would delineate the debate between the scientific establishment, much of which was searching for a pharmaceutical answer for illness, and the mavericks, those arguing for a nutritional solution.

Despite the criticisms of his study, Pritikin was overjoyed with the results of the program. As he and Kern reviewed the work, Pritikin mentioned in passing that a rehabilitation center using the low-fat, low-cholesterol diet and exercise program would be a great success. The thought had been given voice before Nathan realized the significance of what he had said.

11

The Longevity Center
Takes Root

*A*s the Long Beach Study wrapped up, the idea of establishing a rehabilitation center using diet and exercise as therapy took hold of Pritikin. He told his nephew, Dr. Stephen Kaye, of his idea and suggested that Kaye join him in the enterprise. Kaye agreed.

Stephen Kaye was the son of Nathan's sister Ruth and her husband David. He had just graduated from the University of Arizona Medical School in 1974 and planned to enter private practice. Growing up, Stephen had become a kind of protégé to Nathan. Stephen's father had long worked for Nathan, and Stephen would often visit the plant to talk to Nathan about the projects he was working on.

"He loved to teach young people," Kaye recalled. "He approached everything logically and methodically. He became a kind of model for me, the way he thought about a problem and then proceeded to work it out." As a teenager, Stephen became Nathan's "research gofer," getting papers out of the library for his uncle on any number of subjects, from medicine to engineering. In time Kaye also developed an interest in both areas.

Eventually, Stephen went to medical school, where he applied Nathan's ideas to some of his patients while in residency training.

When the Long Beach Study began, Kaye was a natural to assist in the project. He was a young medical doctor who was intimately familiar with Pritikin's approach to health problems. Now, when Nathan was considering opening a rehabilitation center, Kaye seemed like the perfect physician to work with Pritikin.

But the question remained: How could Pritikin publicize the results of the Long Beach Study and open the kind of center he dreamed of? The answer was not long in coming.

In the summer of 1975, Dr. John Kern and Pritikin wrote a series of abstracts–short summaries describing the study and its results–and submitted them to the American Heart Association (AHA) and other medical groups. When an abstract is accepted, there is often the opportunity for the scientists involved in the study to present their results at medical meetings.

Because of his position at the Veterans Administration hospital and other affiliations, Kern was highly credentialed, and thus was listed as the senior author on the paper submitted to the AHA. Two more abstracts–submitted to physical therapy groups, the American Congress of Rehabilitation Medicine and the American Academy of Physical Medicine and Rehabilitation–listed Nathan as the senior author. Robert Pritikin and Steven Kaye were listed as co-authors on all the papers.

The AHA had no interest in the Long Beach Study and dismissed it with a perfunctory reply.

Years later, Nathan would bitterly comment that the American Heart Association published abstracts that same year on such topics as the amount of cholesterol in a guinea pig's liver, employment opportunities for those who had just experienced bypass surgery, and the amount of collagen in a rat's tail. These were more important, Pritikin noted, than a therapy that could get 75 percent of all hypertensives off medication and free of symptoms in six weeks. (That same year, in fact, the AHA had launched a campaign to find a cure for hypertension, a leading risk factor in heart disease and stroke. Approximately 25 million Americans suffer from hypertension, or high blood pressure.)

However, the American Congress of Rehabilitation Medicine accepted the paper and–as fate would have it–asked Nathan, as senior author, to present his findings at their annual medical meeting. The meeting was to be held in November at the Hyatt Regency Hotel in Atlanta, Georgia.

Nathan approached the meeting like a general about to capture the high ground. He had brought his daughter Janet with him to help carry out his plan.

Janet, 26 years of age, had assisted in the Long Beach Study from time to time and was well acquainted with her father's ideas, having listened to them for many years–especially at dinner time. She understood his work and the evidence supporting his basic points. Pritikin's plan was for Janet to try to stir up interest in her father's presentation among newspapers and local radio shows by telling the press that Nathan Pritikin was about to present a radically new therapy for heart disease, high blood pressure, diabetes, and claudication. His new approach would provide hope for tens of millions who currently suffered from these diseases. Janet would also see that reporters had copies of Nathan's speech to refer to later when they wrote their stories.

For his part, Nathan set out to deliver the speech of his life.

There was some initial resistance that would have to be overcome, Pritikin believed. The doctors and physical therapists whom he would be addressing were more accustomed to dealing with the hardware of the physically handicapped than they were to hearing about diet. True, both Pritikin and the therapists expounded the virtue of exercise, but in Nathan's view, exercise was an important but still secondary therapy to proper diet.

The Press Spreads the Word

Pritikin gave his talk on November 19, 1975. He didn't mince words. He stated flatly that a low-fat, low-cholesterol diet could reverse coronary heart disease and that for the millions of people suffering from cardiovascular illnesses, the diet and exercise program used in the Long Beach Study was the best hope for recovery. He also talked about the diet and exercise program's effects on adult-onset diabetes, hypertension, and claudication. All of these illnesses, he said, were caused by dietary factors, and proper diet could reverse them.

Meanwhile, Janet worked the media.

The following day, the lead headline on the front page of the *Atlanta Journal* read: "Heart Disease Breakthrough Offers Hope."

"We beat out Franco's death as the lead story," Nathan recalled triumphantly. The wire services picked up the article, and newspapers around the country trumpeted the remarkable new diet and exercise program advocated by Nathan Pritikin.

Thousands of letters from all over the country poured into Santa Barbara inquiring about the program Pritikin had described. Hundreds more had gone to the VA Hospital in Long Beach but, according to a secretary there, many of them were lost before they could be forwarded to Pritikin. Virtually everyone who wrote to Pritikin wanted to know more about his diet and where they could go to begin such a program.

"And I happened to think," Nathan later recalled, "this would be an ideal time to put it in practice. If I wait for the medical community, it will be 200 years. I better do it myself. In a week's time, I made up my mind."

Suddenly, the potential patients were there waiting. He knew he had to act quickly. As usual, Pritikin decided to go for broke: he would open the Longevity Center on January 5, 1976–a month and a half from the day he gave his speech in Atlanta.

Quickly, he wrote back to the people who had inquired about the therapy and told them he was about to open a clinic using the diet and exercise program he described in his Atlanta speech. The clinic, which he called the Longevity Center, would open in January. If they were interested in attending, they could contact him for more information.

Eventually, nine patients and seven spouses committed to the January program. (Pritikin realized right from the start how important the support of the patient's spouse was in making such radical changes in diet and lifestyle and so he encouraged both patient and spouse to attend the program.)

There was still much to be done.

California law forbids medical doctors from working for a layperson. The law is intended to prevent anyone not trained in medicine from influencing how a doctor treats a patient. Pritikin had to find a way around the law if he was to open his own rehabilitation center that would treat severely ill people. Pritikin decided that he could contract with Kaye to do all the medical tests and physical examinations, while Nathan ran the other aspects of the business, including the lectures, exercise supervision, personal counseling, food preparation, and hotel accommodations. The idea was for Kaye to remain self-employed, but maintain an exclusive contract with the Longevity Center. It was a loose arrangement that Pritikin hoped would work.

Nathan then rented enough rooms and office space at the Howard Johnson's Motor Lodge off Highway 101 near Goleta, a suburb of Santa Barbara, to provide for his patients. Kaye would also operate out of the Howard Johnson's motel, providing on-site access to the doctor.

Ilene agreed to supervise the menu planning and meal preparation, and Esther Taylor, the Pritikins' housekeeper, was enrolled to cook the meals. Nathan decided that each session would run for 30 days, assuming of course that the fledgling program survived for more than one month. (He later changed the length of the session to 28 days.)

Nathan asked Robert to join him. With Robert's scientific background and his experience on the Long Beach Study, he was a natural to eventually work with his father. But Robert needed a break. After six months of working 12-hour days with the Long Beach men, Robert decided that he wasn't ready to jump back into the same routine all over again. Eventually, he would go back to college for a master's degree in business, but meanwhile he needed time to think.

Once his plans for the Longevity Center were in place, Pritikin considered other possibilities to propagate his ideas. He wanted to do more than simply treat people. He wanted to change the way most degenerative diseases are treated in the entire United States, and, indeed, in the Western world. To do that, he would have to change the thinking of the scientific and medical communities. And that could be done only by providing scientific proof of his theories.

What better place to provide such proof, he thought, than the Longevity Center. The Longevity Center seemed to meet all the requirements necessary to make it an outstanding research center: It would have a population of people with a variety of proven illnesses; the treatment his patients received would be limited to his diet and exercise program; and since these people would be housed and cared for under one roof for a period of 30 days, doctors could easily monitor their progress, or the lack of it. If his results were as good as he expected them to be–at least as good as those experienced in the Long Beach Study–he could provide consistent scientific documentation on the efficacy of his program as a treatment of severe illness.

Originally, he envisioned a nonprofit research center that could attract foundation grants from leading institutions. These grants could fund research done at the Longevity Center by eminent scientists throughout the world. But here again, he ran into legal problems. The rehabilitation center would have to be a profit-making enterprise in order to remain a viable business, especially at the outset when it would have little, if any, outside support. The realities of keeping the center alive prohibited Pritikin from joining the rehabilitation center with a research foundation. Instead, he formed a separate entity, called the Longevity Research Institute, whose function would be to conduct research at the rehabilitation center, as well as support the research of outside scientists such as Dr. James Anderson at the University of Kentucky Medical School. He would also hold annual conferences at which papers on diet's relationship to disease would be given. The work of the Longevity Center and its success with patients treated there would be reported also, thus increasing scientific awareness of the center's work.

By late December, Pritikin had formed a board of directors and a board of advisors for the Longevity Research Institute. He had several well-credentialed relatives join the board of advisors. He also had the support of medical doctors who had worked with him on the Low Fat and Cholesterol (LFC) study and other professionals whom he had influenced over the years. These included Dr. Anderson; Dr. Wilbur Currier of Pasadena; Dr. Thomas Bassler of Inglewood, California; longtime friend David Fields of Santa Barbara, who had a Ph.D. in economics; and Leon Perlsweig, the Los Angeles attorney whom Nathan had helped during the Long Beach Study.

Very soon after he had formed his initial board of advisors, Pritikin gained the support of Dr. Hugh Trowell, a British physician who, with his colleague, Dr. Denis Burkitt, did the pioneer research linking the presence of fiber in the African diet with the absence of intestinal diseases. It was Burkitt and Trowell who established the importance of fiber to health. Trowell was listed on the Longevity Research Institute letterhead as a

foreign advisor; he eventually was joined by Burkitt, whom Trowell introduced to Pritikin and who would also become a key supporter of Nathan.

Thus the Longevity Center and the Longevity Research Institute were
born.

Like a magnet that attracts iron filings, Pritikin was attracting the
support he needed to undertake his momentous enterprise. There was a
standing army now, ready to march.

By January 1, 1976, everything was set–or so it seemed.

CHAPTER 12

The "Pritikin Pioneers"

On January 5, 1976, the first nine patients and seven spouses arrived at the newly created Longevity Center. All 16 people would participate in the program equally, though in each case the men were the primary patients, while the wives were in better health.

The 16 "Pritikin Pioneers," as they called themselves, were from as nearby as Santa Barbara, and as far away as Houston, Atlanta, and Philadelphia. Their illnesses were the same ones with which Pritikin had grown accustomed to dealing: heart disease and angina, high blood pressure, adult-onset diabetes, claudication, and arthritis. Of the nine men, seven had been scheduled for coronary bypass surgery by their physicians.

That was the verdict facing Jack Applebaum, a 77-year-old retired dentist from Santa Monica, California. Applebaum had planned to undergo the surgery that very January, but decided in December to attend the Longevity Center instead. He arrived taking 12 to 20 pills per day, depending on how bad his angina pain was. If his condition did not improve during his month-long stay at the Longevity Center, he planned to undergo bypass surgery shortly after he left Santa Barbara.

Ken Robbins, a 67-year-old Houston, Texas, resident, was in much the same shape. An angiogram performed at Methodist Hospital in Houston revealed three severely closed coronary arteries. His doctors scheduled him for triple coronary bypass surgery. He had angina, claudication, and arthritis so severe that walking more than a short distance–from his front door to his car, for example–was out of the question.

Gene Corley was only 45 years old when he arrived at the center. He had had his first heart attack at the age of 38 and had suffered another when he was 44. After that second heart attack, he had had coronary bypass surgery. However, an angiogram done in 1975 showed that the bypass had completely closed and that he had an aneurysm (a sac formation caused by weakness in the wall) in the left ventricle of his heart. He suffered severe angina pain and couldn't walk more than 200 or 300 feet without chest pain. He was taking 17 pills a day when he arrived. His doctors told him that he would soon need another bypass operation.

The others were in much the same shape. They were skeptical, hopeful, and scared all at once. They didn't know what to expect; most of them needed a miracle.

Each patient paid $2,500 for the 30-day session; spouses came for an additional $700. Bypass surgery in 1976 cost between $10,000 and $20,000 (depending on how many arteries were involved), but health insurance covered the costs, in most cases. Pritikin's program was not covered by insurance and, as a result, each patient was clearly risking his money, if not his life. Bypass surgery posed its own risks, of course. The only hope for these Pritikin pioneers was that Nathan had an answer for their illnesses. If he did, then the cost was worth it–but it was still a big "if."

They were housed in the back of the Howard Johnson's Motor Lodge. On the first night Nathan introduced himself and described the program.

As always, Pritikin was upbeat. He laid out the facts about the program and what it would do for them if followed conscientiously. He realized that if his program was going to work, each patient would have to *want* to change–he couldn't force them, nor did he want to. Pritikin believed that given the facts, anyone would change. As far as he was concerned, it was a matter of life and death. As he talked about the program, he introduced some of the staff members.

Dr. Stephen Kaye would provide weekly physical exams and various blood and treadmill tests in his offices (analysis of blood was done by local laboratories). Each patient could also consult the doctor between scheduled visits, while Nathan would counsel every patient personally on his or her specific illness. Ilene would oversee the kitchen and see to their dietary needs, and Esther Taylor would prepare their meals.

Over the period of their 30-day stay, there would be a total of 22 lectures on the relationship between diet and health, including several on food preparation. All smoking would have to stop that very day, Pritikin told them. He explained that smoking rapidly increases the rate of atherosclerosis. "You can't smoke and get well," he said.

When he started to talk about the importance of walking, he could almost feel the collective concern among his patients. Most of the patients dreaded the thought of exercise, even an exercise as seemingly innocuous as walking. As it was, many of them could not walk more than a city block without suffering severe angina, a pain that seemed to press in at the center of their chests like a knife slowly piercing the breastbone. Walking was like opening the door of death. Just talking about exercise inspired fear.

Pritikin assured them that they should not overexert themselves. He advised them to walk as far as they could and then rest. After they had rested, they should walk back to the center. He asked them to stay within a block of the Howard Johnson's for the first few days.

And so it began. They followed a meal schedule that provided eight servings throughout the day, beginning at 7:45 A.M. with a hot grain breakfast. The breakfast usually consisted of oats or cracked whole wheat, with herb tea. A citrus fruit was served at about 9:00, followed by a tossed salad at 10:45. One of a variety of soups was served an hour later and steamed vegetables were served at 12:45 P.M., followed by potato or corn at 1:30. Soup was served again at 3:00, and finally a full dinner at around 5:30. The day was concluded with some kind of fruit snack at around 8:00 or 8:30 after the evening lecture. The multimeal plan was designed to keep people from being hungry and to bring them together for social contact.

After each meal and snack, the patients walked around the block; eventually they graduated to longer prescribed routes, which Nathan had mapped out. The shortest initial path was 0.7 miles; the longest was 3.3 miles. Everyone was instructed to walk along these routes until they felt ready to move on to steeper and more challenging paths. Every walk was clocked and recorded, which helped the patients see their progress and encouraged them to maintain as brisk a walking speed as possible to improve conditioning.

For Jack Applebaum, the program was nothing less than a "last resort." Years later, he recalled in a letter the progression of his illness and his experiences at that first session at the Longevity Center.

> In 1965 I was forced to retire from my practice of dentistry due to angina pains. I was unable to climb the 24 stairs to my second floor office. I had chest pains while walking, excite[d] or after eating a big meal. This condition gradually got worse, especially while walking short distances in the cold weather in Chicago. . . . In 1972 . . . I contacted a cardiologist who was highly recommended. He prescribed medication consisting of 4 Inderal, 4 Isordil for the heart, 2 Esidrix tablets for high blood pressure and 2 Benemid to counteract the uric acid caused by the Essedrix tablets. All in all I was taking between 12 to 20 tablets a day.

In 1975, his doctor recommended bypass surgery.

> I had [a doctor's] appointment for November [1975] and the doctor asked me if I had made a decision as he would like me to go to Birmingham,

Alabama, for the bypass surgery. My wife asked him 'why Birmingham?' He said that is where he would go if he had to have bypass surgery. I told him it was too close to Thanksgiving and that I would decide after the holiday . . . I came back in December and he wanted to make arrangements for the surgery and I told him it's too close to Christmas and the New Year holiday and I would wait until the new year. He said to come back in January. In the meantime an article appeared in the *Los Angeles Times* in December of 1975 soon after I had seen the doctor. The article [quoted Pritikin as saying] that heart condition could be reversed with diet and exercise. I took the article and showed it to my cardiologist and his comment was if I wanted to waste my money that was up to me.

The article Applebaum saw was an Associated Press report of Nathan's November 1975 talk in Atlanta, where Pritikin reported his Long Beach Study results. Applebaum called Pritikin at home, but Nathan was away at the time. Janet took a message and said her father would return the call.

A few days later, Nathan called Applebaum at his Santa Monica home and said he was in Los Angeles and could stop by to talk about his program if Applebaum was interested. Applebaum was.

Once at Applebaum's, Pritikin described the cause of heart disease as an excess of fat and cholesterol in the diet which elevates cholesterol in the blood. This cholesterol, he explained, creates atherosclerotic plaque that clogs the arteries that nourish the heart with blood. When the fat and cholesterol are reduced in the diet, he said, the blood cholesterol goes down and circulation to the heart and other parts of the body are improved.

The Applebaums arrived at the Howard Johnson's motel that January not knowing what would take place there.

"We were very skeptical at first," recalled Muriel Applebaum. "It was the time when all the cults were popular and we really didn't know what to expect." With her husband recently diagnosed as needing bypass surgery, she wondered more than once whether they would even be coming home from Santa Barbara. "I told my daughter where everything was before I left because I didn't know what would happen to us," she recalled.

Despite their concerns, the Applebaums were hopeful, too, at least until Jack Applebaum faced the "little hill."

"There was this little hill outside the Howard Johnson's that we had to walk up, and I couldn't do it," he recalled in 1987. "When I tried, I got terrible chest pains and my eyes started to tear. I came back and told Dr. Kaye and he told me to drive my car up the hill and then walk after I reached the top. But after eating the food and walking for ten days, I was able to climb the hill. And that was a real accomplishment." The hill became Applebaum's inspiration. He had proof of his progress.

Applebaum's condition improved so rapidly and so remarkably that he was able to give up all medication by the third week at the center. "I walked 165 miles during the month, and on my last day I walked 8 miles at two-hour intervals. For me that was great . . . ," he says.

Four years later, at the age of 80, he reported that he was still off all medication, with the exception of an Isordil tablet "now and then" for an occasional angina pain.

In 1987, at the age of 87, Applebaum was still maintaining the program "about 75 to 80 percent of the time." He was walking several miles a week and was still fervently saying that "I wouldn't be alive today if it weren't for Nathan Pritikin."

As of 1987, Jack Applebaum had never had the bypass surgery, and had no plans to have the operation.

For Ken Robbins, a 67-year-old Houston resident, the experience was equally rewarding. Suffering from acute angina and from arthritis in his knee, Robbins had been scheduled to have bypass surgery before he arrived at the Longevity Center. When he left four weeks later, he was walking six to seven miles per day and no longer suffered from either the angina or the arthritis.

Gene Corley was only 38 years old when he had had his first heart attack in 1969. For the next five years, he suffered from arrhythmia and "almost constant angina."

Years later, Corley wrote:

> After a week in the hospital with intense angina, an angiogram indicated that I had a major artery about to close off, so bypass surgery was scheduled. I suffered a massive heart attack several hours before surgery. . . . An angiogram in 1975 showed the bypass completely closed and an aneurysm on the left ventricle. During that year I experienced pericarditis [an inflammation of the sac that encloses the heart] and brief congestive heart failure. After being told that there was nothing else that the medical or surgical field could do for me, I made the decision to try the Pritikin program.
>
> At the beginning of the session I frequently developed angina after walking 300 feet. While at the center, I increased my stamina until I was walking 12 to 15 miles per day, with angina only on steep inclines. Also, I discontinued all my medication while at the center, which had included Lanoxin, Isordil, Persantine, Valium, and aspirin, totaling 17 pills per day. I lost 18 pounds while there, and my problem blood fat levels dropped substantially.
>
> By the time I left the center, I had developed a sense of well-being, both physically and mentally, that I had not experienced in years! My friends and family could hardly believe my change in attitude from complete hopelessness to a truly optimistic outlook toward life.

"Nathan was an incredible motivator," Corley said in 1987. "He'd sit down with a bowl of oatmeal every morning until it got cold while he talked to everyone. He showed a real interest in everyone. He was special to us, and I think we were special to him."

The *Santa Barbara News-Press* photographed Corley, his wife, Martha, and another center patient, Henry Ducot of Modesto, California, actually jogging along the streets of Santa Barbara.

Corley was able to maintain the program strictly for three years without any sign of illness, but he started to drift from the diet after 1980. In 1982, he had a bypass operation. In 1987, he said that he still maintained the program as best he could–though not nearly as strictly as he did in the years immediately following his experience at the center. Still, "I wouldn't be alive today if it weren't for Nathan Pritikin," he said.

By the second and third week of the program, all the patients had begun to feel an extraordinary change come over them. Many patients, who earlier had been afraid to exercise, now began to feel a strange and wonderful confidence in their bodies. Not since they had been youths had they felt the almost intoxicating exhilaration of such physical vitality. As muscle tone improved, as oxygen reached areas of their bodies long starved for breath, as pounds dropped off and new reserves of energy charged through their limbs, the Longevity Center patients began to feel as if they had discovered the fountain of youth. Early fears and skepticism that the program wouldn't work now gave way to a kind of giddy euphoria.

But there was more than simply a physical or biological response to the program–there was a kind of emotional bonding taking place. The Pritikin pioneers were all in the same boat, a boat that–prior to their arrival at the Longevity Center–had been sinking fast. Pritikin's nine patients (the spouses generally were not as sick) may have had different backgrounds and arrived from different parts of the country, but they had one terrible thing in common: they were all being stalked by death. Each of them had his or her own version of the same horror story: steady decay of the body, heart palpitations, angina pain, doctors, growing dependency upon drugs, fear of parking the car too far from their destination, and a consuming dread of the inevitable day when their heart would stop. Death was so close at hand that most of them couldn't even have gas pains without interpreting them as intimations of doom. And now this strange turnaround. Fears that had been with them for years were now being replaced by feelings of exhilaration.

As the weeks went by, the attitudes of the patients toward the program and toward Nathan changed dramatically.

"We became very attached to Nathan. He was such a sweet, gentle person that everyone got attached to him," said Muriel Applebaum.

Mealtimes: Hassles and Humor

While his patients were making remarkable improvements, Pritikin was doing everything he could think of to keep the center from being closed down. Shortly after the center opened, inspectors from the Santa Barbara Board of Health demanded that he stop using the apartment-sized kitchen Howard Johnson's was renting him because it was never intended to provide anything more than coffee and tea service for meetings that took place in the motel. The tiny kitchen had no venting over the stove to prevent fire that might ignite from cooking fats or grease. When Ilene explained that the Pritikins weren't using cooking fats in their food preparation, the health officials dismissed the point as irrelevant. An inspector said that even reheating of food was out of the question in the kitchen. Moreover, the kitchen's dishwasher did not reach sufficiently high temperatures required for restaurant dishwashers. The health department's verdict was simple and harsh: either make the structural changes in 30 days–an impossible task even if the Howard Johnson's and the Pritikins wanted to do such a thing–or close down the operation.

There was only one thing to do: keep the patients in the motel and find a kitchen nearby where they could prepare the meals and then transport the cooked food back to the motel.

For the next two weeks, Ilene searched the surrounding area for a new cooking facility and eventually found one: Angelo's Italian Delicatessen.

Located on busy Hollister Avenue in Goleta, Angelo's deli was the Longevity Center's perfect opposite. Specializing in coffee and pastries, well-marbled meats, a variety of salads, and sandwiches–pastrami, salami, and corned beef were favorites–Angelo's catered to a breakfast and lunch crowd and to neighborhood shoppers. Food was prepared in the kitchen behind the deli counters. Angelo's gave permission to use the kitchen during the times the deli wasn't busy–early in the morning and later in the afternoon.

Each morning around 6:30, a Pritikin breakfast chef arrived to cook the morning's hot cereal, which was then brought to the center. Esther, the Pritikins' housekeeper, arrived at about 10:00 A.M. to prepare the grains, vegetables, and soups. The food was the basis of the program, and as far as Esther was concerned, there was no more important job in the universe.

For a person who saw food as medicine, cooking at Angelo's was, at times, like performing surgery in a barn. As lunchtime rolled around and Angelo's started to crank up the short-order operation, Esther knew she needed to be out of the deli, or opposing worlds of the Longevity Center and Angelo's would come dangerously close to colliding. Sometimes she didn't make it. While Esther boiled her brown rice or steamed her vegetables in the most exacting way she knew, hot pastrami would be sizzling in its own fat on the grill next to her. Soon hot pastrami, corned beef, and hamburgers would be sending fat flying like missiles in all directions, causing Esther to stand guard over her pots as if they were being assaulted.

When Esther finished her cooking, the large thermoses and other food containers were loaded into the Longevity Center's van and driven to the center. Back at Howard Johnson's, Ilene waited nervously. If the food was 10 or 15 minutes late, the patients–who were unaware that their food was being prepared elsewhere and then delivered to the motel–started grumbling. Walking caused them to work up quite an appetite, and everyone took the schedule seriously, especially since time spent waiting for food could have been better spent walking.

This is not to say that the guests were crazy about the food. At the outset of the program, the patients found the food uniformly unpalatable. Applebaum said it was simply "terrible." Another said that the meals were meant to satisfy Nathan's taste buds, which were very unique taste buds, indeed.

Nathan, Ilene, and Esther found that preparing the Pritikin diet for a group was a lot more difficult than cooking at home. A chef was hired to help Esther, but the cooking only got worse. Even Nathan couldn't bear the new chef's food.

"One day we were having soup," recalled Muriel Applebaum, "and Nathan used to eat with all of us." After the group started to eat the soup, each person began to look up and cast suspicious looks at one another, said Mrs. Applebaum. "Nathan tasted the soup and asked, 'My God, what happened to this?'"

The next day, the new chef was gone.

Another day, the menu announced chicken soup for dinner, and everyone looked forward to dinner with great anticipation. "When we were eating the soup that night, no one could find any chicken in it," said Mrs. Applebaum. "Finally, someone called out, 'I found a piece of chicken, I found a piece of chicken!'"

The incident prompted Jack Applebaum to announce that he had a recipe for Pritikin chicken soup:

"Fill a pot with water, put it in the sun, and swing a chicken over it. Serve when ready."

For the next several years, Ilene and Esther would work tirelessly to develop satisfying dishes using whole grains and vegetables and small amounts of low-fat animal foods. They began by making ethnic dishes, particularly Mexican, Italian, and Chinese recipes, and substituting healthful foods for those that were rich in fat, cholesterol, sugar, and salt. It was an effort that required years of trial and error.

"We really wanted to make the food taste good, because we didn't want the people to feel bad about what they couldn't have," said Esther. "But it took a long time to learn to balance the cooking, not too much of one spice, but a balance of tastes."

(Eventually, professional chefs would take over the job of creating Pritikin-style meals and recipes to suit the tastes of the average American.)

Once the first session got going, however, the key issue with the food was not so much the taste but whether it was on time and whether it came in sufficient quantities. As people exercised and began to feel better, their appetites got stronger. They didn't like it when their meals were late and they didn't mind letting people know it. Like hungry people all over the world, they were grateful for the food, and they ate it with enthusiasm, never realizing that the food had been prepared in a world most of them had just left behind.

Pritikin preached that taste preferences were learned, not genetic–otherwise, how could there be such varied cuisine among so many cultures–and that anyone could learn to enjoy simple foods and cooking as he or she ate these foods more. To some extent, he was right: by the second and third week of the program, people enjoyed the food much more than they had during the first week. But at those early sessions, the food had a long way to go before it would be truly enjoyable for most people, as Ilene and Esther knew.

From Despair to Elation

As the vitality of youth seemed to galvanize their bodies and hearts, the patients took on many of the qualities of children. They started to become competitive about their walking distances.

"The patient who had arrived at the center with severe angina or claudication and who was now walking 10 or 15 miles per day was a real celebrity," Ilene recalled. "People were cheering one another on."

Apart from the measurable progress each person made were the myriad accomplishments that could not be measured: the restoration of vitality, personal confidence, a positive outlook on life. People looked and felt years younger. They arrived afraid, their future prospects grim. They left the center feeling that their lives had been restored. Suddenly, they had control of their lives again.

The results from his first session paralleled those of the Long Beach Study. Of the 16 people at the center, 15 lost weight–the largest weight loss being 22 pounds. Everyone was walking a minimum of five miles a day; most were walking ten or more. Blood cholesterol levels dropped 25 percent on the average; high blood pressure, adult-onset diabetes, angina, and arthritis were all being controlled by the diet and exercise program alone. None of the 16 people on the program required medication. All were enjoying what Nathan began calling "normal function," meaning that each of them could live as if they no longer had the underlying disease.

The sessions in February and March were much the same. People arrived with the same fears and skepticism and left with the same physical and emotional renewal. Each session seemed to have its own unique set of challenges, problems and miracles.

Graduation day was filled with tears of gratitude and flights of fancy. People wrote poems to the Pritikins and performed theatrical presentations, most of them parodies of Nathan and his patients. In fact, in the years that followed, Pritikin would be the perennial favorite for jokesters and parodists. He would receive dozens of "honorary doctorate degrees" from grateful center participants, and would have enough poems and skits written about him to rival Santa Claus.

Indeed, most people who went through the center believed Nathan Pritikin had saved or substantially improved their lives.

For the Pritikins, each person's transformation was like witnessing a miracle unfold.

"Nathan and I watched people arrive in fear and, with steady progress, become almost delirious with joy," Ilene recalled. "The group setting required them to spend 30 days together, eating, walking, sharing their fears and their hopes. All of this produced close bonds among people who had previously been strangers. This, of course, is a very rare experience for many adults.

"For Nathan and me, it was so moving and inspiring to watch this cycle of emotions as patients went from fear to elation."

Nathan couldn't get over the change in the attitudes of the patients. The playfulness and competitiveness among the patients caused Pritikin to begin calling the center "summer camp for grown-ups."

As usual, Pritikin made a joke about the events, but beneath his jests were real feelings of accomplishment in his work.

"Nathan would later say that in the past he had been an inventor solving problems with inanimate objects," Ilene said. "Now he would bring his problem-solving skills to people's health concerns. Nothing he had done in the past matched his work at the Longevity Center for sheer joy and satisfaction."

Pritikin wasn't sure where all this was leading, but he was more convinced than ever that this type of program would ultimately replace most drugs and surgery as the treatment of choice for most degenerative diseases.

A Shocking Diagnosis: "Leukemia"

The April session had just begun when Nathan routinely sent off another one of his blood samples to a Santa Barbara laboratory. "We had been running blood panels on everyone," Stephen Kaye recalled. "And Nathan's was among them." Pritikin often asked that his blood be tested to check the accuracy and consistency of the laboratory he was using. However, what came back on April 6 was devastating.

Kaye received the blood reports. He read the report on Nathan and then hurried into Pritikin's office. Kaye sat down on the other side of Pritikin's desk, steadied himself, and said: "I got your blood samples back. I have to tell you that there's a problem. It kind of looks like leukemia."

Kaye and Pritikin went over the report in detail and then began to discuss what to do.

The first thing they decided was to have a thorough examination done at Cottage Hospital in Santa Barbara. Pritikin would have to have a bone marrow biopsy and other tests done to ascertain his condition. Nathan immediately made the appointment, and for a few minutes he and Kaye discussed the kinds of therapies that might be available.

"During the whole time we talked," said Kaye years later, "Nathan completely maintained calm. There was no denial; he was not detached. He held closely to logic, because that was the only tool he had then that could save his life."

Nathan and Kaye went to Cottage Hospital, where Pritikin was examined. Blood tests and other tests were administered. The diagnosis: "acute lymphatic leukemia." It was a death sentence. The most Pritikin could hope for was 30 days, perhaps two months at the outside. There was only one treatment, the examining specialist informed him. He would have to have massive dosages of radiation, which would destroy his bone marrow. The radiation would be followed by bone marrow transplantation, which, the doctor hoped, would eliminate the cause of the leukemia.

Suddenly, it all added up. The imbalance of proteins–the so-called spike–that had been present in Pritikin's blood since 1957 had finally turned to an acute phase. He mentioned to Kaye that he had been feeling tired of late but because of the demands of his schedule didn't think much of it. His latest blood tests showed that he was severely anemic, a consequence of the leukemia, which also explained his recent fatigue.

Pritikin went home and told Ilene of the doctor's diagnosis. The two of them stood in their living room and held one another and cried.

After they got a grip on themselves, Ilene telephoned the children to come home. Ken was at school in the San Francisco area and Robert and Jack were away. Janet and Ralph were in Santa Barbara. The children were told of their father's illness.

"We were all in a state of hysteria," recalls Janet. "The family was in the grip of terrible fear and shock, but then my father and Robert set out to find an answer."

Robert was then dispatched to do a computer search at UCLA medical library on all the available medical literature on leukemia.

Once Nathan plunged himself into the job of finding an answer, an atmosphere of crisis management set in.

"There was no hand wringing, no fatherly goodbyes, no fanfare," recalled Janet. "Just a race against time."

Soon, Pritikin decided that the best place in the area to receive treatment for acute lymphatic leukemia was the UCLA Medical Center, where the finest technology and expert physicians performed the treatment. Nathan and Ilene went to UCLA at the end of April. The Pritikins took a hotel room and expected to be admitted to UCLA Medical Center after Nathan was examined by UCLA physician Dr. David Golde. Golde specialized in the diagnosis and treatment of leukemia.

And then the unexpected and seemingly miraculous thing happened. Golde examined Nathan and changed the diagnosis. Pritikin didn't have acute lymphatic leukemia, Golde said; he had chronic lymphatic leukemia. Though ultimately fatal, this disease was far less virulent than the acute form. Golde said that Pritikin could live another two to three years. Though he was never certain, Golde came to believe Pritikin had a form of leukemia called hairy cell, a chronic leukemia characterized by its small hair-like follicles at the outside of the cell. It is more rare than other forms of leukemia. Golde said that the disease could be treated for some time with drug therapy.

Relief washed over Nathan and Ilene like healing waters. As Ilene later wrote in her diary, "From the death sentence of 'acute lymphatic leukemia,' we were given, instead, a ray of hope, for at least a few years of life to hope for." Golde told them the average survival rate for this disease, was 21 months and, as Ilene wrote, they clung to the "tenuous possibility that in that period of time Nathan, with the best medical help he could muster, would find a way of protracting that survival time into more years."

Golde prescribed a chemotherapy agent called chlorambucil, which had been shown to be effective in the treatment of the illness. Nathan began taking the drug immediately, and over the next few months it did bring his blood proteins and white blood cells into balance.

Nathan was 60 years old and contemplating his own mortality. One afternoon that spring, while he and Ilene sat in their living room, Nathan confided that life had been good to him. He had no complaints. He was satisfied with what he had done.

He read everything he could on leukemia. As was typical of Nathan, he decided it was essential to keep his illness a secret. He believed that people would not understand the true cause of his illness and would wrongly associate his illness with his program. The adverse publicity would destroy his diet and health regimen before it had a chance to demonstrate its effectiveness against disease. He feared that his ideas would never see the light of day.

He and Ilene realized, however, that had they known of Nathan's leukemia, they would never have started the Longevity Center. They would have preferred that Nathan spend his remaining years trying to find a solution to his illness and spending time with the family. But this was not to be. Despite the demands on his time, which he could have been dedicating to finding an answer to his disease, Nathan and Ilene were grateful that things had worked as they had. The Longevity Center had been launched. And like a huge ship that transported people from the colony of the dying to the land of the living, there was no calling it back.

CHAPTER **13**

"Miracles" at the "Lourdes of the Pacific"

*T*he irony for Pritikin was that as death hovered dangerously close, he had at the same time achieved a remarkable integration in his life.

Prior to the Longevity Center, Pritikin's energies were parceled out among several different businesses, half a dozen projects, and his perpetual study of health and medicine. There was never a singular focus, never any one endeavor that towered over all the rest.

But with the birth of the Longevity Center, Pritikin had found the one vocation that would demand all of his varied abilities, his remarkable intellect, his patience and compassion, his dogged perseverence, and his seemingly limitless supplies of energy. Pritikin the healer, the inventor, the revolutionary, the man with a dream for a better world, had finally found a job that would be as demanding of him as he was of himself. As Ilene would say years later, "When the Longevity Center was created, it was as if the many smaller tributaries in Nathan's life had all joined into one mighty river, which carried Nathan toward his dream."

Once his course was set, he went about the business of finding a permanent home for the center. The job was far more difficult than he had earlier imagined. He wanted to remain in Santa Barbara, but one possible site after another fell through. Zoning laws and complaints from potential neighbors–people didn't like the idea of their neighborhood teeming with sick people walking the streets all day–were the principal obstacles that kept him from finding a permanent site. Eventually, he gave up looking in Santa Barbara and arranged an agreement with the Holiday Inn in Ventura, a community 30 miles south of Santa Barbara. He moved the center there in June 1976, but it lasted only two months. The facilities available for meal preparation and for serving were totally inadequate, and Pritikin's people were constantly shunted about. Pritikin never felt welcome–the center was somehow always in the way of the hotel's operation–and by the middle of the summer Pritikin had negotiated another deal, this time with the Mar Monte Hotel in Santa Barbara.

The Longevity Center would remain at the Mar Monte for the next two years, and despite the seemingly endless conflicts between Nathan and Mar Monte owner Buddy Taub, the hotel was, in many respects, ideally suited for Pritikin's Longevity Center. The Mar Monte (which was bought in 1984 by the Sheraton hotel chain) was a large hotel, with 200 rooms, a restaurant, pool, and lounge. Located on Cabrillo Boulevard, directly across the street from the beach and facing the ocean, the Mar Monte seemed to be perpetually bathed in sunlight. Guests of the center only had to walk across the street to be on the beautiful beaches, where they could walk for miles with nothing more to distract them than sunbathers, sea gulls, and the ceaseless lapping of the ocean.

The Mar Monte was a far larger hotel than the Howard Johnson's Motor Lodge and thus allowed Pritikin to occupy more rooms–he needed only about a fourth of the rooms available–and to take on more patients. As a result of the remarkable reports about what was happening at the Longevity Center, more and more people wanted to attend the program. The August session had 50 patients and soon the center would accommodate up to 75 in a single session. By the end of the year, Pritikin would begin overlapping the sessions so that a new month-long program would start every two weeks. With the overlapping sessions, there would be no fewer than 100 people at the center during any given month–and sometimes that number would swell to 150.

Initially, there was only one problem with the Mar Monte: the hotel had begun a thorough remodeling program, which required months of heavy construction. The serenity of Santa Barbara was being shattered daily by the racket of jackhammers, electric saws, welding, and the sound of nails being pounded into wood. Walls were exposed and plaster dust filled the air.

Pritikin worried about the effect of the construction noise on his patients; he was concerned that the constant clamor and disruption might interfere with the health improvements of his patients. But nothing of the kind happened. People continued to improve as quickly and as dramatically as they had before.

One day toward the end of summer that year, Nathan and Ilene crossed paths in one of the hallways of the Mar Monte. Nathan looked up at the ceiling as plaster dust fell and hammers pounded. "This food must be very powerful to make people get well under these conditions," he said to Ilene. They both laughed and went back to work.

There were times when Nathan seemed as surprised as anyone that the program would have as dramatic an effect on health as it did. As the remarkable case histories became more consistent, Ilene recalled Nathan gleefully saying from time to time, "It works, it really works."

By the end of summer, Pritikin was ready to expand his medical staff and began looking around for a new medical director to replace Dr. Stephen Kaye, who had resigned. Dr. Donald Mannerberg, a physician in Houston, Texas, who headed the medical arm of the Kenneth Cooper Aerobics Clinic, heard through a friend that Pritikin was looking for someone to supervise the medical program at the Longevity Center and decided to talk to Pritikin about it. Mannerberg, an internist, had a very traditional background as a physician. He had been practicing medicine for 12 years before hearing about the Longevity Center, and had used nothing but conventional treatment–drugs and surgery–to treat his patients. His experience at the Cooper Clinic had led him to appreciate the benefits of exercise, though he still relied on orthodox therapies in the treatment of disease.

Mannerberg called Nathan that summer for a description of the job. The two discussed the position and Pritikin told Mannerberg about the results he was having with his patients. Mannerberg was intrigued. But before he came to Santa Barbara to talk to Pritikin, he asked a few of his medical colleagues what they thought of Pritikin's ideas. The responses were fairly predictable: Pritikin was a quack and a charlatan, Mannerberg was told. He was advised that if he joined Pritikin, he'd be throwing away his career. Mannerberg, however, saw no harm in at least talking to Pritikin and decided to visit him in Santa Barbara. He arrived "very skeptical" about what he would find. When he sat down with Nathan and went over the patient records, however, Mannerberg became convinced that Pritikin was on to something. He took the job.

"It was the best thing I ever did in my professional life," Mannerberg would say years later. "My experience at the Longevity Center changed the way I practiced medicine and the results we had were amazing."

"Medical Failures" Get Impressive Results

The vast majority of the people who came to the Longevity Center were seriously ill, what Mannerberg and others at the center called the "medical failures."

Pritikin had a statistical analysis done on the center's first 893 patients and the progress they made. The analysis was performed by Loma Linda

University in Riverside, California. The patients' medical histories at admission to the center were as follows:

- Two-thirds of the patients (590 people) suffered from atherosclerotic heart disease and nearly half (423) had had at least one heart attack. (36 had had three or more heart attacks.)
- More than a third of Pritikin's patients (324) had high blood pressure that was being controlled by medication.
- 198 (22 percent) suffered from intermittent claudication (poor circulation in the legs, causing severe pain when walking).
- 259 (29 percent) were obese (20 percent above ideal weight).
- 107 (12 percent) suffered from adult-onset diabetes that was being controlled by drugs or insulin.
- 178 (20 percent) suffered from arthritis, either rheumatoid or osteoarthritis; another 57 (6 percent) suffered from gouty arthritis.
- 393 (44 percent) had positive treadmill stress tests when they were admitted (meaning they demonstrated coronary insufficiency), while another 87 (nearly 10 percent) were borderline or equivocal.

The patients had been through the traditional series of drugs–many were taking 12 pills or more per day for heart disease, diabetes, and other disorders.

Many had been told by their doctors that they needed coronary bypass surgery. Others had already had the surgery but were in danger of suffering another heart attack. By the time they arrived at the Longevity Center, most of these had little hope of regaining anything that resembled health.

"These were the 'death's door' people," recalled David Fields, Nathan's friend and a Ph.D. economist, who was the center's administrator for nearly two years in Santa Barbara. "Some people arrived in wheelchairs; others needed help walking down the block. Most of them were severely ill."

Frances Greger, from North Miami, Florida, arrived in Santa Barbara at one of Pritikin's early sessions in a wheelchair. Mrs. Greger had heart disease, angina, and claudication; her condition was so bad she could no longer walk without great pain in her chest and legs. Within three weeks, she was not only out of her wheelchair but was walking ten miles a day.

Charles Tobolsky, a 69-year-old retired construction worker, was told by his physician in Maple Shade, New Jersey, that he was "a walking time bomb." An angiogram performed at Hahnemann Hospital in Philadelphia showed three severely closed coronary arteries. He was told that he needed bypass surgery to survive. In the meantime, his physicians told him not to walk up a flight of stairs more than twice a day, not to drive at a

(continued on page 161)

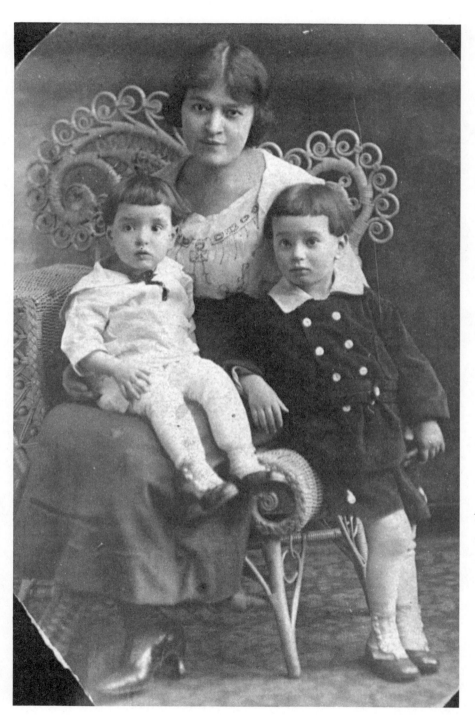

Nathan at age 4 with his mother, Esther, known fondly as Kitty, and his kid brother, Albert, 2.

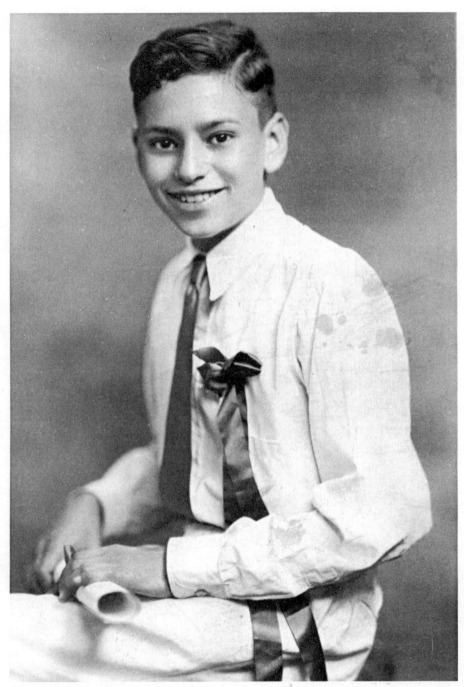

Nathan's elementary school graduation picture in 1929, when he was 14. Nathan began showing promise as a scientist in his elementary school days, even though his father encouraged him to go for a degree in law.

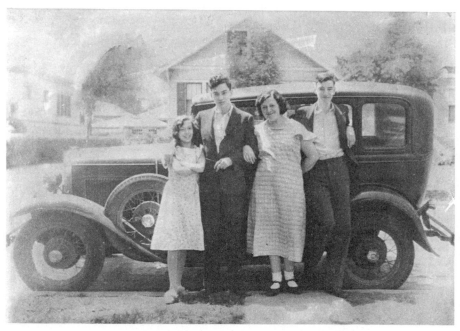

Nathan (second from left) took the family photo, above, in 1934 when he was 18 and an amateur photographer. It didn't take him long, though, to turn professional. Below, he poses on a Chicago street with his business partner, Leonard Dubin, and a symbol of the success of their Flash Foto Company.

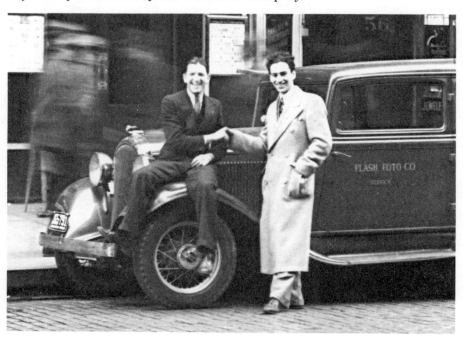

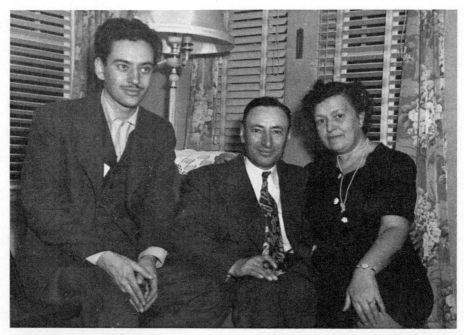

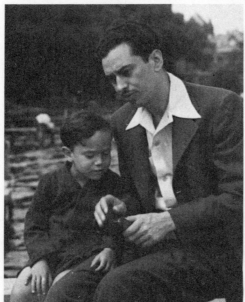

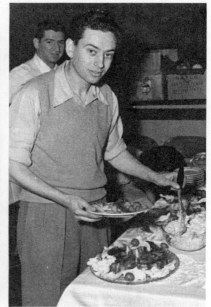

In 1945, Nathan was a man in transition—newly divorced and a single father. At top, he is shown with his mother and father, Jacob and Kitty. Above, left, he shares a pensive moment with his 4-year-old son Jack. Within a few years, however, Nathan was well into another of his successful endeavors—Glass Products. Above right, he attends a party for his staff.

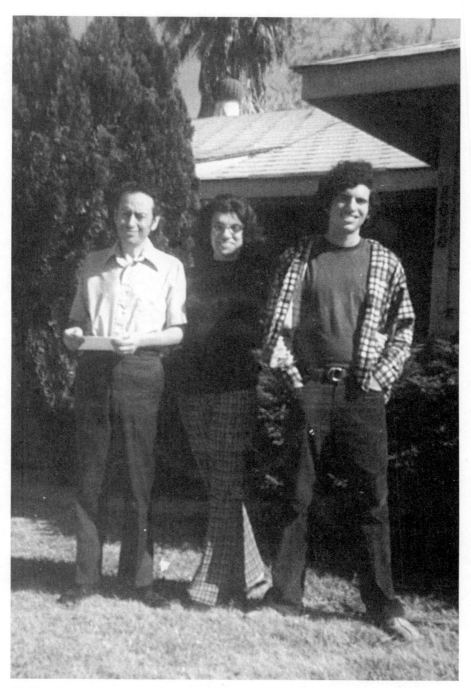

Nathan, his wife Ilene, and their son Robert pose outside the house used as a base for Pritikin's landmark Long Beath Study in 1975. This study was Nathan's first important proof that there is a link between heart disease and diet.

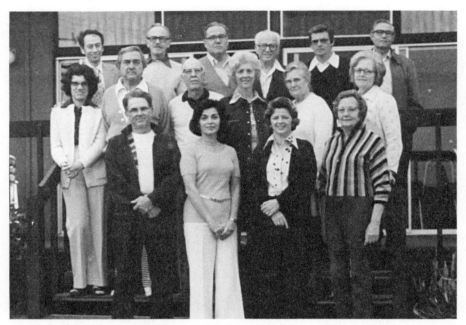

In January 1976, a group of ailing men and their wives became the first en-rollees in Pritikin's Longevity Center. Although they showed impressive results, Nathan's "interference" in the medical world was blasted by doctors nationwide. Ilene and Nathan are to the left in the photo above. Below, Nathan lectures a class on the beach in Santa Monica, after the center's move to its present location in 1978.

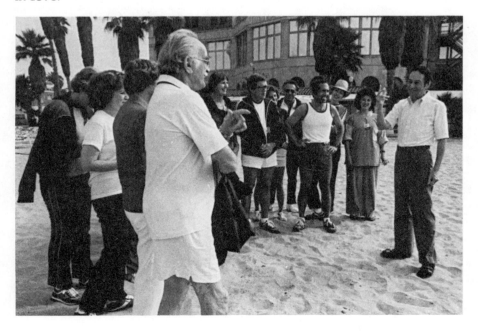

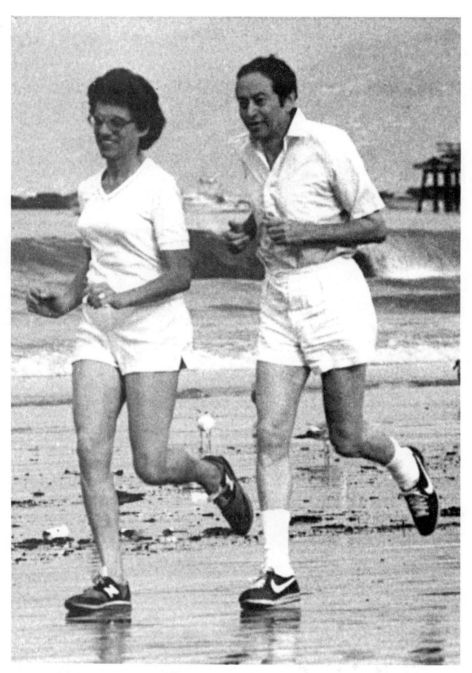

Nathan and his wife Ilene loved daily jogs on the beach. For Nathan, losing his ability to run during the later stages of his cancer was heartbreaking. He never, however, told anyone why he wasn't running anymore. He merely told friends that "running is a thing of the past, now."

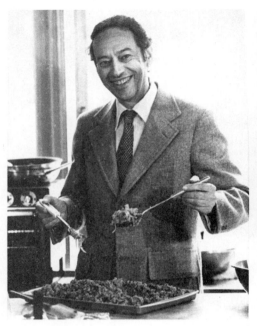 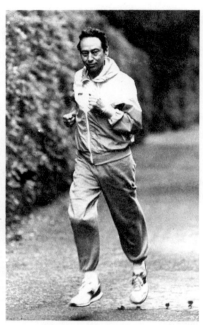

Always his patients' biggest supporter, Nathan often participated in cooking classes, as shown above left. He was also always the picture of health and vitality, as the cover photo for his book The Pritikin Promise, *above right, well illustrated. Below, he is pictured with one of his biggest supporters, former senator George McGovern.*

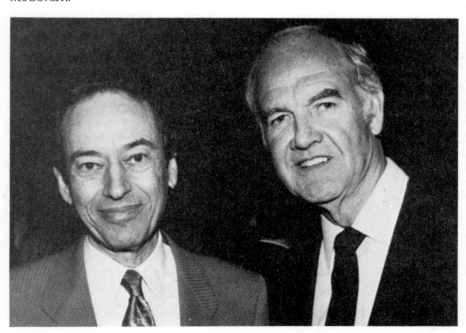

speed greater than 40 miles per hour, and not to drive alone. Worst of all, for Tobolsky, he was ordered to give up his golf game. The swinging of the club and the anticipation of tournaments gave him angina pain and were ruled dangerous to his health. He couldn't walk 100 yards without chest pain. He was given a variety of medications, including nitroglycerin for his angina.

Tobolsky also suffered from diabetes, which he had had for the past 13 years. He was taking Orinase and Diabinese to help control the disease.

Being told to give up golf was shattering. "Emotionally, I was devastated," Tobolsky wrote two years later. "Many times, under certain conditions, I had periods of crying due to my feelings of utter impotency."

In June 1976, Tobolsky read an article in the *Philadelphia Inquirer* about heart disease. The article mentioned Pritikin's claim that diet could be an effective treatment. Tobolsky contacted Nathan and decided to go to Santa Barbara to try the program. Before he left for the center, he asked his cardiologist about the Pritikin program. The doctor "ridiculed it," Tobolsky recalled, and called the Longevity Center "a racket."

In August of that year, Tobolsky was at the Longevity Center eating the Pritikin diet and taking his daily walks. By the time he left, he was off all medication, including that for his diabetes, and was walking eight to ten miles per day.

When he returned to New Jersey, his cardiologist at Hahnemann Hospital refused to look at his records from the Longevity Center and "dismissed me." The doctor also wrote a letter to Tobolsky's personal physician to do the same, in order to avoid any responsibility in the event of Tobolsky's death. His personal physician, however, remained impressed by what Tobolsky had accomplished at the Longevity Center.

Four years later, at the age of 73, Tobolsky was still maintaining the diet and playing golf. He was also competing in tournaments. In 1980, Tobolsky wrote to Nathan that "I have won golf championships at my golf club and every man that I have beaten [has been] many years my junior, some more than half my age. . . . "

Duane E. Bluhm had his first heart attack in 1959 at the age of 37. After suffering his third heart attack in 1976, he retired at the age of 54. He couldn't walk down the block without suffering from severe chest pain. In the summer of 1976, he heard about the Longevity Center and was one of 75 people in the September session. When he arrived, he was taking nine pills a day for his heart disease. Three weeks later, he was walking 15 miles a day and was off all medication.

One after another–so many of the stories were the same. They arrived seriously ill, and, in many cases, incapacitated. They went home feeling reborn.

"For the first time in my professional life, I could take people off medication and make them well," Mannerberg recalled years later.

Loma Linda confirmed Mannerberg's assertion. The university found that:

- The average drop in cholesterol was 25 percent. Of those who arrived at the center with a cholesterol level between 260 mg.% and 279 mg.%–at very high risk of having a heart attack–the average patient's cholesterol level when they left the center was 190 mg.%, well below the high-risk category. Pritikin was, in essence, cutting in half the risk of having a heart attack.
- Of the 218 confirmed hypertensives taking drugs to control their high blood pressure, 186 (about 85 percent) left with normal blood pressures and off all drugs.
- Half of all the adult-onset diabetics using insulin when they arrived left the center with normal glucose levels and no longer needing insulin injections; of those taking oral drugs for adult-onset diabetes, 80 percent left the center drug-free.
- Seventy percent of those who arrived taking medication for gout left free of severe symptoms and off medication.

Reports of Pritikin's successes were spreading quickly throughout late 1976 and in early 1977. That year the Air Line Pilots Association and the Aviation Insurance Agency, Inc., began sending pilots who had been grounded because of poor health to the Longevity Center. The Federal Aviation administration sets health standards for airline pilots, and each year pilots are required to undergo physical examinations to determine their health status. Those who fail the physicals–often for high blood pressure, diabetes, or angina–have their flying privileges revoked. Unless they regain their health, their careers as pilots are usually over.

The Aviation Insurance Agency sent more than a hundred grounded pilots from all the major carriers to the Longevity Center, with remarkable results. "Nine out of ten pilots who went to the center returned to pass their physicals, and had their flying privileges restored," Dr. Charles Gullett, a physician at the Aviation Insurance Agency said in 1986. "Every pilot we sent who had a positive attitude toward the center was returned to his job after taking the program." Indeed, the Gray Eagles, Retired Airline Pilots Association, dubbed the Longevity Center the "Institute for Miracles" for saving the careers of so many pilots.

Additional Inspiration

Pat Walters was a waitress at the Mar Monte coffee shop when Pritikin opened his center there. Each day she watched the Longevity Center guests and staff, and thought about what was going on over there in the large dining room next to the coffee shop. As she poured coffee and offered cheeseburgers to her customers, Pat Walters got a daily education in the Pritikin program by watching the progress of the Pritikin patients and overhearing bits of information from the guests as they passed in the hallway.

Ms. Walters was in her late thirties and had already raised nine children. She was a gregarious, warm, energetic woman with a shrewd eye for sizing up a person's character.

One day in the spring of 1977, Pat Walters walked up to Ilene Pritikin and asked for a job with the center. Ilene talked it over with Nathan and they hired her to act as liaison between the staff and the guests. Ms. Walters supervised the dining room and mingled with the guests, listening to their complaints, noting their requests, giving encouragement, cheering them on when they walked an extra mile. Pat Walters was the perfect den mother and troubleshooter. Every little request was noted and attended to: Another pillow mysteriously arrived in the room of the person who had mentioned that he hadn't slept well the night before; Nathan would inquire about a particular person's problem, after Pat Walters had overheard the person talking about it; one of the recipes served would be modified at the suggestion of one of the patients. Pat Walters saw it as her responsibility to make people a little happier while they changed the very foundations of their lives.

"These were very successful people who came to the center," Ms. Walters recalled in 1986. "They were highly educated, self-made men and women who came to Nathan. In many cases, they were captains of large industries, entertainers, people in government, who were used to being powerful. Now, all of a sudden, their disease had made them weak, and it was a humbling experience. These people were scared to death. Many were inoperable. Nothing could be done. And Nathan was basically telling them that 'you may be the richest man in the world, but now you've got to eat like a peasant.' They came willing to do anything, to eat anything, just to get well. My job was making that transition from sickness to health a little easier, a little more comfortable."

Pat Walters described the atmosphere of the center as being like that of watching a baby learn to walk. "Some people arrived who couldn't walk the length of the room, and then you start seeing these people make progress. At the beginning, someone would say that he had slept all right last night. Then someone who had arthritis would say, 'Look, I can move my fingers," and then another person would say, 'Look how far I walked today; I walked a whole mile and didn't have to stop once.' People were getting standing ovations for coming off medication. The camaraderie was incredible."

Nathan was in his element. He lectured daily and saw patients for individual counseling in his office. In between patients he talked on the telephone to sick people all across the country, telling them what to eat for their particular conditions and giving suggestions for their doctors. His correspondence with people who could not come to the center was voluminous. He sent letters to scientists and doctors describing the results of the program. He requested that the scientists come to Santa Barbara and examine his records; he asked doctors to refer patients to him. He also wrote to members of Congress requesting that the lawmakers fund research examining the relationship between diet and health.

In addition, Pritikin gave lectures locally on diet and health to lay and medical audiences. In lectures at Cottage Hospital, he invited physicians to examine his patients and their records to see for themselves the effectiveness of his program.

"This was Nathan's reason for being," Pat Walters recalled. "He had the ability to forget himself and his problems and be more concerned about the other person's problems. People would stop him in the hall or the dining room and talk about their problems and he would give advice until they were satisfied. He loved to puzzle over people's diseases."

All of Pritikin's years of study were finally being put to full use.

A Man of Incredible Knowledge

According to Don Mannerberg, Pritikin's knowledge of medicine rivaled that of most medical specialists. "Nathan could hold his own in a discussion with specialists in heart disease, diabetes, and many other fields," said Mannerberg. "He was brilliant. He also had a photographic memory. He could recall studies or medical information better than anyone I had ever met."

Dr. Monroe Rosenthal, who began at the Longevity Center as a staff physician and eventually became its medical director, recalled that Pritikin's "medical expertise was equal to any M.D.'s. His library at Santa Barbara was incredible. Professors of medicine at Harvard didn't have access to literature Nathan had."

David Fields, Pritikin's administrator, was an acquaintance of one of the premier diabetes researchers in the United States. Fields invited the diabetes researcher and Nathan for dinner one night so the two could share their ideas. Pritikin and the researcher talked for four hours that night, debating their respective points of view. The scientist, who favored the use of drugs in the treatment of all types of diabetes, refused to concede to Pritikin that diet could be more effective in the treatment of many diabetics. When the two parted company that night, Fields took a short walk with the scientist and asked him, "What do you think of Nathan's ideas?" Years later, Fields recalled the scientist's response:

" 'Dave,' he said, 'I've studied diabetes my entire professional life and nobody in the country knows more about this illness than I do. And I've never met anyone who knew more about diabetes than Nathan Pritikin. But do you know what would happen if I started prescribing a diet for my patients? They would stop coming back. Because they want a pill, or they want insulin. They don't want a diet. That's why they come to me, because I give them what they want.' "

Pritikin was aware that this type of thinking was an obstacle but realized that in the last analysis, laypeople could alter the direction of medicine by demanding new approaches to disease. To change medicine, he would have to change the thinking of the average patient.

CHAPTER **14**

Pritikin
versus the Medical
Establishment

*P*ritikin's move into the doctor's domain of health care had all the audacity and bravura of an old western melodrama in which an unknown loner rides into town and takes on the local gang.

It wasn't long before the fireworks started to fly.

Shortly after the *Santa Barbara News-Press* ran a story on the Longevity Center in March 1976, a local physician wrote a long letter to the newspaper condemning the center and Pritikin for his claims. The letter, in part, is reprinted here.

> Regarding your story "Longevity Center Claims Reversal of Heart Disease" which appeared in the News-Press on March 14, I, as a physician in this community, feel compelled to state my views concerning Mr. Pritikin's approach to coronary artery disease ... [Ellipses printed by newspaper.]
>
> To simplify the prevention of coronary artery disease to merely lowering cholesterol and exercising is nonsense. According to the MRFIT [Multiple Risk Factor Intervention Trial] government study on heart disease, coronary heart disease is a "multifactorial condition."
>
> Furthermore, many risk factors have been identified, but these are not all of equivalent importance in population groups or individuals. Those considered to be of greatest influence are age, sex, hypertension, high cholesterol, diabetes, and cigarette smoking. I am certain that Mr. Pritikin doesn't claim to be able to control the first two (age and sex).
>
> Instead of charging $2,500 per "patient," which can only be afforded by a very minute portion of our population, Mr. Pritikin might do better to promote teaching sound nutrition to teenagers while they are acquiring their eating habits and before damage occurs, rather than prey on the fears of the older population who are looking for instant cures.
>
> It is entirely possible that the person who goes to the "Longevity Center"

with a positive attitude that he will be helped will exhibit some short-term changes. He is ripe to suggestion. His chest pain may temporarily lessen. There could be less leg cramps. As with an effective diet, there would be weight loss.

But it is not scientific to conclude that these people have been "cured." I have seen patients in my practice who have low cholesterols (below 160 mg.%) who in spite of that have had massive heart attacks and others with very high cholesterols who did not. To approach coronary disease from only one aspect is myopic!

The cause of coronary artery disease or hardening of the arteries is probably not cholesterol, but more important, a defect in the wall of any artery which causes the cholesterol to be deposited. When we find out just what causes this defect we may have a cure. The center takes a band-aid approach....

"Name on file."

Pritikin responded to the doctor–whom he referred to as Dr. X–with his own detailed reply.

He began by pointing out that the MRFIT study, done by the National Heart, Lung and Blood Institute at a cost of over $100 million, "hopes to demonstrate whether a reduction of heart disease deaths can be effected by lowering three risk factors: elevated cholesterol, elevated blood pressure, and smoking."

One of the major goals of the MRFIT study was to lower cholesterol level by 10 percent in *six years*. Pritikin was able to accomplish that in six *days!*

Pritikin wrote:

In the last 30-day session, 12 drug controlled hypertensives started with average blood pressures of 141/82. After 30 days, these patients no longer are on drugs and their average blood pressures are 119/67–a 100 percent reversal of hypertension by our program, even though some had been drug-treated for years.

Chest and leg pains are due to insufficient blood supply. As the pain disappears and adequate blood flow returns in response to our program, the improvements can be quantitatively measured by EKG tracings. Since Jan. 5, ten candidates for coronary bypass surgery have all improved so much that none requires surgery, including some whose vein grafts have closed. These improvements are confirmed by electrocardiograms taken during treadmill testing.

As for the doctor's statement that cholesterol is probably not the cause of heart disease, Pritikin countered that the *Journal of the American Medical Association* (JAMA) had reported that 80 percent of heart disease deaths have at least one of three risk factors: elevated blood cholesterol, smoking, and high blood pressure (JAMA, 227:1243, 1975). He marshaled numerous studies, all of which showed that elevated cholesterol was a major cause of most heart disease.

He pointed out that he had been giving free lectures on the subject of diet and health regularly since 1964 and had recently lectured at Cottage Hospital in Santa Barbara.

Finally, Pritikin stated that he had invited physicians to come to his center to examine his records on several occasions, and that Dr. X was still welcome.

The physician's letter to the editor was significant because it represented the views of many physicians and scientists who believed that dietary fat and cholesterol had little or nothing to do with heart disease. They believed other factors, such as aging and some mysterious defect in human arteries, were the principal causes of this disease. As a result, these health professionals viewed Pritikin not only as wrong, but dangerous. He was using diet and exercise as a therapy, when many physicians believed that such things had little to do with the cause of the disease, much less the cure.

Pritikin's rebuttal to Dr. X was effective, however, and from that point on his enemies changed their tactics. Shortly thereafter, a letter was circulated within the medical community stating that doctors should be on the lookout for any information that could be used to "get" Pritikin. The letter fell into Nathan's hands and was circulated among the professional staff at the Longevity Center. Everyone at the center was suddenly on guard.

California Challenges His Credentials

By the late spring of 1976, Pritikin was informed that the California Board of Medical Quality Assurance had launched an investigation of him on two counts: first, that he was practicing medicine without a license; and second, that as a layman he was breaking the law by employing physicians. Both counts were possible felony charges. The Board of Quality Assurance supervises the practice of medicine in the state of California and has the power to investigate doctors who offer false or dangerous therapies, or laypeople who practice medicine without a license. Investigations are usually launched after a complaint–often made by a local physician–is filed with the board. Once a charge has been investigated fully and the board is satisfied that a criminal act has been perpetrated, the evidence is then turned over to the county district attorney for use in prosecution. (A doctor found offering unsubstantiated treatments could lose his or her license.)

The investigation of Pritikin was already under way when Dr. Don

Mannerberg arrived in August 1976 to run the medical arm of the center. As Mannerberg saw it, there was only one way to avoid prosecution: Nathan had to be careful how he counseled people, and an entirely new corporate relationship would have to exist between the doctors and the center.

Mannerberg would work with the investigators for the next two years, assuring them that Pritikin was not diagnosing patients or prescribing medicine. Pritikin was turning over all patients to the medical staff for testing, diagnosis, and treatment, said Mannerberg. In addition, Mannerberg sought legal help in establishing a corporate structure that would make the medical doctors working with the center a separate entity, that contracted its services out to Pritikin's Longevity Center. Mannerberg and his five-physician staff called their new corporation De Novo, meaning "the new" medicine.

After nearly two years, the investigators seemed satisfied, but the message to Pritikin was clear: he was on notice and being watched.

"I don't think Nathan ever appreciated how vulnerable he was to being shut down in those early days," Mannerberg said in 1986. "He was really operating on the edge."

In fact, the charge of practicing medicine without a license would shadow Pritikin for the rest of his professional life. He insisted on seeing patient records and counseling patients personally. Often he firmly disagreed with medical doctors over how to proceed with a patient's treatment. This brought Pritikin into regular conflict with the physicians on his own staff, even those who respected him deeply but saw his involvement in a patient's therapy as jeopardizing the center. Still, many of the Longevity Center physicians over the years did not take kindly to being instructed by a layman.

Said Dr. Rosenthal, a staff physician and later director of the Longevity Center's medical department: "It was very difficult for most physicians to accept the fact that someone who was not an M.D. could tell them what to do."

As in all other aspects of his life, Pritikin tended to "live dangerously," despite the probe by the Quality Assurance Board. Not only did he want to counsel people, but he also wanted to treat anyone who walked in off the street, no matter how sick the person was. He had an unshakable confidence in his program and his own abilities, and he believed that as long as the program was carried on properly, it could help almost everyone.

"We were really proud of the treatment we were providing," recalled Mannerberg. "Although we were treating seriously ill people, we only had one death during the two years I was at the center. And that was an 86-year-old woman who died in her sleep of a ruptured aneurysm."

Still, Pritikin's medical staff was often justifiably cautious. Had the Longevity Center had any deaths that seemed suspicious to the investigators, the state board would surely have ended Pritikin's career in health care.

It was because of the success the program had achieved that Pritikin had such confidence in it, but his differences with his medical staff over who could be helped by the program would remain a fundamental part of his life at the center right up to the time of his death.

In the spring of 1976, Nathan was invited back to Cottage Hospital to talk to local physicians about his program. The lecture came shortly after Pritikin's exchange of letters with Dr. X, and Nathan was clearly a hot topic within the Santa Barbara medical community. Some might have thought it was like walking into the lion's den, but Pritikin seized any opportunity to spread his message.

Pritikin presented the evidence linking diet to a variety of illnesses, including heart disease and diabetes. When his presentation was finished, he asked for questions. At that point, one physician stood up and began berating Pritikin for his views. The doctor became increasingly angry as he bitterly denounced Pritikin. The situation might have gotten out of hand were it not for the fact that Pritikin remained absolutely unruffled. Another doctor who was present in the audience–a physician not connected to the Longevity Center–recalled Pritikin's response to the doctor's angry attacks.

"Nathan was cool," the doctor said. "He never lost his composure. He stuck to the facts of his talk and never got personal. In fact, in all the years that I watched Nathan, I never once saw him lose his temper or composure."

Pritikin let the doctor exhaust his criticisms and then calmly let the meeting come to a close. He never addressed the physician's personal attacks.

Nathan's battle with local physicians was essentially a tempest in a teapot in comparison to the larger front he was about to open. In fact, as soon as he started the Longevity Center, Pritikin took on the largest medical institution in the country, the National Institutes of Health (NIH) and its enormous subdivision, the National Heart, Lung and Blood Institute (NHLBI).

Criticism Goes National

Pritikin began his national campaign to change the way medicine treated heart disease by sending Democratic Congressman Robert Leggett, of California, information on his program and the scientific evidence that supported the use of diet as a means of prevention and treatment of illnesses.

He also sent his Long Beach Study and three patient reports from people who had recovered from serious illnesses using the Pritikin program.

Nathan wrote to Leggett: "In our experience, angina can be reversed so rapidly, no longer requiring drugs, even in many patients with severe angina, that coronary bypass (open heart) surgery is no longer considered. In addition to the possibility of death due to the operation, the bypass closure problems [from continued accumulation of cholesterol deposits in the arteries] need to be taken into account, since 20 percent of all bypasses are reported to close in the first 12 months."

Leggett, in turn, sent Pritikin's material to Dr. Robert Levy, director of NHLBI, and asked that Dr. Levy respond to Pritikin's points.

Right from the start, Levy dismissed Pritikin's claims as unsubstantiated and anecdotal. Levy wrote back to Congressman Leggett that Pritikin's diet and exercise program had resulted in "some expected changes" in patient conditions, but "it will still need to be seen how many of the patients who have undertaken the 30-day live-in diet-exercise program under Mr. Pritikin's direct supervision continue on this regimen as long as a year afterward."

Levy wrote: "Patients can show symptomatic improvement in their disease and some of this improvement can be found under supervised exercise regimens. While the drastic dietary program would be likely to lower plasma cholesterol, it would not be possible to accept the evidence presented as proof of reversal of atherosclerosis."

On February 3, 1976, Levy wrote to Leggett, saying: "We believe that some of the improvement in symptoms and exercise tolerance is understandable; however, these data are not sufficient to establish that specific improvement in the underlying atherosclerosis from the diet-exercise regimen has resulted. . . ."

These two issues–the question of whether people could stay on the diet and the fact that reversal of atherosclerosis had never been proven in humans–became the basis for critics to dismiss Pritikin's work.

In 1976, scientists had yet to conduct a definitive study showing reversal of atherosclerosis in humans on a low-fat, low-cholesterol diet. Reversal had been shown on such a diet in monkeys, but many scientists maintained that there was no "final proof" that what was happening to monkeys was happening in humans, too.

But in the early rounds, Levy went still further. Revealing his lack of knowledge of nutrition and the Pritikin diet, Levy wrote, "It also would require close medical supervision to assure that such a diet devoid of animal products supplies adequate mineral and vitamin requirements."

Undaunted, Pritikin wrote back to Leggett, answering each point of criticism raised by Levy. "Dr. Levy characterizes the three case histories as having improvement of angina and stress treadmill test," wrote Pritikin. "It would be more correct to say elimination of angina and a completely normal stress treadmill test. These results in spite of two cases each with a 100 percent occluded coronary artery. . . .

"Dr. Levy might be interested in knowing that a diet devoid of all animal products, which we do not advocate, is more than adequate in every mineral and vitamin requirement. If the fruits and vegetables are washed, then vitamin B_{12} would be required. Animal products are lacking in vitamins A, C, E, and most minerals." Pritikin concluded his letter with a pointed remark.

"Medical supervision would be required only in a diet high in animal protein. A million U.S. citizens die each year from cardiovascular diseases on this diet, and the medical cost is enormous. ..."

Leggett, too, would not be put off. On February 25, 1976, the congressman wrote a stinging letter to Dr. Levy, stating: "I do believe that [Pritikin] is conducting continuous medical research with an outstanding cadre of professionals. While his success could be ignored by your institute, I do believe you have an obligation to investigate, albeit an unconventional procedure."

Levy had no alternative but to follow the congressman's request to examine Pritikin's work.

On March 8, Levy wrote back to Leggett stating that he would be "pleased" to take Pritikin up on his invitation to have NHLBI representatives visit the Longevity Center. "It would be an important medical contribution if the benefits reported are achieved" he stated, "and particularly if they can be sustained beyond the period of supervision within the Longevity Research Institute."

On March 31, 1976, Levy sent four medical consultants and a staff member from NHLBI to the Longevity Center in Santa Barbara to review Pritikin's records. None of Pritikin's results seemed to impress the visiting scientists.

On June 29, Levy wrote back to Leggett reviewing the investigators' findings. He conceded that there had been "a significant decline" in blood cholesterol levels, "some weight loss," and "some improvement" in blood pressure among the patients at the Longevity Center. However, "It is unlikely that many persons would be willing and able to continue such dietary restrictions very long after leaving the supervised environment provided by Mr. Pritikin's staff. ..."

[A year later, in 1977, Pritikin would get Loma Linda to begin doing follow-up studies to determine the extent to which people maintained the program once they left the center. Loma Linda employed professional survey takers who used both questionnaires and telephone follow-ups. The survey found that 80 percent of the Longevity Center alumni had stayed on the program approximately 80 percent of the time. However, the data would be regarded as "soft" to most scientists, particularly to those at NHLBI, because it did not evaluate blood lipid levels and because people could say that they no longer ate certain foods, even if they had given them up that very day. In short, all Pritikin had was the word of his alumni that they were staying on the diet. And that wasn't enough for most scientists.)

Levy stated that the diet "does not appear to be practical for most persons to follow" and that "NHLBI cannot endorse or recommend the program. . . ."

Levy went on to say that if Pritikin would like to conduct research as to whether his diet was actually reversing atherosclerosis, he could apply for a grant at NHLBI, which would be reviewed for possible approval.

In short, as long as Pritikin had not proven reversal of atherosclerosis, or that people could stick to his regimen to sustain its benefits, Levy pronounced Pritikin's work meaningless.

Pritikin argued that there was an enormous amount of good that could be done for people without having "final proof" that the diet was reversing the underlying atherosclerosis. NHLBI seemed impervious to this point, however.

On July 30, 1976, Levy wrote to Leggett: "To gain scientific or medical acceptance for the potential value of the Diet-Exercise Program, Mr. Pritikin would first have to show that a significant proportion of participants in the 30-day program can be maintained on such a regimen after leaving the controlled supervision his staff provides. If these participants can continue such a program for a year it would be possible to determine whether the symptomatic improvements observed in the supervised environment are sustained."

Nathan wanted Levy to survey his alumni to see what compliance was being observed, but Levy had no interest in such research. NHLBI had already poured more than $250 million into two major diet-related studies studies–the MRFIT (mentioned in Dr. X's letter to the editor) and the Lipid Research Clinics Coronary Primary Prevention Trial, or LRC, for short. Unfortunately for the American taxpayer, MRFIT (as we will see later) would prove to be an enormous waste of money and a major embarrassment to NHLBI and the American scientific community. The LRC study, on the other hand, would vindicate Pritikin.

McGovern Senate Committee Shows Support

Robert Levy and other scientists at NHLBI may not have been impressed with Pritikin's work, but another man in the federal government was. That man was Democratic Senator George McGovern of South Dakota. McGovern was chairman of the Senate Select Committee on Nutrition and Human Needs, which had begun hearings in 1968 on the problem of hunger and malnutrition in the United States. McGovern had initiated the hearings after seeing a CBS television network documentary on hunger which reported that as many as 25 million people in the United States were malnourished. The scene that moved McGovern the most showed children in a school cafeteria going without lunch because they had no food or money to buy it. McGovern set to work. Five years later, he and his committee had helped to create such federally subsidized programs as the School Lunch program, which guarantees that no child in school would go without lunch; the WIC program, which provides food for women, infants and children who cannot afford it; and the Food Stamp program, which provides federal subsidies for low-income people to purchase food.

After these programs had been enacted, the Senate Select Committee stumbled upon the issue of nutrition and its relationship to illness. From 1973 to 1978, the subcommittee listened to expert witnesses tell them that six of the ten leading causes of death in the United States–including heart disease, the common cancers, and diabetes–were all linked to the typical American diet. The principal components in the diet that were causing these illnesses, McGovern's committee found, were fat and cholesterol.

By 1976, the Select Committee had listened to hundreds of witnesses and formulated its basic ideas. And then they found out about what Pritikin was doing. Pritikin was putting into action what many scientists were just beginning to acknowledge.

"In a sense, Nathan's work corroborated ours," recalled McGovern in 1986. "We were looking for support for the testimony we were getting from our expert witnesses. The closest thing we could find in support of what the experts were saying was the Pritikin program."

McGovern was not aware of Pritikin's work when he directed the committee through a labyrinthine search of the scientific literature, but their paths were destined to intersect.

"We came at our ideas from independent routes, but we confirmed each other's findings," McGovern said. "I went out to Santa Barbara and spent three or four days with Nathan. You couldn't help but be impressed with what he was doing."

In the spring of 1977, the Select Committee published *Dietary Goals for the United States*, a landmark document recommending that Americans change their eating habits to include more fish, whole grains, vegetables, and fruits. *Dietary Goals* also urged people to reduce fat and cholesterol, salt, sugar, and refined grains, such as white bread. The committee recommended that people consume fewer total calories in order to control or reduce weight, consume only moderate amounts of alcohol, if any, and stop smoking.

Dietary Goals was the first government report that actually addressed the quality of the typical American diet. And it came as a shock to many areas of the food industry, including the meat, dairy, and egg producers, who raised a furor over the subcommittee's recommendations. The controversy over the report gave rise to a great deal of publicity, which helped to awaken people to the threat posed by a diet high in fat, cholesterol, sugar, salt, and refined flour products.

Despite the McGovern report and the early press reports on the Pritikin program, the scientific establishment was in no way ready to give credit to Nathan. By the end of 1976, the NIH–and much of the scientific community–had closed the door on Pritikin. As far as many establishment scientists were concerned, his work was a dead issue.

But not quite. For Pritikin had just begun to fight.

15

A Counterattack—
and Worldwide Fame

*I*f Pritikin had any hope of being accepted by the medical establishment, he quickly became disabused.

The American Heart Association (AHA) joined in the fray by openly criticizing Pritikin's program in the press. AHA nutritionist Mary Winston called Pritikin's diet "unrealistic" and stated that, "Until he [Pritikin] shows us more than anecdotal evidence, there is nothing to evaluate his work on."

But getting his work published in the scientific press was another matter.

"Trying to get our data published was terribly political," said Dr. Hans Diehl, director of research at the Longevity Center. "We were being turned down because of who we were."

Nathan had hired Diehl, a health researcher from Loma Linda University, in the summer of 1976 to organize the data the center was collecting and get it published in reputable scientific journals. However, Diehl's first paper on diet's effects on high cholesterol levels, diabetes, and angina was turned down by every journal he submitted it to.

The paper was eventually published in the book *Western Diseases*, by Dr. Denis Burkitt and Dr. Hugh Trowell, two eminent British scientists. Burkitt and Trowell had earlier allied themselves with Pritikin by becoming advisory board members for Pritikin's Longevity Research Institute.

Pritikin and Diehl continued to try to publish the results of their work in the scientific press, but it would be years before medical journals would even consider a paper coming out of the Longevity Center.

Pritikin was not the type to wait around patiently for acceptance from the medical community. He was a born promoter, a man who could magically inspire hope or rage, depending upon who he was talking to and what effect he wanted to achieve.

The very first newspaper coverage Pritikin received for the center was from his local paper, the *Santa Barbara News Press*. The second was a national paper–the *National Enquirer.*

From the standpoint of credibility, the publicity from the *Enquirer* was hardly ideal (Pritikin was competing with the latest UFO sighting). But the exposure was enormous. The *National Enquirer* story reached five million readers from all over the country and many of those people passed the article on to friends. Mail poured in to the Longevity Center from people in all corners of America.

Soon, other newspapers and magazines started writing articles about Pritikin. And Nathan took full advantage of the forum to launch a few well-placed volleys of his own.

He called the McDonald's hamburger empire "a busy organization bent on destroying our population. . . ." He said that "if the Russians had to formulate a drink to wipe out the American public, they'd have invented Coke." He called ice cream "a chemical feast. It's a case of completely destroying an already dangerous milk product." As for pizza, he told a reporter that "I can't imagine the Italians could have invented this suicide dish, because they are such nice people."

Pritikin harshly criticized the American diet and the medical establishment for failing to alert the public about the dangers of a diet high in fat, cholesterol, sugar, and salt.

"There's supposed to be something so sacred about the American diet," Pritikin told one reporter, "and the American public is supposed to be so stupid that they would not change one iota of the diet. That's what they [the scientific establishment] would have us believe, at least."

He pulled no punches when it came to telling the press that his program, for many, could be an alternative to bypass surgery.

"We know we have a possible alternative to coronary bypass operations," Pritikin told reporter Benno Isaacs in *New West* magazine. "We predict 90 percent success. We've had almost 100 percent, but I'm only saying 90. Imagine. There are about 50,000 to 100,000 people who go through coronary bypass surgery each year–at a cost of nearly $1 billion annually– and with what we now know about diet and exercise, many of them really don't have to have this operation!"

He repeated over and over again that "it's ridiculous that a million people should die each year from heart disease. Probably hundreds of millions of people in the world exist on the low-fat diet and they simply do not get heart attacks."

Pritikin mercilessly castigated the medical establishment for its attachment to drugs and surgery. He boldly stated the reason surgery is pushed more than diet is because some doctors were more interested in the money they made in open-heart surgery than with other, less lucrative therapies.

Pritikin was not alone in calling attention to the promiscuous use of bypass surgery. The famous Dr. Christiaan Barnard, who pioneered the heart transplant, said in 1976 that "the reason the bypass was done so frequently in the United States was that it is a simple operation and a money maker."

(In 1981, a cardiac surgeon writing in the *New England Journal of Medicine* estimated that the average surgeon doing coronary bypass operations was making $350,000 a year on that operation alone. In 1976, there were approximately 80,000 bypasses performed in the United States, each one costing between $10,000 and $20,000. Three years later, there were nearly 100,000. In 1984, Dr. Joseph Boyle, outgoing president of the American Medical Association [AMA] called on doctors to police their profession with greater scrutiny in order to weed out physicians whose incomes, in Boyle's words, were "outrageous.")

"The National Institutes of Health knows full well what diet can do against heart disease, yet they call for more studies," said Pritikin.

Dr. Robert Levy of the National Heart, Lung and Blood Institute countered Pritikin's public relations effort by dismissing him in the lay press.

Levy told the *Washington Post:* "You prove something by controlled scientific studies. We would hope we could do that some day. I consider it inappropriate to put those anecdotal claims in the press and the lay press at that, not the scientific press."

Burkitt's response to such an argument seemed trenchant. "To say you must uphold action until the case is fully proven is a totally indefensible stand. It's like refusing to throw a life jacket to a drowning man because you're not certain it can save him."

Pritikin argued publicly that doctors would not change until laypeople demanded a new type of health care—one that emphasized prevention and relied more on diet and lifestyle. For many years, Pritikin maintained that this could not be accomplished without a major overhaul of the medical establishment.

"It's kind of like having a king on the throne who is a bad king," Pritikin once said. "You have to take the king off the throne before you have a new government, and new ways of doing things."

This overhaul of health care could be accomplished only by educating medical doctors, scientists, and the lay public on the efficacy of diet as a treatment against degenerative disease. People had to understand that drugs and surgery—while occasionally necessary—had severe and often negative side effects, Pritikin argued. More importantly, they did not get to the root causes of the disease; diet and exercise did.

"Our hope is to educate enough people to start a grassroots movement," he said.

Though he was eminently quotable and even entertaining, Pritikin did make one tactical error when he claimed that his diet could reverse atherosclerosis in the coronary arteries. In fact, there was little scientific proof of this, and no "final proof" that it was taking place in humans. (A handful of studies had purported to show reversal of atherosclerosis in the coronary arteries of humans, but these were largely dismissed by established researchers as unreliable or poorly done.) Scientists simply didn't know what was happening in the coronary arteries of people on a low-fat, low-cholesterol diet.

Pritikin drew an enormous amount of criticism from doctors and scientists for this assertion. For those who were looking for ammunition to use against him, the reversal statement was all they really needed. For years, scientists critical of Pritikin would use his unsupported claim to dismiss him.

By the end of 1977, Nathan modified his claim to say that his patients were "restored to normal function," meaning that their health had been restored to the point that they could live their lives without the symptoms of heart disease and other degenerative illnesses. He could prove that by showing that blood pressure and cholesterol levels had returned to normal, and that treadmill stress tests demonstrated improved blood flow to the heart. In addition, people could perform better in all aspects of life. They physically felt better.

Still, there were those who believed that even his most far-fetched statement might well be true.

Said Dr. William Castelli, director of the Framingham Heart Study and Harvard Medical School professor: "My feeling is that if angiograms were performed on his patients, Pritikin would be able to show reversibility [of atherosclerosis]."

Dr. Peter Wood, deputy director of the Heart Disease Prevention Program at Stanford University, told *New West* magazine in 1977: "I wouldn't be the least bit surprised if all his claims turn out to be true."

"60 Minutes" and Stardom

Despite Pritikin's increasingly controversial stands, it soon became apparent that dismissing him was going to be impossible, especially after October 16, 1977, when he became an overnight celebrity. That was the night the popular television magazine show "60 Minutes" broadcast its first of two telecasts on the Longevity Center.

According to staff members who were at the Longevity Center in

1977, the "60 Minutes" team initially arrived in Santa Barbara to do an exposé on Pritikin and the center.

"After they had been there for a while, they told us that they originally intended to do the show with Mike Wallace doing his investigation with hidden cameras and the whole bit," recalled Don Mannerberg. "It was only after they had been here a while and seen what we were accomplishing that they changed their minds and had Morley Safer do the interview."

"There was no doubt about it," recalled Dave Fields. "They came to investigate us and expose us as charlatans."

Regardless of the original intention, the show could not have provided a more glowing report.

The "60 Minutes" piece examined three patients with serious heart disease who were told by their doctors they needed open-heart surgery to replace clogged arteries. The three patients were Max Eisenberg, a 58-year-old Chicago travel agent; Dan Allen, 54, who ran a shrimp business in Texas; and Clair Shaeffer, a 54-year-old New York electrical contractor. The "60 Minutes" report called all three "fairly hopeless cases."

Max Eisenberg talked about his inability to walk 200 or 300 yards without taking two or three nitroglycerin tablets. He talked about his fears of death and the effects of his disease on his marriage "due to my fear of having sexual intercourse." Dan Allen chose the Longevity Center as a last chance against bypass surgery. Clair Schaeffer had been so distressed by his illness that after he had suffered a heart attack the hospital staff "took me out of intensive care up to the 15th floor, and that night I woke up with terrific pain. I didn't even want to try to get a nurse. I just tried to get out the window. I didn't want to go on. Fortunately, I didn't get the window open."

All three patients were flown to the Miami Heart Institute by "60 Minutes" to be examined by a physician, appointed by the show, who would ascertain their conditions. There was little that could be done for them. At the Miami Heart Institute, Dr. David Lehr diagnosed the three as being fairly typical heart disease patients. On camera, Lehr expressed his frustrations with the limits of what traditional medicine could do for heart disease patients.

"Well, you go systematically through a whole battery of drugs," said Lehr, "some of which are very new, newly developed drugs like Inderal and the Isordils, that it reaches a stage after you've gone through those last rites of medications and the patient still has pain and the patient may or may not be amenable to surgery, then you're frustrated, you're stopped. You really have nothing more to offer other than sympathy."

This was the state the three "60 Minutes" patients were in when they arrived at the Longevity Center. After showing Lehr, the program cut to Pritikin. Said Nathan: "We can take the most serious heart disease [patients] and return them in many cases to normal function, and bring them to such normal function that they can operate completely as if they had no problem."

"60 Minutes" followed the three men through the program as they ate the diet and took their daily walks. The show reported that each man had improved his ability to walk from mere yards to ten miles per day without chest pain. Four months later the three were reexamined by Lehr, who proclaimed them "remarkably improved, clinically." The underlying disease had not disappeared, according to electrocardiogram tests, but all three had been able to give up their drugs, dramatically increased the amount of activity they could do without chest pain, remarkably lowered their cholesterol levels, lowered their blood pressures, and lost weight. In short, each of the men said he could resume his normal life once again.

The show was a bombshell. The Santa Barbara telephone operators could not handle all the calls directed to the center. Phone lines coming into Santa Barbara were jammed for days.

In addition to the "60 Minutes" broadcast, major newspapers, including the *New York Times* and the *Washington Post,* did articles on Pritikin and his program. The *Washington Post* article quoted the British medical journal *Lancet* as saying that although there was not enough human data to support the claim of reversal of atherosclerosis in the coronary arteries, animal studies had shown that such a claim is possible on a low-fat, low-cholesterol diet. In other words, Pritikin's boldest claim might not be as crazy as some scientists would have people believe.

All across the country, magazines and newspapers began reporting the Longevity Center's program. Pritikin's fame spread to other continents, including Australia, Europe, and Africa. The Umhlanga Rocks *Times* of South Africa did a story quoting one of his patients as saying that Pritikin "deserves the Nobel Prize."

Pritikin had been launched. Within a matter of months, his name became a household word among people who were ill, or knew someone who was.

What was clear at this point was that those who sought to dismiss the diet-health connection as meaningless now had a formidable enemy. Nathan was not just another diet proponent. He possessed certain abilities that made him unique and, from the standpoint of his antagonists, difficult to deal with.

First, he had a thorough command of the medical and scientific literature relating diet to health. Moreover, he was fluent in the physician's tongue. But he was also a unique blend of professional scientist and layman, a man who had spent nearly 40 years as an engineer, searching for solutions to very practical problems. His was not a life spent in an ivory tower, removed from the common man. On the contrary, Pritikin saw himself as the common man. For four decades, the experts had been telling him that his ideas were empty, and for as many years he had been proving the experts wrong. Though he possessed rare abilities, Pritikin had no identification with an elite professional class, but looked upon the medical and scientific establishment with skepticism.

It was this combination of engineer and common man–plus a penchant for stating things boldly–that served him so well with the lay press. Pritikin was able to make complicated subjects understandable for lay audiences and journalists. He was a master teacher. He possessed the ability to translate technical and abstruse subjects into easy-to-understand language, and give his listeners the sense that they, too, had an understanding of their health concerns.

And then he went one great step beyond. He applied the available knowledge in a therapeutic setting.

"Nathan made the quantum leap from theory to practice," recalled Dr. Hans Diehl. "He had tremendous ability to motivate people to eat a diet and follow a simple lifestyle. He had a very clear concept of the diet he wanted people to follow and he was able to communicate it to people. When I came to work at the Longevity Center, I couldn't believe people would follow such a diet, but after a few weeks of listening to Nathan and watching the results he was having, I realized that it could indeed be done."

This was an unprecedented accomplishment. No one had taken the science of nutrition and used it to treat so many illnesses so successfully.

This singular achievement made him a powerful adversary to the medical and scientific community. The lives of thousands of patients who went through the Longevity Center served as living proof that his program worked. These people formed an ever-increasing army in support of him. Pritikin forced the scientific world to reexamine not only the role diet plays in the onset and treatment of disease, but also the way the medical establishment approached the problem of treating degenerative disease.

And somehow, he came along at just the right time.

Science Forced to Take Notice

When Pritikin arrived on the scene, the scientific world was concentrating most of its efforts on finding a biochemical answer to heart disease, cancer, diabetes, high blood pressure, arthritis, and other degenerative illnesses. To most scientists, nutrition and diet were not considered important or exciting areas of study. Prompted by the discovery of antibiotics and the so-called wonder drugs of the 1930s and 1940s, scientists envisioned the day when drugs could be invented to cure every known illness. The microscopic world was far more tantalizing than the world of nutrition and diet.

In a remarkably revealing statement, Dr. Donald S. Fredrickson, director of the National Institutes of Health (NIH), described the attitude of scientists toward diet research versus other therapies. In 1978 Fredrickson, who as director of NIH was arguably the most powerful scientist in the country, told Senator George McGovern's Senate Select Committee on Nutrition and Human Needs:

"The major thing that moves science today is technical opportunity. Immunology has moved like a rocket because there are techniques for measuring antibodies and their relationship to disease and to health. And when we get techniques for measuring nutritional status that are far more microscopic than they are in regard to whether you had a coronary or you have a tumor of the bowel, then we will begin to see movement there, too. And that is the crucial thing that determines the movement in science."

The study of nutrition was an altogether unwieldy subject for most laboratory scientists. One high-ranking scientist, formerly of the NIH, described why: "Drugs and surgery fall more in the nature of modern science. We don't really know that much about nutrition today and the hard-nosed scientist stays away from nutrition because its very hard to isolate what [a nutrient like] calcium might do. But with Pritikin pushing diet, all of a sudden NIH had a problem, because diet is not a laboratory problem–it's not a virus or a germ–it's a cultural problem, a lifestyle problem, and that's beyond the capabilities of basic biomedical science."

To most physicians, especially in the late 1970s and early 1980s, nutrition was an altogether foreign discipline. According to an AMA survey reported in 1979, only 30 of the 125 U.S. medical schools questioned had required nutrition education courses. After investigating medical school curricula, Democratic Senator Patrick Leahy of Vermont discovered that medical school students were given more instruction in how to set fees than they were in nutrition education.

Physicians and scientists had little, if any, appreciation for the scientific studies being done by a minority of researchers over the previous 60 years. Once confronted with this information, the scientific world rebelled. They demanded more proof–even "final proof"–and in the meantime maintained that the link between diet and health was only a "hypothesis."

And yet, there was a vast amount of scientific evidence accumulated that testified to the efficacy of diet in the prevention and treatment of illness.

In assessing that evidence, Dr. Jeremiah Stamler of Northwestern University Medical School, wrote in 1978:

"The terms *hypothesis* and *theory* both have precise meanings in the language of science. The Random House unabridged dictionary states 'A *hypothesis* is a conjecture put forth as a possible explanation of certain phenomena or relations, which serves as a basis of argument or experimentation by which to reach the truth,' and 'A *theory* properly is a more or less verified or established explanation accounting for a known fact or phenomena.'

"Given the vast body of consistent information from many research methodologies on the relationship between lifestyle [including diet] and atherosclerotic disease, it is inappropriate to use the term hypothesis in speaking about this general area of knowledge."

Stamler pointed out that if other sciences were held to the same rigors as the research connecting diet to heart disease, "the entire bodies of knowledge acquired in modern times by geology, astronomy, and evolutionary biology would have to be classified as hypothesis rather than theory, since they rest almost exclusively on observational, rather than experimental, data. It would have to be the hypothesis of gravitation, not the theory of gravitation; the hypothesis of relativity, not the theory of relativity; the hypothesis of evolution, not the theory of evolution."

In short, diet was being scrutinized more rigorously than most other scientific studies, and, by far, more rigorously than most drugs rushed onto the market.

The evidence linking diet to illness, therefore, faced several enormous obstructions within the scientific community: it was foreign to many physicians and scientists; the methodologies used in the study of diet and health did not fit into the scientific laboratory model; and in their ignorance of the research and nutrition's potential as a therapeutic tool, many scientists and doctors clamored for more research, and even "final proof," before they would acknowledge the benefits of a low-fat, low-cholesterol, high-complex carbohydrate diet.

Pritikin simply caught most doctors and scientists by surprise.

"Very few people realized what diet and exercise could accomplish until Nathan came along and did it," said one NIH scientist.

In the absence of any real appreciation for the efficacy of nutrition, and the enthusiasm for biochemistry, the claims made by Pritikin seemed outlandish at first. Many scientists had to see the proof before they would accept him.

"Levy was doing what any hard-nosed scientist would do," said Castelli years later. "He needed to see the hard evidence before he was willing to recommend that diet replace existing therapies."

But as Stamler pointed out, the key question was: How much evidence did the scientific world need before action could be taken?

Pritikin presented one other issue that tended to complicate matters for the scientific world: he possessed no degrees.

In a world that spins on the twin poles of higher education and prestigious credentials, Pritikin was an anathema. His very existence within the world of health care drove many doctors to fits of rage. It was as if he bypassed the accepted channels and somehow managed to beat everyone to the top.

As an NIH scientist explained, credentials are not mere ribbons on an inflated chest; they are essential to the livelihood of scientists.

"Credentials are fundamental to getting grants and moving your career ahead in science," said the NIH researcher. "Unless you are a well-established, credentialed scientist, your chances of getting a grant and doing your research are limited because there is so much competition for grant money, and there isn't that much to go around. Credentials are a means of evaluating who the person is, so naturally, people take these things very seriously. It's very important to stay within the club and watch your p's and q's. Of course, this shapes the kinds of studies that are done. Now here comes Nathan, who is not a doctor or a credentialed scientist, and he contradicts the medical community. The first reaction to him was 'How dare he say anything?' And he made it even more difficult by going right to the public. And it was perfectly timed, because the public was ready for it."

Like revolutionaries everywhere, Pritikin broke the rules. Naturally, he incurred the wrath of those who lived within the rules and expected to benefit by them. But unlike revolutionaries who come from within the system, Pritikin was a complete outsider, and as such, an embarrassment to those who maintained that the system itself was necessary to produce qualified scientists and, more importantly, answers to society's illnesses. Pritikin's success called into question some of the fundamental methods and attitudes scientists and doctors had come to accept and live by. In that way, his very existence was a healthy thing for the health care system, and those it served.

Soon Nathan Pritikin represented the dividing line for many scientists and doctors. As he became increasingly popular and publicized, he received an attendant amount of contempt and reverence from professionals and laypeople alike. He became so controversial that many scientists in established positions could not associate themselves with him for fear of losing their jobs.

One well-known scientist, who had been listed on Pritikin's board of advisors for the Longevity Research Institute, was approached by his superiors and told flatly to disassociate himself from Pritikin. Another admitted that he refused to put Nathan's name on a study Pritikin had contributed to because it would have hurt the scientist's credibility and his chances of getting future work published in scientific journals.

There would be other defections. From the time he opened the Longevity Research Institute, Pritikin held annual meetings at which leading scientists presented papers on their work. Among the speakers at the meetings were Trowell and Burkitt, as well as Dr. James Anderson, from the University of Kentucky Medical School. One year, Pritikin invited one of the top researchers in cardiovascular disease to speak at the Longevity Research Institute's annual meeting. The researcher agreed to give a paper, and the arrangements were made for his presentation. However, just days before the annual meeting was to be held, the scientist was told by his superior that if he spoke at Pritikin's Longevity Center, his funding would be cut off. The researcher told Pritikin he couldn't make it.

In 1978, UCLA scientist Dr. James Barnard, who had published in the scientific literature for more than a decade, was hired to do research for the Longevity Center. Barnard conducted a study using Pritikin patients and then sent his paper off to a number of scientific journals, all of which rejected it. Barnard was shocked that the paper had been rejected. He told Nathan that he believed the paper had been rejected because Pritikin's name was on it. "We can fix that," Pritikin told Barnard. "Take my name off it." Barnard did and submitted it to another scientific publication, the *Journal of Cardiac Rehabilitation*, one of the leading scientific journals reporting the work in cardiovascular disease research. There it was accepted. Only when Barnard was proofreading the galleys before publication did he put Nathan's name back on the study. He then called the editor of the journal and told him that he had mistakenly left Pritikin's name off the study and was now placing it back on the paper. The editor agreed.

The hazing of Pritikin would continue. However, as he became more successful and gained wider publicity, the opposition to him became less and less effective. That didn't stop his critics from trying.

CHAPTER **16**

More Stories of Hope and Success

*I*n May 1978, Pritikin moved the Longevity Center to a large hotel on the beach in Santa Monica, 90 miles south of Santa Barbara. The center would be the sole occupant of the new facility.

Despite his success in Santa Barbara, Pritikin never felt at home at the Mar Monte Hotel. He and Mar Monte owner Buddy Taub ran into endless disagreements over how much rent the Longevity Center should pay. In early 1978, Taub raised by half Pritikin's monthly rent of $51,250. Pritikin decided it was time to look for a new home for the center. Longevity Center employees demanded that Pritikin remain in Santa Barbara and Pritikin himself preferred to remain there, since Santa Barbara was his home. However, after scouting Santa Barbara and neighboring Goleta for months in search of a permanent location, nothing turned up.

In March 1978, Los Angeles businessman and real estate developer David Roberts approached Pritikin about forming a partnership. In exchange for shared ownership in the center, Roberts would provide a large facility in Santa Monica, previously owned by the Synanon drug rehabilitation group. Though badly in need of refurbishing, the building was perfect. It comprised 130,000 square feet, with 125 guest rooms, a large, modern kitchen, an enormous dining room, a ballroom that seated 500, a theater with a stage, a gym, a swimming pool, and numerous offices and larger rooms that could be used for classes and medical offices. The building was located right on Santa Monica beach, where participants had only to walk out the back door to be in front of the ocean. In April, Pritikin and Roberts agreed to become partners, and in May, Nathan moved the center en masse to Santa Monica. Pritikin offered all his employees the same jobs in Santa Monica, but the move was unwelcome and most of his 50 employees chose not to join him.

Once in Santa Monica, Pritikin's staff burgeoned. Eventually the center's staff would swell to 250, including cooks, housekeepers, kitchen and dining room attendants, nutritionists, exercise physiologists, a couple of research scientists, and ten full-time medical doctors.

In order to ensure that the program was run properly in Santa Monica, Nathan and Ilene moved into the new facility and remained there from Monday through Friday night, when they returned to their home in Santa Barbara. Ilene continued to supervise the kitchen, menu plans, and food preparation talks. Nathan ran the program, counseled patients, gave lectures, and maintained his frenetic pace as public spokesman for the use of diet as a treatment for disease.

By living in the center five days a week, the Pritikins had fully given themselves over to the program. It was their life from early morning till late at night.

"I would go up to our room at the end of the day," Ilene recalled. "Nathan would still be seeing patients or giving a lecture. At first we ate our meals in the dining room, but soon Nathan would be besieged by people and it became impossible to eat, so we began to eat in his office and later, in our room. After dinner, Nathan would often lecture, and see people who had questions, and eventually he would come up to our room. He would have to make some phone calls then, and by the time he was finished he was exhausted."

Ever since the "60 Minutes" broadcast, Pritikin was more and more in demand for speaking engagements and for television interviews. Many medical and dental groups requested that Pritikin provide lectures on his approach to degenerative diseases. Dental societies, in fact, became one of the leading supporters of Pritikin and his program.

"Dentists understand the relationship between health and what you put in your mouth," Pritikin once commented. "My ideas are not so foreign to them."

With the increase in the number of guest rooms and available space, the Longevity Center took on more patients. And the remarkable case histories grew more numerous.

No More Pain, No More Pills, No More Wheelchair

Minnia Biener, of Elizabeth, New Jersey, was one of several patients who arrived at the Longevity Center in a wheelchair in 1978. In 1980, she wrote to Nathan to wish him a happy birthday and to describe her remarkable recovery:

> My life has a new meaning and I have new joy in living. For eight years I
> was confined to bed with severe pain, unable to walk and dependent on the
> use of oxygen. During that time I was hospitalized seven times, suffering

three myocardial infarctions [heart attacks]. I had the additional problem of being a diabetic and high blood pressure victim.

Many times I entertained the thought of death. There seemed to be no purpose in living with pain and causing distress to my loved ones. When I reached a point where the Demerol pills which I had been taking for pain were no longer too effective, panic set in. In desperation I called my doctor and pleaded for some course of treatment, other than complete bed rest, heart medication and Demerol. His response was he regretted nothing more could be done and his exact words were "you better face it, you are not going to get better; learn to live with it."

It was in a state of depression that I first saw "60 Minutes" on CBS presenting Nathan Pritikin['s] Longevity Center Program. I began to have a glimmer of hope which became stronger when I saw the David Susskind program on the air with five former patients of the Longevity Center. Each one of these handicapped heart patients were returned to normal function because of you. It was during this program it seemed to me you were reaching out to me with the message "don't despair, you can be helped." I felt the excitement of optimism run through me, and in my mind I was on my way to Santa Monica.

And so it was that a short time later, full of hope and expectation, I arrived at the center in my wheelchair. I was in that chair for five days when you approached me and wheeled me over to a secluded area. It was then you started me on my first walking lesson. From that point on, I felt you were taking a personal interest in me, encouraging me each time we met.

Later on, as I met other patients, many of them expressed the same feeling that your interest in them was personal. You can't imagine how grateful we all were for your compassion and your caring attitude.

It seemed like a miracle to me at the end of two weeks, I was walking for a period of ten minutes. I walked with pain in my unused legs, but I walked.

When I arrived at the center, I was loaded with medication. I took 160 mg. of Inderal [for hypertension] daily, 100 mg. of Cardilate [for angina pain], 100 mg. of Apresoline [for severe hypertension], 250 mg. of Diabinese [for diabetes], 5 mg. of Valium [for anxiety] several times a day and Quinamm for leg cramps. Also 30 mg. of Dalmane for sleep.

Upon my first visit to Dr. [Sam] Cherney [Longevity Center physician], he immediately took me off Diabinese and gradually reduced the Apresoline to zero. He cut down on my Inderal. After a few days I was able to eliminate the Valium, Dalmane, and Quinamm.

When I left the center, I was completely free of pain, no longer had leg cramps, and only took a reduced amount of Inderal and Cardilate. At the end of my four weeks, I was walking a quarter mile four times a day, with a great feeling of well-being.

When I came home, I was delighted with the reaction of my doctor. After a thorough exam, including a cardiogram, he said with surprise, "Minnia, for the first time in years, your cardiogram is normal and I am elated." I continued making progress. My lifestyle changed. We moved to Florida, where I walk two miles every morning at 6:30, every day with a feeling of gratitude to you. For the first time in eight years, I am leading a normal social life . . . I am president of a 450-member women's club. I have been able to do the choreography for a home talent show, a far cry from being unable to walk at all. People find it hard to believe I was incapacitated.

What do I believe in? I believe in "Miracles" and I believe in "Nathan Pritikin."

With great affection and gratefully yours,
Minnia Biener

Minnia Biener turned 74 in 1987 and she was still following the Pritikin program, walking about a half mile per day and riding her stationary bicycle. In 1987, Mrs. Biener recalled the details of her walking lesson with Nathan.

"He came up to me and turned to my husband and said, 'Do you mind if I take Minnia for a few minutes. I'll bring her right back.' And he took me over to the side and he said that the carpet was very thick so if I fell I wouldn't hurt myself, but he wouldn't let me fall. He had me take a few steps while he held on to me, and after that he said, 'Now, I think you're ready for the gym.' And that's when I started to work with a physical therapist on the treadmills."

At the end of two weeks, Mrs. Biener was walking about a half mile to a mile per day. About that time, Pritikin came up to her and asked if she would tell her story to the rest of the Longevity Center participants at his lecture that day.

There were about 250 people in the room when Nathan asked Mrs. Biener to stand up and tell her story.

"I told everyone that I was making progress. And I'll never forget the look on his face when I spoke. His smile was so broad, it was something."

Not everyone Pritikin was counseling at the time actually came to the center. On a regular basis, Pritikin advised hundreds of people who never set foot in the center, either because they couldn't afford it or because Pritikin told them they didn't need it. In fact, much of Pritikin's day was spent on the telephone with people calling for health advice.

Hypoglycemia Symptoms Gone

Stan Keller had been an attorney in the entertainment business for nearly 20 years before contracting hypoglycemia that eventually became so severe that he could no longer conduct his practice. He became deeply depressed, devoid of energy, and suffered from cold sweats and dizziness. For the next 14 years, he went to a series of doctors, psychotherapists, and nutritionists without any sign of relief. In 1978, he was eating a high-protein diet and taking massive doses of vitamin and mineral supplements.

He held to this program religiously, though it gave him little relief and he still was unable to return to work.

Keller's wife, Wilma, had read Nathan's book *Live Longer Now*, and her brother, a dentist, had recommended she call Nathan to ask his advice about Stan. Wilma did. She explained her husband's severe symptoms and the diet and vitamin therapy he was on.

For the next hour, Pritikin outlined a diet and exercise program for Stan Keller that, in Wilma's words, "gave us the life back."

Stan Keller followed the program outlined by Pritikin and in ten days was well again, having regained his energy and lost all the symptoms of his hypoglycemia.

Pritikin might never have heard from the Kellers again if Wilma hadn't decided two weeks after her husband started the program that she wanted to work for Pritikin.

The Kellers had had a long involvement as social activists and Wilma was about to begin working for Edmund "Jerry" Brown, who was then governor of California. But having seen in her own experience what Pritikin was accomplishing, Wilma Keller decided she was going to work for him.

Short, spry, and energetic, Wilma Keller was as emotional as Nathan was reserved. She had enough energy and enthusiasm to bring a smile to the face of the most bitter misanthrope and a glimmer of hope to a lost depressive. And indeed, she did manage to land a job at the Longevity Center.

At first she went to work for Dr. Hans Diehl, director of research at the center, but Wilma wanted to be closer to Pritikin. She felt her abilities would be better used on "the front lines," where Pritikin was dealing firsthand with the sick. Wilma asked Pritikin if he didn't need an assistant in his own office. He already had a very competent secretary, so he asked Wilma, "Can you do a newsletter? Do you have any experience at that?"

"No," Wilma said.

"Do you take dictation?" he asked.

"No," Wilma answered.

"Do you have any secretarial skills that we might use in the office?" asked Pritikin.

"No," said Wilma.

Pritikin seemed perplexed. He didn't know quite where to place her.

"I'm a people person," said Wilma. "I could help you with public relations and be a buffer between you and the people who want to see you. I could organize your time and your appointments. Let me have a three-month trial with you and I'll create a place for myself that will help you."

Perhaps because of her enthusiasm and because he hated to say no, Pritikin agreed. Wilma's title was secretary, because Nathan had no idea what she was going to end up doing when he agreed to hire her.

But in the six years that followed, Wilma Keller became an indispensible girl Friday for Nathan, shepherding people in to see him, organizing alumni meetings, keeping in touch with former patients, and organizing fund-raisers for research. Pat Walters, who had risen to program coordinator at the Santa Monica center, and Wilma Keller became the center's motivational one-two punch. While Pritikin and the professional staff administered the intellectual nuts and bolts of the program, Ms. Walters and Ms. Keller provided the enthusiasm and the emotional support so many patients needed.

Eventually, Stan Keller also came to work for Nathan as his legal advisor.

With the center now in a larger facility and taking a higher profile, the risks to Pritikin and his staff were enormous. But Pritikin's success against the seemingly incurable illnesses was, at times, uncanny. He continued to attract those with severe heart disease, high blood pressure, type II (adult-onset) diabetes, gout, claudication, and arthritis. But there were also many related illnesses, some of them seemingly intractable after years of treatment. A woman in her late sixties arrived after being unable to speak or walk for several years. She was virtually comatose. Her success on the program was so remarkable that by the time she left the center she was thinking lucidly, as well as walking and talking. On the concluding night of her session, a birthday party was given for a man named Harry in the ballroom of the center. At the end of the evening, the woman got up from her chair and walked across the ballroom floor to the amazement of everyone present and wished Harry a happy birthday in a voice loud enough to be heard by the entire crowd.

Woman's Sight Returns

Nancy Washburn, a 29-year-old nurse who had been a diabetic since childhood, had lost the sight in both her eyes as a result of hemorrhaging caused by the diabetes. Mrs. Washburn had undergone as many as 5,000 laser treatments in her right eye and nearly 6,000 in her left eye before she lost the sight in both eyes. Surgery was performed that restored her sight temporarily, but subsequent hemorrhages left her blind in both eyes after the operations.

Her doctor attended a medical meeting in Los Angeles at which Nathan lectured. After Pritikin's talks, Mrs. Washburn's physician discussed her case with Nathan. Pritikin believed the program would help Mrs. Washburn recover her sight and asked the doctor to have Mrs. Washburn call him. While Nathan did not believe he could wean Mrs. Washburn of her dependency on insulin (juvenile diabetes is extremely intractable, even with improved diet and exercise, Pritikin found), he did believe the program might help her with her sight and perhaps reduce her insulin needs. He also believed he could help her avoid the many side effects, including kidney damage and heart disease, that are so common with diabetes. Mrs. Washburn called Pritikin and enrolled in the March 1983 session at the center.

When she arrived at the center, Nancy Washburn could see no images. The sight in her right eye was permanently gone. Her left eye was incapable of seeing the details of objects. Even in a well-lighted room, everything was an opaque blur. Occasionally, very intense colors such as red would emerge as a hazy image, but the source of the color could not be ascertained.

Each day, she ate the food and walked on the treadmill, talking to the people whom she could not see on either side of her. She walked for hours and miles, hoping that she might eventually regain her vision in her left eye. Nathan was hopeful as well, but he thought it might take months for her circulation to improve so that blood could pass through the tiny capillaries that nourish the eyes. Once this occurred, Pritikin believed the sight in her left eye could be restored.

As the weeks went by, Nancy Washburn experienced no improvement in her sight but saw a marked improvement in her vitality, blood values, and kidney function. The swelling that had been chronic before she came to the center was receding and her insulin requirements were being reduced.

Still, when the program concluded, she went home with her sight no better, but with Pritikin's encouragement to be patient and to continue on the diet and exercise program.

Three months after she concluded the program, the sight in Mrs. Washburn's left eye began to return. At first, she could only make out images on the periphery of her vision, but gradually the clarity worked its way in toward the center. Four months after she began the diet and exercise regimen, Nancy Washburn could see again.

She had also reduced her insulin needs by 25 percent and, according to her physicians, her kidney functions had stabilized. In 1987, Nancy Washburn's sight in her left eye was 20/40, which was corrected to 20/20 with eyeglasses. She had a driver's license and was a practicing nurse.

A Folk Hero

Reports of these and other remarkable recoveries made Pritikin a national celebrity in the popular media. Articles about Pritikin and the Longevity Center turned up in such widely circulated magazines as *Time,*

Newsweek, New York, Woman's Day, Family Circle, Runner's World, and many others. The center was uniformly portrayed in an extremely positive light, and it wasn't long before the Longevity Center was being called the "U.S. version of Lourdes."

It soon became obvious that Pritikin was not going to just fade away, that his was not another "fad diet" like so many others before him. In response to the growing public pressure to investigate Pritikin's program, Dr. Robert Levy and a team of physicians and scientists from the National Heart, Lung and Blood Institute (NHLBI) descended upon the Longevity Center to examine Pritikin's data on July 18, 1978–two years after NHLBI's original review.

According to a transcript of that meeting, the discussion once again centered on patient compliance. Levy dismissed Pritikin's 1977 Loma Linda compliance studies because they had been conducted by telephone interviews, which were not scientifically valid. (People could say they no longer ate meat or dairy foods because they had given them up on the day of the telephone call, Levy said.) As one scientist said, Pritikin's evidence of compliance was "very soft." Levy maintained that Pritikin had not proven that people could stay on the diet and as a result NHLBI could not recommend that doctors begin using diet and exercise in place of drugs and surgery as a treatment for heart disease, or anything else, for that matter.

There was still the question of what exactly was taking place in the coronary arteries of patients on a low-fat, low-cholesterol diet. No one had proven scientifically that diet could reverse coronary atherosclerosis. Levy concluded that Pritikin and his staff should conduct a prospective compliance study, that is, a study that would designate a group of patients at the outset of the program and follow them for several years to see how well they remained on the program. That would be an expensive and tedious project, but it was the only sort of proof the scientific establishment would accept, according to Levy.

Pritikin was undaunted by the latest meeting with Levy. He was having a growing impact on the American public without the assistance of the federal government. And in the end, it would be the public that changed medicine. Laypeople could do this simply by demanding that medicine pay greater attention to diet, both as a means of prevention and treatment.

Something else was happening. NHLBI may have been officially unimpressed with Pritikin's work, but he had clearly grabbed the lead in the fight to make diet an important issue in the minds of laypeople, and indeed, a growing issue among medical doctors and scientists.

In fact, the more NHLBI tried to belittle Pritikin's work, the more Pritikin appeared to be the man trying to help people in the face of resistance from powerful institutions. This was clearly the perception of the national media, for whom Pritikin was fast becoming a kind of folk hero.

It was only three months after Levy and his scientists left the Longevity Center that "60 Minutes" struck again. On October 22, 1978, "60 Minutes" broadcast what CBS correspondent Morley Safer called a "medical checkup" on the same three patients the television show had reported on before: Max Eisenberg of Chicago, Dan Allen of Texas, and Clair Shaeffer of New York City.

The show opened by updating the audience on the medical histories of the three men and their remarkable functional recovery as a result of the Pritikin program.

"Well, that was a year ago, and we reported at the time all three were in good shape, on the diet and virtually free of medication," reported Safer. "We took a lot of criticism at the time from doctors who said a few weeks or a few months means nothing. Some said most patients would not stay on the diet, it was too severe. And anyway, with the carefree life of the center, they were bound to feel better temporarily. Fair enough. There was still no track record on Clair Shaeffer, Max Eisenberg, and Dan Allen."

The show then reported that all three men had continued to remain on the diet religiously and had continued to improve in virtually all areas of their lives. As it had done a year before, "60 Minutes" flew the three men to the Miami Heart Institute to be reexamined by Dr. David Lehr. Lehr had examined the men before and after their visits to the Longevity Center and was now in a position to determine how much improvement had been made during the previous year while the men maintained the diet and exercise program on their own.

Safer asked Lehr, "Would you dare to say that they're cured?"

"A functional cure, yes," said Lehr. "A scientific standard set by medicine by the tests we use, no." He went on to say that large studies have to be designed using large groups of people with documented heart disease to see if it really holds for more than 3 people. "If it holds for 40 people, then maybe the government will get in and do it on thousands of people," he said.

Safer asked, "Dr. Lehr, what would happen, do you think, if everyone in this country overnight went onto a–changed their lives and stayed with this sort of diet and this sort of exercise?"

"Well, overnight, the next morning, nothing would happen," Lehr replied. "Over a period of years, the population, if they dropped their cholesterol and other fats to levels of 150 [mg%. per deciliter of blood] and the triglycerides way down, we might see cardiovascular disease drop off the face of the earth, our earth, much like those populations in the world that eat this diet who don't have the diseases now."

The show cut to Max Eisenberg, who summed up the benefits he derived from the program.

"I don't panic any more," said Eisenberg. "When I used to have pain, I panicked. 'I'll drop dead!' Now I don't. I have faith. I know my capacity. No more fear."

Like the first show, this one had an explosive impact. In the weeks that followed, Pritikin and the Longevity Center were deluged with calls and letters wanting more information about the diet and exercise program. Producer Harry Moses, who produced the show on Pritikin, told Wilma Keller that the program had generated more mail than any other so far broadcast by "60 Minutes."

Whatever Pritikin's critics might have been saying, the "60 Minutes" broadcast conveyed a simple yet profound message: Nathan Pritikin was making people well, and while there were many questions yet to be answered, there was little doubt that the program worked.

It was a message anyone could understand.

CHAPTER 17

Personal Troubles

*F*rom every outward measure, Nathan had achieved enormous success. Someone else in his position might have relaxed and let the ship continue on course. But Pritikin was driven. As he and the center gained wider public acclaim, Pritikin seemed all the more taken up by his larger goal: to change the way medicine treated degenerative disease. Pritikin was so focused on this larger goal that the allures of fame, power, or prestige seemed lost on him. In fact, Pritikin was completely out of touch with any sense of celebrity, either his own or someone else's.

From 1979 on, the Longevity Center became a mecca for powerful people in the fields of entertainment, business, and government. But Pritikin, who was so totally out of touch with the popular culture, had to be informed by Wilma Keller or Phyllis Major, his secretary, who a particular person was. Rather than try to cultivate an advantage among the rich and famous, Pritikin went through his day as if wearing blinders.

"Everyone was the same as far as Nathan was concerned," recalled Wilma Keller. "He didn't know, nor did he care, if someone was rich or famous. Once, I had to tell him who Barbara Streisand was."

Moreover, as increasing demands were made upon his time, he seemed forever in a hurry. Pritikin literally ran around the Longevity Center, going from one appointment to the next. Once he was in his office or listening to a patient, he was entirely focused, but between destinations one had to keep up with him while he jogged en route.

"Nathan was always in a rush," recalled actor Lorne Greene, who attended the Longevity Center. "If you wanted to talk to him, you had to keep moving. It was not a sedentary conversation, it was a moving conversation. But he would come up with a lot of interesting details while he was moving away. He never left you without something. But everyone wanted to see him. He was *the* man, and the others were pale in comparison."

Business Goes Bankrupt

While he was attending to the illness of hundreds each month, Pritikin had plenty of his own troubles to cope with–including personal bankruptcy.

After Pritikin started the Longevity Center in 1976, he devoted less and less time to his other businesses, especially Photronics. Meanwhile, Photronics fell deeper and deeper into debt. Pritikin decided to siphon the profits of the Longevity Center into Photronics to keep the company afloat. But the business needed more, and Pritikin was forced to borrow money to make the Photronics payroll and keep the company going. In a desperate attempt to keep the company alive, he obtained a large loan by using his home as collateral. But Photronics was doomed, and at the end of 1978, the company went bankrupt.

In January 1979, one of Nathan's major creditors called in his loan and threatened to foreclose by taking possession of his house. In order to avoid losing his home, Nathan placed his personal finances in Chapter 11 of the bankruptcy code, thus giving him a little time to settle his debts with the profits of the Longevity Center. The courts assessed Pritikin's total debt at $1.23 million, while his personal assets were $1.25 million.

While Pritikin tried to reorganize his finances and pay off his debts, his stockholders at Photronics sued him in order to grab a percentage of the Longevity Center, which they claimed Photronics owned because Pritikin had once signed a contract stating that all of his future inventions were the property of Photronics.

Nathan's attorney, Howard Parke, argued that Pritikin had turned over only the rights to electronics-related inventions. The legal battles hung on for months, while the fate of Pritikin's control of the Longevity Center, his home, and his personal finances hung in the balance. A superior court judge finally agreed with Pritikin and ruled that Photronics had no claim on the Longevity Center. It took Pritikin nearly a year to get out from under the Chapter 11; he paid 100 cents on the dollar on debts that eventually amounted to $1.5 million.

Nathan's Secret Illness

Despite the enormity of his financial problems, Pritikin's main concern was elsewhere. His cancer had begun to show signs of returning.

Pritikin's leukemia had been in remission since 1976, with the help of the chlorambucil chemotherapy agent he had been taking intermittently since he was diagnosed at UCLA. Nathan did not want to take the drug, however, and in 1979 he discontinued it entirely.

There was every reason to stop the chemotherapy, as far as Pritikin was concerned. He felt well, had seemingly limitless energy, and felt no need to slow down. He maintained what can only be described as a torrid schedule. He had been taking only small doses of the chlorambucil, and was regularly in conflict with his physician, Dr. David Golde at UCLA, over how much of the drug he should be taking. Nathan argued for reduced amounts and usually got his way, since he was the one controlling the amount of the drug he took.

Despite his abundant energy, however, Pritikin had begun to look ill. His skin was pale and a little yellow. People regularly asked him about the pallid cast of his skin. He would say that his work prevented him from getting much sun. Upon meeting Pritikin, one doctor noticed the yellow color of his hands and asked him if his hemoglobin was low. Pritikin acknowledged that it was, but that he was monitoring it and it was well within normal limits.

In fact, Pritikin's hemoglobin tended to be at the low end of normal, usually hovering at about 10 mg.% (normal hemoglobin ranges from 10 mg.% to 14 mg.%). His hemoglobin remained in the low-normal ranges throughout the late 1970s and early 1980s.

From 1976 onward, Nathan sought to keep his illness a secret by using the alias Howard Malmuth when being treated. He chose the name because, as he said, it was easy for people to forget. He desperately wanted to keep his illness from the general public because he feared that, as an exponent of health, he would lose all credibility if his illness became public knowledge. He did not want to have to explain that he had con-tracted the blood disorder before he had changed his diet. Only Pritikin's doctor at UCLA was supposed to know who Howard Malmuth was, but word leaked out and news of Nathan's leukemia circulated as a rumor in Los Angeles medical circles throughout the late 1970s and early 1980s.

In 1979, a doctor approached Wilma Keller and told her that Pritikin suffered from leukemia, but Wilma refused to believe or repeat the statement. That same year a patient at the Longevity Center, who was from the Los Angeles area, approached Pritikin and bluntly asked him if he suffered from cancer. Nathan's response was that his blood was being treated for a protein problem, which was being controlled by medication. That was all Pritikin said and the patient seemed satisfied.

For his part, Pritikin always wished he looked healthier. His energy and endurance were his only outward signs of good health, and indeed people tended to overlook the color of his skin and marveled at his seemingly limitless vitality. Still, Nathan was not a self-conscious person, and the issue of his appearance was always a small one for him. No matter whether his cheeks were pale or rosy red, Pritikin knew that his knowledge and hard work were his most important personal assets in spreading his message. As for the program, its basic effectiveness spoke for itself in the lives of those who adopted it.

But his illness shadowed him like a terrible debt that could only be paid with his life. After he was diagnosed as having hairy cell leukemia, Pritikin stayed continually abreast of the scientific literature related to his disease. He maintained a steady correspondence with Golde, who was sending Nathan scientific papers on his disease. In the meantime, Nathan's son Robert had done a computer search at UCLA medical library and Nathan was having it continually updated with new and additional scientific papers. As he had with his heart disease, Nathan kept detailed records of his blood tests and other tests. He made graphs and charts, trying to relate the tiniest symptom to his behavior patterns, particularly his diet and exercise routines. But no path presented itself, and Nathan confessed to Ilene that the leukemia bored him for its lack of interesting research.

Pritikin let no one know his inner concerns about his disease.

"Nathan lived in his own private world. He was incredibly detached about his disease," Ilene recalled. "He would make his observations and keep his records, but no one really knew what his inner thoughts were about his illness. When the children or I would ask him, he would always reassure us by saying that he was feeling well and that an effective treatment would be found. And we always believed him, because he always seemed to have the answers for everyone."

But Pritikin was not finding an answer. As the center became more successful and he more in demand, he devoted less and less time to finding a solution to his leukemia. Ilene would press him to spend more time investigating his disease. He would pacify her by saying he was going to do that at his first opportunity. But something always came up to claim his attention. The demands on him were quickly becoming enormous, and he gave himself over to them entirely. He was pushing in another direction, trying to convince the world that heart disease, diabetes, certain forms of cancer, arthritis, and gout could well be eliminated by adopting a more simple diet.

In the spring of 1980, his hemoglobin started to drop precipitously. It got below 9 mg.% and then fell to 7 mg.%. Golde insisted that he have his spleen removed. A splenectomy is performed to improve the blood count, which, in Nathan's case, meant increasing the number of red blood cells and hemoglobin. Pritikin resisted the operation. He didn't like the idea of losing an organ and thought he might be able to find an alternative to his falling hemoglobin. But his blood count was dropping fast and for once he had no ready answer.

In July 1980, Pritikin was admitted to UCLA Medical Center under the alias Howard Malmuth and underwent surgery to have his spleen removed. The operation proved successful: Pritikin's red cell count shot back up and his hemoglobin went back to 10 mg.%.

Once again, Pritikin kept the treatment a secret. Within weeks of the operation, he was back at the Longevity Center and was as busy as ever.

However, from 1980 onward, there would be a growing perception among those at the Longevity Center that Pritikin's schedule was becoming increasingly demanding, and perhaps getting out of control. He was trying to do too much in too short a time, they would say.

Years later, when people had the luxury of hindsight, many would look back and speculate that Nathan must have realized that within him a biological clock was ticking, always reminding him that despite his seemingly limitless energy, he did not possess limitless time.

CHAPTER **18**

A Man in Demand

*I*n October 1979, Grosset and Dunlap published *The Pritikin Program for Diet and Exercise*. The book, written with Patrick McGrady, provided a simple and straightforward discussion on the effects of diet and exercise on health. It contained more than 200 pages of recipes and menu suggestions, and a section directed to health professionals on the scientific basis of the Pritikin program. It was, in short, the perfect manual for anyone interested in the regimen. That turned out to be quite a lot of people. The book sold more than 350,000 copies in hardback and another 1.74 million in paperback. The hardcover edition would stay on the *New York Times* bestseller list for more than a year. The book would be published throughout Europe and in Australia, where it started an active and sizable Pritikin movement that included Australian Prime Minister Robert J. Hawke.

Grosset and Dunlap arranged an extensive media tour for Pritikin, which lasted through 1981 with the publication of *The Pritikin Permanent Weight-Loss Manual* (Grosset & Dunlap, 1981), which also became a bestseller.

With the publication of these two books and the subsequent media tours arranged by his publisher, Pritikin became one of the most in-demand interview subjects on both radio and television in the country. In less than a month–May 11 to June 5, 1981–Pritikin appeared on 27 television programs all across the nation, from the "Today Show" in New York to "Good Morning Houston" to "Seattle Today." In addition, he was interviewed on another 23 radio programs, and by nearly as many newspapers and magazines. On most of these days, he rushed from one studio to the next.

That year, Pritikin appeared on more than 50 television programs– many of them national shows, such as "Merv Griffin," "Mike Douglas," and

"Good Morning America"–and more than 50 radio programs.

In addition to the book tours, Pritikin was being asked by lay and medical groups to give presentations on his diet and exercise program. These became so numerous that he told Ilene that, if he wanted to, he could begin a whole new career just on the speaking circuit. In 1979 and 1980, he provided diet and health lectures to 32 medical groups alone, including talks at major hospitals and medical centers from coast to coast. He was also asked to speak to doctors at American Heart Association meetings.

In a three-month period in 1981–from September 10 to December 7– Pritikin gave 21 lectures coast to coast in such cities as San Francisco, Kansas City, Boca Raton (Florida), Santa Monica (California), San Diego, Secaucus (New Jersey), Far Rockaway (New York), New York City, New Orleans, Milwaukee, Chicago, Glendale (New York), and Long Beach (California).

In addition to all of this, Pritikin was the featured speaker for numerous dental groups and university audiences, including lectures at the University of Pennsylvania and Georgetown University.

One of the groups he particularly enjoyed speaking before was medical students, whom he lectured at Yale and UCLA medical schools. Pritikin saw this as his opportunity to influence young doctors before they became entrenched in orthodox practices; talking to medical students was a way to shape the future of medicine.

When he wasn't giving public lectures, Pritikin maintained a 12-hour day at the Longevity Center. Since he lived at the center from Monday through Friday, his days began early and ended late.

According to his secretary, Phyllis Major, who prepared a lengthy report on Pritikin's typical work routine in 1982, Nathan began his day at 6:30 each morning, when he did a four-to five-mile run along the beach. After his run, he ate breakfast. Pritikin's typical breakfast consisted of brown rice and sliced bananas. He loved rice and although his choice of grains varied, brown rice was his favorite.

Pritikin did not believe his diet was at all austere. In fact, he and Ilene had adapted so many ethnic dishes, made with a wide variety of spices, condiments, and sauces, to the Pritikin regimen that he considered his diet varied and satisfying.

Whenever he ate in restaurants, he usually chose Italian or Chinese cuisine because he could get pasta, rice, and plenty of vegetables. Pritikin was unusually demanding in a restaurant. He knew just what he wanted and how the food was to be prepared, and he didn't leave any doubt in the waiter's or waitress's mind.

"My dad was the kind of guy who had waiters hopping when he came into a restaurant," said Robert. "He would say, 'Here's what I want and here's how I'd like it prepared.' Because he was so clear about it and because people liked doing things for him, he generally got what he wanted."

When Pritikin found himself in a restaurant that offered only typical American fare, he kept the meal simple.

"One time Nathan and I went to lunch on business," recalled his attorney, Howard Parke. "We went to a local restaurant and there wasn't much on the menu he could eat, so he ordered a small dinner salad, which arrived with wilted lettuce, and he had an ear of corn with nothing on it, and I thought, 'How can he eat that?'"

Actor Lorne Greene and his wife Nancy accompanied Nathan on an airplane trip from Louisiana to Los Angeles in 1980. When the stewardess began serving lunch on the flight, "Nathan took out a small brown paper bag from his briefcase," recalled Greene. "He took out a couple of slices of whole wheat bread, added some lettuce and a sliced tomato from the salad on his tray, and made himself a sandwich. I thought, 'Yes, that's probably the way to do it.'"

Though he stuck to his diet rigidly, Pritikin did have a powerful appetite.

"Sometimes Nathan would get these irrational food cravings," recalled Phyllis Major. "He would eat a whole loaf of bread or a whole package of rice cakes or several bananas. He would suddenly get this enormous appetite that had to be satisfied."

Nathan especially enjoyed desserts and became fond of "fruit smoothies," his version of ice cream, that he and Ilene made in a food processor.

Pritikin did eat fish and on social occasions, when there was nothing else available, he would eat chicken, but otherwise he maintained a vegetarian diet that centered on whole grains, potatoes and vegetables.

After he finished eating breakfast, his day began. At 7:30 Pritikin was making long distance phone calls to the East Coast. Two mornings per week, at 8:15, he gave lectures to the patients at the center. On the other mornings, he saw patients and would continue seeing them throughout the rest of the day. Between patients, he took telephone calls. He received no less than 40 calls per day, and according to Phyllis Major, "On several occasions I tallied as many as 60 to 70 incoming/outgoing calls" in a single day.

Pritikin ate lunch at his desk and continued working. He would invariably have to move a pile of papers to clear a space for himself.

"Papers were always all over the place when Nathan was at his desk," recalled Ms. Major. "I tried to organize him but he couldn't have someone else organize his work. He had to have everything that he was working with out in piles, but he had no trouble finding anything. He relied on his memory. He didn't take notes, but he had an incredible memory; he could always remember where a particular piece of paper was in one of his piles on his desk."

Pritikin maintained a relentless pace through the course of his day. When he wasn't at work in his office or giving a lecture in one of the lecture rooms at the center, he literally ran from appointment to appointment.

Pritikin finally stopped for dinner at 7:00 P.M. Dinner would be brought up to him in his room, number 415. Each night, he would make several phone calls. He would leave notes for Phyllis Major to follow up on the following day. Three times per month, he would give evening lectures to the center participants.

In addition to all of this, Pritikin had several projects going that he kept abreast of constantly. In 1977, he started having his own bread baked according to his recipe for Longevity Center patients. By 1981, Pritikin had the Intercontinental Baking Company marketing several of his whole grain breads in supermarkets under the Pritikin name. He also had a line of soups, salad dressings, and sauces sold in supermarkets. At the same time, Pritikin had Dick Brotherton, his son Robert's college friend, working on one of Nathan's ideas for packaging Pritikin meals that would not need refrigeration and rehydration once the package was opened. The project never came to fruition, though Nathan poured more than $200,000 into the food-packaging idea.

Meanwhile, Pritikin started three new centers. In 1978, he opened another Pritikin center in Orlando, Florida (the center was eventually relocated to Hallandale, Florida), featuring the same live-in, 26-day program, with a professional staff and medical doctors. He would open a vacation program in Hawaii in 1979, which provided hotel rooms, classes in the Pritikin diet, and Pritikin meals, but no medical facilities. (The program closed in 1986.) In 1982, he started another center in Downingtown, Pennsylvania. The Downingtown program was, after Santa Monica, the largest of the Pritikin centers. It took in 45 patients per 26-day program, and like Santa Monica, it had a full professional and medical staff. Pritikin made regular monthly trips to the Downingtown center to give lectures, welcome new participants, and congratulate the graduates. The Downingtown and Florida centers would eventually offer both 26- and 13-day sessions.

Though Nathan addressed a wide variety of challenges during any one day, he especially enjoyed seeing patients.

"I think that seeing patients was the most fun for him," said Phyllis Major. "He liked to hear about a patient's progress. He had a sixth sense about what the problems were, too."

Pritikin's commitment to his work was nothing short of awesome in the eyes of his staff. Those who worked closely with him were inspired by the amount of work he took on each day.

"We really thought we were doing something special when he was at the center." said Ms. Major. "It was like being part of some very special mission."

Despite Pritikin's obviously compulsive nature, he maintained a calm exterior.

"Nathan was driven, yet he was always calm," said Ms. Major. "He never seemed frazzled or high-strung. He calmly went about his business, but with such a singular focus. He was always going straight ahead."

As an employer, Pritikin never criticized nor complimented a person for his or her work. Pritikin drove himself relentlessly, thus creating a formidable example. According to his staff, this caused those who worked for him to try to please him and even to be appreciated by him, but no outward sign of appreciation was ever forthcoming. In this sense, Pritikin was a difficult man to work for, because he rarely acknowledged the efforts others were making. Just as he could not tell people of his love for them, he was equally reticent when it came to saying thank you.

He valued loyalty in his staff above everything, however, and he gave the same in return. Whenever someone criticized a person to whom Nathan was loyal, he simply turned away or refused to believe the critic.

"Nathan couldn't bear gossip," said Phyllis Major. "In every office there's always the office politics and gossip, but every time some type of gossip came up in conversation, Nathan would make himself scarce."

Nathan and Ilene

While Pritikin's staff was galvanized by his high energy and relentless work routine, his daily life left little time for his family. Though Ilene stayed at the center during the week with him, she saw little of Nathan. Their only real time together was in scattered hours over the weekends, and their 90-minute drives to and from Santa Barbara.

In 1980, when Nathan contracted with Grosset and Dunlap to write the *Pritikin Permanent Weight-Loss Manual,* Ilene decided that the center had become too demanding. She stopped going to Santa Monica and instead remained at home in Santa Barbara, where she worked on the book with other staff members at the house. Nathan would continue to live at the center from Monday through Friday for the next three years.

The year 1980 marked a turning point in their lives. Six years had passed since they had embarked together on their adventure in health care. It was 1974 when Nathan and Ilene worked feverishly on his first talk before a medical audience. That speech, given to the International Academy of Preventive Medicine in Miami Beach, Florida, marked the first real recognition Pritikin received in his new career. From that point on, Nathan and Ilene were a team. They complemented each other: Nathan, the visionary, ever-expansive leader; Ilene, ever-grounded, steady, and devoted. Together, they worked to achieve the same daily goals, reaching toward the same larger dream.

In 1975, Nathan and Ilene celebrated his 60th birthday and the success of the Long Beach Study, the first real proof that his program worked.

Years later, Ilene recorded her memories of that 60th birthday and the gift she gave Nathan.

"To commemorate his 60th birthday, I sought expression for my deep feelings about him and my happiness in being his life partner in a new way, by trying my hand at poetry. Carried away by the spirit of creativity, I did all but make my own paper and ink, writing my lines in my best script on vellum pages embellished with my primitive illuminated decoration, then binding the pages between hard covers. A private gift, reflecting our private world."

The poem, entitled, "For Nathan, at 60," read as follows:

> The cliffs of our lives are eroding,
> Time crashes against their face
> Each grain, a sentient moment
> Freed, gently wafts to the base.
>
> No mere debris, this talus
> Our past lies embedded there
> Transmuted rock, but not mute
> These particles once were aware.
>
> Put your arms around me; gaze at our landscape
> I love our cliffs, yours and mine
> The soft slope of memories at its foot
> At its crest (for you!), a fragrant pine.
>
> That precipice that rends the sky
> I'll still dare to risk with you
> Though mountain climbers we are not
> (It's clearly "folie à deux").
>
> Later, when we've wearied some
> We'll explore the memory slope at the base
> Our private "dig"–terra unique
> We're the only "scholars" who can map the place.
>
> Eroding cliffs, a growing slope
> Vital forces complementary
> Is it presumptuous to say the same
> Of the two of us, you and me?

From 1975 to 1980, Nathan and Ilene struggled together to spread a message they both fervently believed in. What had originally been "Nathan's crazy idea about diet," as Ilene had thought back in the late 1950s, turned into their mutual mission. For Ilene, those five years were filled with struggle and happiness. They met the world and its seemingly endless challenges together. His successes were her successes; his failures her failures. There was no separating the two of them. The difficulties they had faced together had tempered them as one.

But by 1980, things had changed.

"By the time of Nathan's 65th birthday, our 'terra unique' was no longer a private landscape," wrote Ilene. "It was as peopled as a Breughel painting of a peasant fair and just as full of vitality. In those five years in which he had moved from quiet scholar to very visible reformer of the American lifestyle, it was a source of profound joy for him–as it was for me–that his impact on the health of so many was so beneficial. I prepared to commemorate his special day in the most appropriate way I could conceive. I wrote to all the people who had gone through the Pritikin Longevity Centers, suggesting to each that they send Nathan a birthday letter, telling him how their health had changed as a result of following his program. There was an avalanche of heartwarming letters in response, as I had expected. Nathan could have had no finer birthday present.

"One grateful writer put it this way: 'When one man is responsible for saving another man's life, it seems only fitting that he should know about it.' "

The two very different birthday gifts served as a metaphor for how their lives together had changed. Five years before, the gift was a private expression of love. By 1980, Ilene joined her love with that of the many who had been helped by her husband.

Nathan had been taken over by his work. And so Ilene stepped aside. She remained at home in Santa Barbara, helping him to write his books and awaiting his return each weekend. Very often, his media trips interrupted his weekends at home, but like everything else, Ilene accepted this.

Nathan kept telling Ilene that he would phase himself out of the center as soon as he could find someone to take his place. In the meantime, the two of them dreamed of buying a recreation vehicle and traveling. But each Monday, Nathan was in the car and off to Santa Monica where his work awaited him.

"Every time he went out our front door," Ilene recalled, "he belonged to the world."

AMA Launches Attack

The year 1980 started off with another volley of cannon fire between Pritikin and the scientific-medical establishment. The January 4, 1980 issue of the *Journal of the American Medical Association* (JAMA) carried a review of the *Pritikin Program for Diet and Exercise* in its "Questions and

Answers" column. The review, written by nutritionist Therese Mondeika, a registered dietitian, was prompted by a letter asking the journal its opinion of "the merits" of the Pritikin program. Ms. Mondeika used the letter as an opportunity to bitterly attack Pritikin's ideas.

After describing the program, Ms. Mondeika wrote:

> The diseases addressed by the Pritikin program are highly complex, multifactorial, and inadequately understood. In addition to diet, some of the risk factors associated with degenerative diseases are smoking, overeating, inadequate exercise, and alcohol consumption. Genetic inheritance also may play a role. The program deals with many of these risk factors and therefore may have some beneficial effect. However, claims of spectacular reversals of serious illnesses or of prevention of disease in symptom-free adherents of the program have yet to be established scientifically. Until then, the Pritikin hypothesis regarding diet and disease must be considered experimental.
>
> The book contains many erroneous statements. For example, the discussion of proteins contains a statement that unrefined, minimally processed grains, roots, vegetables, and fruits are much better sources of protein than meat, fish, eggs and milk. It is further stated that all natural food grown contains all the amino acids, "essential" and "nonessential" in sufficient quantities to satisfy human requirements. These statements conflict with scientific fact. The Pritikin diet formula is also advocated for pregnant women and burn victims. Considering the increased need for protein during pregnancy and in patients with extensive burns, following this advice would be contrary to proper nutritional care.
>
> Food additives, according to the program, should be avoided. The authors point out that some 3,500 new chemicals have found their way into our food–and "that our bodies simply aren't ready for them." White flour is not recommended because of the "dangerous chemicals used in the bleaching process." Such inaccurate statements throughout the book do not qualify it as a reliable source of nutrition information.
>
> This book, the authors state, is intended primarily for those who consider themselves healthy or who have minor problems such as mild hypertension or borderline diabetes. Persons taking prescription drugs are warned not to attempt the Pritikin program without medical supervision. One wonders, then, why the *Pritikin Program for Diet and Exercise* was published in book form and written for the layman.

The AMA then published a press release that quoted Ms. Mondeika's criticisms. The press release ran the headline (in capital letters): "DIET BOOK OFFERS UNSOUND ADVICE, AMA EXPERT SAYS." The release was turned over to the Associated Press, which in turn wired the story to newspapers all over the country. The typical headlines in newspapers from coast to coast read: "Diet Plan Claim Hit in Article"; "Nutritionist "Challenges Pritikin Diet"; "Pritikin Diet Plan Questioned."

The *Chicago Sun Times* added to the AP story by calling into question Pritikin's credentials. The story ran under the headline: "AMA Expert Assails Pritikin Diet." The JAMA article, which the story was based on, did not mention Pritikin's lack of credentials, but the *Sun Times* stuck on a paragraph at the end of the story that read: "Critics also have challenged Pritikin's credentials. Not a physician, he spent most of his life as an independent entrepreneur developing electronic gadgetry."

The *Sun Times* version of the story was picked up by other newspapers and widely circulated as well.

Pritikin responded to the JAMA article with a lengthy and well-documented reply. He addressed each of Ms. Mondeika's criticisms with the scientific evidence supporting his statements.

He wrote that Ms. Mondeika "disagrees with my claim that vegetable proteins are as good a source of protein as animal protein. Orthodox nutritional dogma based on the work of Osborne and Mendel is probably the source of her views. Their influential and standard-setting body of work was based on studies with rats whose nutritional needs differ from humans both in regard to the quality and quantity of protein requirements. Rats thrive poorly on human milk, which has one-fourth the protein of rat milk, but your babies and mine do splendidly on it.

"Much research demonstrates the adequacy of vegetable proteins as compared to animal proteins. J. Knapp and co-workers (*American Journal of Clinical Nutrition* 26:586-90, 1973) show that infants from 5-14 months old suffering from diarrhea and admitted to a hospital in Corpus Christi, Texas, fared better on vegetables and grains than on [cow's] milk in their post-recovery period. Not only were there no growth rate or nitrogen retention differences among the babies, but the percentage of urea excretion was lower in the vegetable protein group."

Pritikin went on to list four more studies, two published in the *Journal of Clinical Nutrition*, another done at Purdue University and yet another done at Duke University, all showing superior protein metabolism in humans on vegetable diets as opposed to animal protein.

He commented that high levels of protein on a diet rich in animal foods increases the body's loss of calcium and causes osteoporosis. "Eskimos eat 25 percent total calories in protein, mostly in animal protein, and consume up to 2,500 mg./day of calcium," Pritikin wrote. "They have even more osteoporosis and breast cancer than do American women, whose rates of these diseases are among the highest in the world. . . . Bantu women have almost no osteoporosis or breast cancer, yet the 10,000,000 Bantus in South Africa live on a 12 percent protein diet, primarily vegetable protein, with only 350 mg./day of calcium. Bantu women bear an average of nine children and breastfeed up to two years. My dietary guidelines parallel the Bantu diet, nutritionally. . . . "

Pritikin also noted that animal protein sources are rich in fat and cholesterol, which lead to illness and thus make them less than ideal in comparison to vegetable sources.

As for JAMA's criticism of Pritikin's concern about additives, Nathan wrote: "The remaining 'erroneous statements' attributed to my book by your reviewer have to do with concern I expressed over a food supply adulterated with some 3,500 chemicals and with chlorine-bleached flour and with my stated preference for unadulterated food and stone ground whole-wheat flour. Does the AMA really prefer the former? I find that hard to believe!"

Pritikin concluded his letter by saying that the "AMA has done a disservice to its readers and the American people with its reckless and indiscriminate attack on the *Pritikin Program for Diet and Exercise.*" But, he said, the physicians who were familiar with the diet would "not be misled."

JAMA refused to print Pritikin's rebuttal.

Pritikin received a number of letters from doctors who were outraged by the JAMA review. One doctor, from Anchorage, Alaska–who mailed Pritikin his reply to the JAMA article–wrote to Ms. Mondeika, saying: "I hope I am over my 'rage' at your article in January 4, 1980 issue of the Journal." The physician recounted his frustrations with medicine when he had to treat both his parents for heart disease with drugs, only to find that his parents got progressively worse. At a loss, the physician bought a copy of *Live Longer Now.* In his letter, he stated:

> I found it to be equally as good if not better than most of the books we used in medical school as regards these adult-onset degenerative diseases. At least it had a logical reason for the onset and propagation of the diseases. I began going to the medical library to look up the references to read, Xerox, and study to be sure that Mr. Pritikin wasn't just dreaming up some wild ideas.
>
> I contacted Mr. Pritikin and he sent me some reports on work that had been done at the newly begun "Longevity Center."
>
> In May of 1976, after much difficulty, I persuaded my father, an old dyed-in-the-wool pill-pushing physician, that he was going to take mother to Nathan Pritikin's Longevity Center for a month. She was "off her rocker" [the physician's mother had had two heart attacks and had suffered from apparent senility], had angina, and arthritis. Most of the time she didn't know my brothers or me, where she was, or you name it, she didn't know. In retrospect I am not certain how much of this was iatrogenic [caused by medical treatment] due to her husband but if it was it was because he was trying to keep up with her complaints of hip, shoulder, and chest pain using the "shotgun" theory of therapy. That plus what other doctors were prescribing. . . .
>
> One month later mother was home and back among the living at age 74. She wasn't 'hitting on all eight' but she was hitting on seven and when she

went she was hitting on less than one or two. A remarkable change for the better, and she was off the heart medication. No chest pain, virtually no arthritis, and mentally very acceptable. The only problem was how to stay on the food program. We have done moderately well over the last four years, but it would have helped if one could have walked into a restaurant and said "Give me your Pritikin special" and known that the amount of fats and oils were at a minimum. . . .

The physician then went on to explain to Ms. Mondeika the scientific basis of the program. The doctor concluded his letter by saying:

Medical doctors can't think or discuss nutrition because they aren't taught that and dietitians/nutritionists can't discuss disease because they aren't taught that, and both are taught that the relationship between the two, nutrition and disease, is only casual and "forget it." Shake yourself loose from the Ivory Tower, do a little more reasoning, do a little research, do a little studying, keep an open mind, and let us see if we can't bring both camps together in a meaningful relationship. . . . Nathan is probably the best educated man in both disciplines of anybody in this country or the world. He is the Einstein of the medicine-nutrition field and I think he deserves recognition for that and I think he deserves a lot of it as well as the wholehearted support of the medical community. . . .

Interestingly, six months later, the American Dietetic Association (ADA) published a position paper on diets based solely on vegetable foods and stated that "The American Dietetic Association recognizes that most of mankind for much of human history has subsisted on near-vegetarian diets. The vast majority of the population of the world today continues to eat vegetarian or semi-vegetarian diets for economic, ecologic, philosophical, religious, cultural, or other reasons."

The ADA reported that "well-planned vegetarian diets are consistent with good nutritional status. . . . Furthermore, a total plant dietary can be made adequate by careful planning, giving proper attention to specific nutrients. . . ."

Pritikin was not advocating a total vegetarian diet–though he had long pointed out that much of the world subsists very well on such a diet–since he permitted the use of small portions of fish, poultry, and other low-fat animal foods.

The JAMA attack on Pritikin did little to slow him down, however.

No matter what the opposition, Pritikin believed implicitly that it was just a matter of time before most Americans would eat a Pritikin-like diet. In February 1980, he testified as an expert witness on health before the Senate Subcommittee on Health and Scientific Research, and told the senators, "I am certain, in five years' time in this country, 50 percent of the people in this country are going to be on a large aspect of this diet."

It was that kind of confidence that propelled Pritikin into his most ambitious–and certainly his most audacious–project as a health promoter. In January 1980, Nathan launched a campaign to convert the town of Natchitoches, Louisiana, to the Pritikin program.

A Good Idea Goes Bad

Located on the Cane River, just 70 miles south of Shreveport, Natchitoches (pronounced Nackitash) is one of the state's oldest towns, having been settled in 1714 by the French and Spanish. Its many 19th-century houses and cobblestone streets reflect not only the town's charm but also its strong ties with the Old South.

Louisiana Governor Edwin Edwards had been convinced by a close friend that the Pritikin program could wipe out most cardiovascular disease and adult-onset diabetes if it was adopted by a large population. Edwards became excited about the idea of applying Pritikin's program on a large scale and chose Natchitoches as a test site for "Project Life," as Pritikin's experiment came to be called, because of the exceptionally high mortality rate from heart disease and stroke among its 19,000 citizens.

The goal was to reduce the mortality rates from heart disease and stroke by 10 percent in one year. Ruston, Louisiana, about 70 miles northeast of Natchitoches, was designated as the "control" group, since it was about the same size as Natchitoches. Ruston residents would receive no information about diet and health and would therefore serve as a comparison population.

The governor provided $40,000 in public funds; Pritikin contributed another $15,000. He then hired local sociologist C. B. "Lum" Ellis, Ph.D., and his wife, Donna Ellis, Ph.D., to educate the town in the Pritikin diet and exercise program. Lum Ellis organized a group of volunteers who, with Longevity Center nutritionist Christine Newport, provided cooking classes, public lectures, and radio and television shows. A local bakery agreed to provide Pritikin bread–baked according to Nathan's specifications–and store owners stocked up on Pritikin staples, including grains and nonfat dairy products.

No one thought it was going to be easy. Natchitoches was famous for its meat pie–made with a deep-fried crust and lots of fatty beef and gravy. The specialties that were favorites among the local citizens were fricassees, crawfish, fried chicken and fried chicken steaks, cajun specialties, and shrimp jambalaya. Not exactly in the Pritikin line.

Nathan's diet of whole grains, vegetables, fruit, and low-fat animal products seemed as foreign to these people as Tokyo. But Pritikin thought he could win over the good people of Natchitoches with five promises that could be realized by anyone who faithfully followed the Pritikin program.

The big five, as Lum Ellis liked to call them, were: longevity, better sex, clearer thinking, feeling better each day, and saving money (between $1,500 and $2,000 annually, according to the Longevity Center).

"If those five things won't fly, nothing will," said Ellis.

Pritikin also developed a point system to provide incentive: eliminating eggs was worth 9 points, avoiding butter and margarine was worth 4 points, eliminating cream was worth 3 points, and so on. The people of Natchitoches were asked to score a total of 90 to 100 points to graduate to good health.

The study began on January 21, 1980, a day the governor named "Nathan Pritikin Day" in the state of Louisiana. It was kicked off with a gala banquet at Northwestern State University in Natchitoches, where volunteer chefs provided local citizens and various dignitaries–including the governor himself–with what was meant to be a Pritikin feast. The banquet turned out to be the first of a series of disasters.

The meal started off with a broccoli bisque, which, to everyone's horror, was scorched. Nathan, Ilene, Governor Edwards, and Lum and Donna Ellis all sat together at the same table. After she began eating the soup, Donna Ellis turned to her husband and whispered, aghast, "The soup is scorched, Lum!" She then looked over at Ilene and Nathan, both of whom were having trouble getting the soup down. Soon Nathan stood up and announced that the soup had been burned and that people should not eat it.

Later on, someone said the soup tasted like "boiled cigarettes," a quote that was picked up by the wire services and reported around the country, and from there, it was all downhill.

Governor Edwards–in an obvious attempt to play it safe before the voters of Natchitoches–was now backing off his wholehearted endorsement of Pritikin and later told the press that, "I think I'd just as soon die ten years earlier as eat that stuff–but it is a noble experiment." That quote was also widely reported.

Lum Ellis was an affable and well-liked man around town. He had grown up in nearby Jonesboro, Louisiana, and became a Baptist minister in town before he moved to Natchitoches and became the president of the Natchitoches Chamber of Commerce. He eventually taught sociology at Northwestern State University in Natchitoches, and remained an active and popular member of the community.

Ellis was an enthusiastic spokesperson for the Pritikin program. He spoke with real inspiration about the benefits of the program, including the ones he had experienced: he had lost 25 pounds and had seen his cholesterol level drop from 250 mg.% to 170 mg.%. He felt like a new man, he said, and, judging by the way he looked, people believed him. But convincing others to change was another matter.

"We approached the problem of changing people's diet from the point of view that human behavior is learned," Lum Ellis recalled years later. "If you grow up liking steak, you can learn to like other things." But getting the people of Natchitoches to go through that learning process wasn't easy.

"We were up against four things," Ellis said, "The first one was culture, which was a big battle. Eating is a social kind of experience and fatty foods are ingrained as part of the Louisiana culture. These people grew up eating this diet; it is the diet of their parents. And their parents before them." Lum Ellis explained that trying to change the way some of the local people were eating was like trying to make them go against their own heritage.

The second problem the Pritikin program faced was the opposition from the food industry, namely, the beef, egg, and dairy industries. The local and national cattlemen's associations were so infuriated by Pritikin's study that they sponsored association meetings in Natchitoches and hired a medical doctor from an out-of-state university to come into town and expound the virtues of cholesterol and fat-rich foods. Pritikin suggested a debate between the cattlemen's doctor and either himself or a physician familiar with the Pritikin program, but the cattlemen's doctor refused.

The food industry proponents didn't stop there, however. They attacked Ellis and Pritikin viciously in the press and in local talks sponsored by the group.

"You'd have thought I was a communist," said Ellis, after personally being attacked by spokesmen for the cattlemen. The food industry also got local politicians involved in the battle against Pritikin, denouncing the whole program as a public relations tool.

The third big problem facing Pritikin and Ellis came from local doctors. "There are more ignorant doctors than the law allows," Ellis recalled. Local physicians argued in favor of the local diet and pronounced Pritikin's program a fraud.

"The real problem was that anybody who is not a physician who talks about health and wellness is getting on their [the doctors'] turf and they don't like it," said Ellis. "There are a lot of doctors who especially don't like it when you talk about prevention because all they're interested in is prescribing drugs and using a knife."

The fourth major problem the program faced was the sizable amount of illiteracy and poverty present in Natchitoches. "For the people who can't read, a recipe doesn't mean a thing," said Lum. "Unfortunately, the poor have the highest morbidity and mortality rates from these diseases, but it's very hard to change these people because they're very attached to their fried chicken."

"The poor people would come in and say, 'I'll do anything to get rid of my high blood pressure, but don't make me give up my fried chicken,'" Donna Ellis said. "But it was the fried chicken and all the other fatty foods that were killing them."

Pritikin made Natchitoches famous for the study. All three major television networks reported Pritikin's project. Television and radio shows from all over the country came to Natchitoches to do reports. "Canada's version of the 'Tonight Show' flew me up there to be interviewed," recalled Lum Ellis. In addition, the major newspapers and magazines–including *Time* and *Newsweek*–did articles on the program. Despite the opposition and some early setbacks, Pritikin was still full of confidence, telling *Newsweek* in March, "We're going to demonstrate that any population in the country can change its diet and improve its health."

But such was not to be. The Associated Press circulated a story that was printed across the country that quoted a local store owner as saying, "If I got to eat something that chokes me, I'd just as soon stay fat." The Rockford, Illinois *Register Star* ran the story with the headline, "Fried Chicken Wins over Pritikin Diet."

Many of the press reports characterized Nathan as a "California nutritionist," or "guru," out to make a fast buck on the publicity, even though the publicity was overwhelmingly negative. Calvin Trillin satirized the project in *The New Yorker.* Wrote Trillin: "Except for the fact that he has been caught wearing a necktie, Nathan Pritikin, who claims that he can reverse cardiovascular disease through diet and exercise, has most of the characteristics common to the sort of self-ordained Southern California health savants who sometimes manage to energize in me an otherwise dormant affection for the American Medical Association. . . ."

Countered Lum Ellis: "Nathan was the most unpretentious, unpromoting person I ever saw."

Still, to newspaper and magazine writers eager to fit Pritikin and his project into a formula article–either humorous or critical–Nathan became the "California guru" using unfounded claims to foist an unpleasant diet on the innocent folks of Natchitoches. Any good that he might have been doing was lost under deadline.

But in the last analysis, Pritikin had brought the whole problem down on himself. He had vastly underestimated the difficulties of changing the eating habits of a regional population, especially those so vastly different from his own. Once again, his poor judgment regarding human behavior– and especially the emotional aspects of long-standing dietary patterns– had gotten him into trouble. Natchitoches was not Santa Barbara or Los Angeles or New York or Chicago. It possessed none of the cosmopolitan attitudes nor tastes of a big city. Its culinary tradition went back to the eighteenth century. That tradition was reinforced not just by time but by family ties.

By the end of 1980, when it was apparent that the "noble experiment" was not going to effect a 10 percent reduction of cardiovascular disease deaths, Governor Edwards lamented that Pritikin would have found it easier to convert people "in other parts of the country where the food is no good anyway."

There was a silver lining in the dark cloud, however. A test group of 15 people who were followed closely by physicians throughout the study recorded remarkable improvements in health. On the average, the group lost 17.8 pounds, experienced a decrease in blood cholesterol of 23.4 percent, saw diastolic blood pressure drop 8.4 millimeters of mercury (mmHg) and systolic pressure fall by 28 mmHg, and experienced a decrease in serum triglycerides of 77.5 mg.%.

In addition, Northwestern State University did a followup study and found that 34 percent of those surveyed in Natchitoches had increased their exercise habits as a result of the program. The survey also found that 32 percent had changed their diets to include fewer fat- and cholesterol-rich foods.

"I got a lot of people exercising," Pritikin would say later in a humorous acknowledgement of his failure to achieve his loftier goals.

"I think we had a serious impact," said Lum Ellis. "The people of Natchitoches became more nutritionally conscious and now the daily media is supporting that consciousness. It's being reported every day that diet affects health. But back when we started the project, it was entirely new to people. The problem was that Nathan was three decades ahead of everyone else."

CHAPTER 19

Nathan— and Others— Sound Off

From 1980 onward, Pritikin continued to be in high demand for television and radio interviews. This was a rather remarkable phenomenon because Pritikin often was terrible on television. He occasionally came across as angry and, at times, so aggressive that he bordered on being offensive. Sometimes he crossed that border. In 1981, Pritikin appeared on a popular New York television show and attacked a leading diet proponent by saying his diet was killing people. That statement landed him a multi-million-dollar lawsuit. (The suit eventually was settled out of court.)

On March 27, 1984, Pritikin and Mount Sinai's Virgil Brown appeared together on Ted Koppel's "Nightline." Pritikin was so intellectually aloof that he threatened to turn a national program into an esoteric medical debate. After listening to Pritikin talk for a few minutes, Koppel warned that the discussion threatened to go over the heads of his audience.

Pritikin felt badly about his performance on "Nightline" and admitted as much to Wilma Keller after he returned to Santa Monica.

"He was kind of sheepish when he first came up to me and said, 'I didn't do so well, did I?' Then he made a joke and we both laughed."

While Pritikin gained many supporters for his direct way of speaking, those who were close to him were wary of the effects of his sharp tongue.

"We were continually trying to get my father to moderate his attacks," recalled his son Ken. "We tried to get him to understand that his attacks were not always having a beneficial influence and that sometimes they were backfiring, but in the beginning he couldn't bring himself to keep from criticizing institutions which he saw as contributing to the spread of disease."

Lorne Greene tried to help Pritikin improve his performance on television by coaching him on his presentation and his breathing. But the task proved to be impossible. After working with Nathan for about an hour one day, Greene walked dejectedly out of Pritikin's office, throwing his pencil into the air in a gesture of surrender. As he passed by Wilma Keller's desk, he muttered that Pritikin was "hopeless."

"Nathan was too busy," recalled Greene. "Someone from Washington or from Timbuktu would be calling. The phone constantly was ringing. He had no time to improve his style."

The fact that Pritikin was well aware that he was being abrasive in many of his television interviews led some people to believe that his approach was calculated to gain the greatest amount of publicity for his cause.

"Had my dad gone along and made moderate statements, his message would never have gotten the kind of publicity he wanted it to have," said his son Robert. "In many ways, my dad's approach was brilliant promotion."

Despite the threat of lawsuits or personal criticism, Pritikin did not hesitate to launch another salvo in the press at the next opportunity. And sometimes he went right for the jugular. "I'm more and more convinced that the National Institutes of Health is the marketing arm of the pharmaceutical industry. NIH knows full well what diet can do," he stated.

The substance of Pritikin's criticisms were as follows:

● That millions of dollars were being spent on unnecessary research. In the case of the National Heart, Lung and Blood Institute (NHLBI), which was being funded by the U.S. government, millions of dollars in taxpayers' money was being wasted.

● That NHLBI was not doing anything to alert the public to the hazards of the American diet. He believed that calling for more research before alerting the public to the dangers of the American diet was almost criminal.

● That the dietary recommendations by the American Heart Association (AHA) and other scientific groups didn't go far enough, and therefore would be ineffective in the prevention or treatment of heart disease.

● That rendering diet therapy ineffective, drugs and surgery remained the preeminent means of treatment for heart disease and other degenerative illnesses. These approaches were not the ideal methods of treatment, however, since they had severe side effects. Sometimes, these side effects were fatal.

Despite his polemics, Pritikin clearly served an important function. The scientific establishment had proven entirely unable to police itself, he claimed, especially in its failure to make consistent and clear statements on diet's relationship to health. From 1977, when *Dietary Goals* was first published, to the middle '80s, the public statements made by scientists were often very confusing and sometimes even irresponsible.

Government Report, Study Discredited

In May 1980, the Food and Nutrition Board of the National Academy of Sciences published a report stating that fat and cholesterol did not pose a health threat and that people need not restrict consumption of foods rich in fat and cholesterol to avoid disease. Dr. Alfred E. Harper, a biochemist who chaired the Food and Nutrition Board, told the *New York Times* that the board "wanted to allay apprehension about diet," and stated that "People should not be afraid of food and what they eat."

The report contradicted virtually everything that had been known about the relationship between fat, cholesterol, and heart disease.

The scientific community at large reacted to the report as if it were a leper come home. Even Dr. Robert Levy of the NHLBI criticized the report, telling the *New York Times*, "It's true that not all the facts are in, but to recommend doing nothing in the meantime is inappropriate. The existing information indicates that Americans should hedge their bets and seek a diet lower in saturated fats and cholesterol, at least until more evidence is available."

Other scientists were less diplomatic. They pointed out that the board had heavy ties to the food industry. Two of the six members on the board were food company executives. Other members had served as paid consultants to the food industry, including the egg producers. The *New York Times* reported that Harper earned up to 10 percent of his income as a consultant to the Pillsbury Company and Kraft, Inc. Kraft, of course, is a major producer of cheese and other high-fat and -cholesterol dairy products. Dr. Robert E. Olson, who wrote the final report, was a paid consultant to the American Egg Board, which sponsored consumer information on eggs.

The National Academy of Sciences committee had no cardiologists, epidemiologists, or public health experts on it, and did not take into consideration any human population studies that link diet to heart disease.

The report was a sham.

These revelations exposed the enormous conflict within the medical and scientific communities over diet's role in the cause of degenerative disease. More damaging was the fact that the public now saw hard evidence of how industry ties seemed to influence the outcome of information that directly affected the average American's health.

Unfortunately, the controversy would continue.

In 1982, the NHLBI announced its long-awaited findings from its Multiple Risk Factor Intervention Trial. The study, known as "Mr. Fit" (MRFIT), took ten years and cost the American taxpayers $115 million. In the end, however, the huge experiment turned out to be a colossal waste of money and became a worldwide embarrassment to the vaunted American scientific establishment.

At the outset of the study, 12,866 men, ranging in age from 35 to 57, were randomly selected over a four-year period. The men were all at high risk of having a heart attack or stroke. All of the men had at least one of the three leading risk factors for heart disease: they either smoked, had high blood pressure, or had an elevated cholesterol level.

The men were divided into two groups of about 6,400 each. The first group received "special care," which consisted of counseling to stop smoking and reduce fat and cholesterol in the diet. The goal was to reduce their cholesterol level by 10 percent, a reduction so small many wondered "Why bother?" since it would clearly do little toward preventing heart disease deaths.

If the dietary advice didn't work, those with high blood pressure were given drugs to lower blood pressure. The "special care" group was encouraged to take the drugs if their blood pressures did not come under control. Unbeknownst to the scientists, the drugs would turn out to be an unexpected but major cause for concern.

The second group, composed of 6,438 men, received no special advice outside of the "usual care" received from their physicians, which could include general dietary advice to reduce weight, and drugs. The drugs were not emphasized, however, as they were in the "special care" group.

Both groups were followed for the next six years at 22 clinics across the country.

The results left scientists scratching their heads.

The study showed that there was no significant improvement of health in the "special care" group as opposed to that of the "usual care" group.

There was no significant difference between the groups with regard to deaths due to cardiovascular disease. And the total mortality from all causes was actually 1 percent higher in the "special care" group than in the "usual care" group.

In short, the NHLBI "special care" did little or nothing to lower mortality rates.

In fact, the study revealed there were more deaths among those with high blood pressure and abnormal electrocardiograms who took the antihypertensive drugs than among those who did not take the drugs. The study found that the more the drugs were emphasized, the higher the mortality rate seemed to be.

After reviewing the data, Dr. Jeremiah Stamler, chairman of the Department of Community Health and Preventive Medicine at Northwestern University in Chicago, sounded a warning about the use of drugs in the treatment of high blood pressure.

"Hypertension must be controlled," Stamler said. "It's bad news–a major risk factor in heart disease. But the lesson is to treat the patient nonpharmacologically, using lifestyle interventions. Then, if you must prescribe drugs, use as low a dose as possible."

In every way, MRFIT revealed that the so-called special treatment was an utter failure. Despite the "special care," there was little difference between the two groups in lowering blood pressure and blood cholesterol and in cigarette cessation.

For all the time, money, and careful planning put into the study, the outcome was embarrassingly simple: the best treatment medicine could provide had little positive effect on heart disease. Even worse, the study showed such treatment might also be dangerous.

The scientific community turned on itself when the study's results were announced.

The *Journal of the American Medical Association* (JAMA) editorialized that the results of the study actually backfired, contradicting many cherished medical practices. "The results fly in the face of current medical dogma and practice," JAMA stated. The journal pointed out that since nutrition had suddenly become an important subject in the lay press, many people had been changing their diets without their doctor's advice, prejudicing the results of the study, since no one could guarantee that the "special care" group would get more or better nutrition advice than the "usual care" group. In other words, the word on diet and cigarette smoking was out. As a result, the study, with its enormous costs, could no longer be well controlled.

The prestigious British medical journal *Lancet* wrote that. "One can only offer sympathy to the investigators, who have so painstakingly conducted and analysed this vast effort to so little scientific profit. The results prove nothing, and we must turn elsewhere to answer the question, Does prevention work?"

The *Medical Tribune* wrote: "But what sticks in the craw is the [fact that among people with ECG abnormalities and high blood pressure] fatal outcome from coronary heart disease was more common in the SI [special care] group than in the UC [usual care] group."

The study revealed how far behind the times the scientific establishment really was. For $115 million, NHLBI and its collaborators proved nothing, except perhaps that current drug therapy and special care by physicians was dangerous to one's health. The average person was probably better off going into a bookstore and buying a $15 best-selling diet and health book.

Heart Association Makes Bold Moves

In comparison to these fiascos, the American Heart Association looked like an angel of mercy. The AHA had a long history of telling the American public to reduce its level of fat and cholesterol to prevent heart disease and other cardiovascular illnesses. But even the AHA would not be spared the image that they were woefully behind the times.

Pritikin was a constant thorn in the side of the AHA. On television and radio shows, in newspapers and magazines, in speeches before lay and professional groups from coast to coast, Pritikin launched one broadside after another at the organization. He was often invited to speak at local AHA meetings in large cities around the country. He never missed an opportunity to tell the AHA members what he thought about their dietary recommendations.

Pritikin once summarized his feelings about the AHA's advice.

"It's like cigarette smoking," Pritikin said. "The Surgeon General doesn't recommend that people reduce smoking, he says stop smoking. Heart disease is the same way. We shouldn't be giving people a diet that will do them no good and tell them that it will make them better. We should give them a diet that will prevent disease and reverse the symptoms and let them decide if they want to follow it or not."

Not surprisingly, the AHA felt the sting of Pritikin's attacks.

During the years that Pritikin mounted a public campaign for better dietary recommendations to the general public, the AHA several times revised its dietary statements.

The AHA originally had recognized the link between diet and health in 1957, and endorsed the concept of cholesterol-lowering diets in 1961. In 1973, the AHA recommended that Americans reduce their consumption of fat from 45 percent to 35 percent of total calories. People were urged to eat no more than 300 mg. of cholesterol per day, and to increase their consumption of naturally occurring complex carbohydrates from fruits, vegetables, and grains.

In 1978, the AHA lowered its recommendation on fat, stating that fat should make up no more than 30 to 35 percent of the total calories in the diet. The organization held fast to its recommendation that no more than 300 mg. of cholesterol be eaten per day.

In 1984, the AHA changed its dietary recommendations once again, this time offering "a progressive approach," or a three-step, phased program that gradually reduced fat intake from 35 percent of calories to 30 percent and finally to 20 percent. Carbohydrates were to be increased in the same way, from 45 percent to 50 percent and then finally to 55 to 60 percent. Cholesterol was to be reduced from 300 mg. to 250 to 200 mg. and then to 100 mg. per day. In short, the AHA's ideal diet had 60 percent of its calories from complex carbohydrates and 20 percent from fat, with only 100 mg. of cholesterol per day. In other words, the AHA diet was getting progressively closer to Pritikin's. Nathan had been saying since the 1960s that the ideal diet should be composed of 80 percent complex carbohydrates, 10 percent fat, and 100 mg. of cholesterol per day.

In 1986, the AHA got even closer to Pritikin, again recommending a phased-in program that lowered fat still further and recommended more complex carbohydrates. In one of the great ironies in the battle between Pritikin and the scientific establishment, the AHA used one of Nathan's published studies as support for its recommendations.

By the early 1980s it was clear that Pritikin had captured the high ground and it was just a matter of time before the scientific community was forced to acknowledge the essential soundness of his program.

CHAPTER 20

Big Hopes, Little Time

*I*n the summer of 1983, when he was 68 years old, Pritikin realized that his cancer was beginning to reassert itself. It happened slowly and at first almost imperceptibly. He normally ran about five miles each day, sometimes more when he had the time, but by autumn he started to fatigue after three miles and had trouble going beyond that distance. Instead of filling him with energy, running was making him increasingly tired during the day.

Nathan consulted his physician, Dr. David Golde at UCLA, who performed another series of tests. These tests revealed that Pritikin had two separate malignancies. Golde diagnosed him as having hairy cell leukemia and what he termed a non-Hodgkin's lymphoma, or a malignancy of the lymph system. The malignancy in the lymph system was characterized by the presence of macroglobulins (abnormally large protein molecules) that were beginning to proliferate, thus crowding out the other cells. Meanwhile, the white cell count in his blood was also increasing. His hemoglobin at the time was remaining steady at around ten grams, about four grams below normal.

The year before, Golde had recommended Nathan see a second physician, Dr. Ken Foon, of the National Cancer Institute in Washington, D.C. Foon specialized in biological therapies for cancer, such as the use of antibodies and interferon. One of his particular interests was the development of highly specialized antibodies for patients with leukemias and lymphomas.

Ever since he met Nathan in 1982, Foon had been attempting to create antibodies for Nathan's illness. Nathan met with Foon periodically throughout 1983 and 1984 to check on Foon's progress.

Upon meeting Nathan, Foon was immediately impressed by Pritikin's medical knowledge.

"Nathan was the type of person that one would have to describe as a zealot," Foon wrote in 1985. "Whatever he did, he did fully, thoroughly, and with an enormous energy. His interest in his disease led him to explore every possible avenue." Foon stated that Nathan was "so bright and well-read" that Foon could discuss the science of leukemia with Nathan as if he were talking to another expert.

In 1983, however, Foon was a long way from perfecting the antibodies he wanted to use to treat Nathan.

Golde urged Nathan to begin taking the experimental drug interferon to treat his disease. Interferon had been shown to increase the red blood cell count and bring the red and white cells into balance in patients with hairy cell leukemia. But Pritikin was undecided. The literature seemed weak to him, and he wanted to know more.

He had stopped the chemotherapy agent chlorambucil in 1979, and had his spleen removed in 1980, but he had avoided any treatment since then. He didn't like taking drugs of any kind and wasn't in a hurry to begin a new therapy now. Golde continued to supply Nathan with all the available information about interferon while Pritikin considered his options.

Meanwhile, other symptoms began to surface. By November, the cancer started to block his lymph system, causing his lymph nodes to swell. The swelling, which became acute in the groin area, would cause the lymph nodes to become as large as two inches in diameter. It also caused his ankles to swell, especially after standing for any length of time. At night, he would lie down and elevate his feet, which somewhat reduced the swelling and the discomfort. By December, the swelling had become so great that he had to give up running.

Those who worked closely with Nathan began to ask him why he had stopped running.

"Oh, running is a thing of the past, now," he would reply, almost wistfully. But Ilene and the children knew how much he loved to run, and, in the words of his son Robert, Nathan's inability to run "was eating him up inside."

He kept his pain a secret. He shared his inner world with no one, not even his family. Whenever Ilene or one of his children would come to him with their concerns about his health, he would calmly assure them that all was well and that he had things under control.

Years later, his daughter Janet wrote of her father's behavior each time she told him of her concerns for his health.

"My father's way was to remain low-key, unflustered," recalled Janet. "His calm, reassuring words would placate our fears and bolster our hopes.

"There were times, however, when my aggravation with his behavior became very strong. Occasionally his attitude smacked of a kind of denial of the seriousness of his situation, and I was afraid that his taking the matter too lightly could ultimately hurt him. But then, this tendency of his was inextricably tied to his eternal optimism. This optimism was no façade; it was real. Mostly I saw it as a good thing, because it gave him the strength and serenity to forge ahead, often under terrible odds. And needless to say, it was always nice to hear that rose-colored report from him about whatever we asked, even if it didn't come true."

Nathan had been keeping his own detailed blood records between 1976 and 1980, but then he abruptly stopped, apparently losing interest in keeping track of his disease after the 1980 splenectomy improved his blood count. There are no more charts or graphs among his files, no more of his meticulous note-taking on his body signs. However, he continued to have regular blood tests, which in 1983 showed that his hemoglobin hovered at borderline. Despite the low hemoglobin, Pritikin felt his condition had improved since the splenectomy. But there was more to it than that.

The scientific studies on leukemia that he had been so diligently keeping track of were not leading anywhere. As Pritikin's son Robert indicated, the scientific evidence linking diet to heart disease was far more advanced when Nathan began to study the illness–even in the early 1940s–than the study of leukemia. There was something altogether logical about the process of atherosclerosis. Leukemia, on the other hand, was more peculiar and unpredictable. None of the leukemia studies seemed to suggest a possible solution and too many studies contradicted one another. Pritikin continued to read the research that Golde sent him. He had his brother Albert doing library work for him, too, but between 1980 and the fall of 1983, Nathan was clearly placing his emphasis elsewhere.

No one knows whether Pritikin had already decided that his days were numbered at this point, but his secretary, Phyllis Major, clearly saw a change come over him in 1983. Pritikin began taking on more work that year; he seemed to let go of anything personal in his life. He was not a social person to begin with, but he possessed a lightness of spirit that gave him an amiable, approachable air.

But by summer, Phyllis became aware of an altogether new intensity and seriousness about Pritikin.

"There was a quality of 'too muchness' about him," she recalled. "He was trying to do too much. He took on too much during the day. He was reaching out too broadly. There was a sense that time was running out, though nobody knew why he was behaving this way. He also seemed to be teaching everyone automatically."

At home, he tried to play down the dangers. He told Ilene and the children that if things suddenly got bad, he would begin the interferon treatments, which, even if they didn't effect a cure, would slow the disease process long enough for him to come up with another therapy.

His family believed that he could come up with a cure for his leukemia while at the same time devoting prodigious amounts of energy and time to his other projects–a testimony to what they thought of him.

"Nathan had had the answers for so many people that we just believed that, with the best medical assistance, he would come up with another answer for his own disease," recalled Ilene.

Said Janet: "Dad had been like a cat who always landed feet-first after a fall. Things could get very tense and it could be a close call, but somehow he would find a way to pull a rabbit out of a hat at the most critical times. This kind of larger-than-life thinking was an affliction we all suffered from to a degree in relation to my father."

To Thousands, "a Hero"

By 1983, Pritikin had achieved nothing less than hero status in the minds of those who knew him well, worked with him, or came to him seeking a recovery from illness.

Indeed, Pritikin was often referred to in the press–including *Time* and *Newsweek*–as a "guru" to the thousands of people who followed his program. The word could not have been more appropriate. He was the focus of so many people's psychological projections that, as the years went by, he increasingly was regarded in spiritual or mystical terms.

"Nathan had an ability that is referred to in the East as 'one-pointedness,'" recalled Phyllis Major. "What that means is an ability to focus entirely on a single object so that all other distractions are eliminated. One almost becomes one with the object that one is concentrating on. You couldn't help but be impressed with his ability to focus. While everything else was falling apart around him, he was utterly calm, because he was concentrating on the thing that was right in front of him."

"Nathan never talked about religious or spiritual matters," recalled legal advisor and former patient Stan Keller. "But because he was so giving, people at the center would always see him in spiritual terms. One time a rabbi from New York City came to the center and, after watching Nathan, the rabbi said that he wanted to make Nathan an honorary rabbi. And in his unassuming way, Nathan said, 'If it makes you happy, be my guest.' And so he did. We had a big ceremony at the center that was translated from the Hebrew and Nathan was made an honorary rabbi. And after that he went back to work."

In 1983, Keller arranged a meeting between Nathan and the famed Indian guru Muktanada, who had encouraged one of his disciples to seek Pritikin's help in overcoming a recent heart attack. Nathan, Keller, Muktanada, and a couple of Muktanada's disciples met at the guru's ashram in Los Angeles. Pritikin and Muktanada sat opposite one another on pillows. The two talked about diet and health.

At one point Muktanada stated that while diet and exercise were helpful, there was also "karma" that had to be taken into account.

"What's karma?" Nathan asked.

Muktanada pointed to Keller and said: "Ask your friend on the floor." Keller told Nathan that karma meant that "When it's your time to go, you go." To which Pritikin responded, only half in jest, "Oh, no–you get on my diet, you'll live forever!"

Everyone laughed.

Muktanada assured Nathan he was eating a diet very similar to Pritikin's. After they had talked a while longer, they parted, but not before Muktanada hugged Nathan and told him, "Mr. Pritikin, you and I are on the same path."

Because he had improved or restored the health of literally thousands of people, he was often revered as a miracle worker.

Muktuk Marston, a retired Army officer and explorer who organized military expeditions of Alaskan Eskimos during World War II, came to the center after suffering a heart attack at the age of 87. He needed cardiac shock treatments and a long list of drugs to keep his heart pumping. Marston, who had lived a remarkably adventurous life, was not the type of man who could accept dependency of any kind. Large, gruff, and imposing, Marston was used to living life on his own terms. But after suffering the heart attack, he couldn't walk more than 100 feet without gasping for breath and having to rest. He'd rather die than be bedridden and dependent upon drugs, he said. His wife insisted that they come to the Longevity Center, and Marston agreed.

On the day he arrived, Marston met a man who had a gangrenous foot and who had been ordered by his physicians to have his leg amputated. Two days before the operation was to be performed, the man chose to come to the Longevity Center instead. Over the next month, Marston watched as the gangrenous foot gradually became well. Meanwhile, Marston was astonished by his own improvement. He was walking greater distances each day and rapidly regaining his health. By the time the 26-day session was over, Marston was walking more than a mile a day and the man with the gangrenous foot was completely healed.

"His foot was as clean as a baby's foot," Marston said. "That's a miracle. I don't care what you say about it. This program is doing the same damn thing that that great man [Christ] was doing 2,000 years ago. This man Nathan is doing the same thing right here, now, curing people who had given up."

For his part, Pritikin never talked about the respect he was accorded by those who came to the center and those who worked for him, but on several occasions he confided to Ilene that he had come to understand how religious movements got started, that is, by a charismatic figure with a revolutionary idea.

Pritikin never lacked for young protégés. He drew great satisfaction from teaching young people, especially young doctors and scientists. In fact, he had an incalculable impact on the careers of hundreds of young doctors, including his nephew, Dr. Stephen Kaye. Many of the young physicians he influenced never met Nathan, but heard him lecture or followed his work. However, dozens of others sought Pritikin out and studied his program firsthand. Dr. John A. McDougall, author of the *The McDougall Plan* and *McDougall Medicine,* derived his inspiration to go into the study of nutrition from Pritikin. Dr. Stephen Inkeles became board-certified in nutrition and internal medicine after he read Pritikin's book *Live Longer Now.* Inkeles eventually came to work at the Longevity Center and was one of the physicians Pritikin pointed to as an example of the doctor of the future, using diet and exercise as therapy against some of the most dread diseases.

Pritikin introduced a new kind of medicine that was based almost entirely on nutrition and exercise, and many young physicians, concerned about the side effects of drugs and looking for ways to prevent disease, jumped on the bandwagon as if it were an answer to a long-awaited prayer.

In the late fall of 1983, Nathan stopped going to the center each week. He worked out of his study at his home in Santa Barbara, where several of the bedrooms in the house had been converted into offices for those who worked for him there.

That year, Nathan had placed the center in the hands of his son Robert and its chief administrator, Kevin Wiser. Under the new arrangement, Nathan was still close enough to keep a hand in things and he visited the center several times per month to give lectures, talk to patients, and congratulate the graduates.

What occupied most of Pritikin's time was the Pritikin Research Foundation. Nathan had a staff of five people going full-time in his home, working with him on his books, research, and myriad other projects. Among the people working for him were Nan Bronfen, a nutritionist and writer; Nell Taylor, Nathan's secretary and librarian; and Nathan's brother Albert. Nathan also had Dr. Miles Robinson working on position papers, doing research in the medical literature, and writing sections of his books. Robinson, who moved to Santa Barbara after becoming interested in Nathan's work, was a former Washington-based physician and medical consultant on the staff of U.S. Senators Paul Douglas of Illinois and Edward Long of Missouri.

Meanwhile, Nathan continued his remarkably active schedule of public lectures, and television, radio, and print interviews. He also worked feverishly on a series of projects, including his new book, *Diet for Runners*.

Special Advice for Runners

As one who loved running himself, Pritikin maintained a long-standing interest in the sport, particularly endurance running. He drew his example from the Tarahumara Indians of central Mexico and other native peoples who were capable of running incredible distances (the Tarahumara men are able to run 100 miles without stopping). Pritikin maintained that the best diet for runners is one low in fat, cholesterol, protein, and simple sugars. The ideal diet, he said, is made up primarily of complex carbohydrates–from whole grains, vegetables, and fruits–which provide long-term energy and endurance. In short, the Pritikin diet. Such a regimen, which is supplemented by small quantities of low-fat animal products, is rich in vital nutrients and low in fat.

Pritikin was the first to sound the alarm to runners who eat too much fat or diets deliberately rich in protein. In *The Pritikin Promise*, Nathan warned runners that vigorous exercise coupled with a high-fat diet could lead to heart attack and death. He cited the case of Goodloe Byron, 49-year-old U.S. Congressman from Maryland who had run six Boston Marathons. Byron had been warned by his physician that despite his apparent good health, he had failed a stress treadmill test and had a cholesterol level of 305 mg.%–dangerously high. Byron ignored the doctor's warnings and on October 12, 1978, he died of heart disease. The pathologist doing the autopsy on Byron stated that the atherosclerosis in the coronary arteries was "extensive and diffuse" and that Byron clearly had died from the illness.

Pritikin went on to warn that high-fat and high-protein diets are extremely dangerous to athletes. Excess protein gives rise to high levels of ammonia in the bloodstream. Ammonia molecules, which are highly toxic, join to form urea, which can cause gout and damage the kidneys. Since large quantities of water are necessary to rid the body of urea, high-protein diets also result in dehydration, Pritikin said. Athletes, particularly, must be concerned about dehydration because any reduction in the water content of the body throws off the cooling system, thus increasing the risk of heatstroke.

High-fat diets and atherosclerosis are the underlying cause of ventricular fibrillation, a kind of heart attack that results when the heart is unevenly oxygenated and then placed under stress during exercise. The uneven oxygen flow changes the electrical currents in the heart and results in uncoordinated beating. As the heart muscle is exercised during running, more blood and oxygen are required and, as a result, the uncoordinated beating becomes more pronounced. Ventricular fibrillation is often the result and is very often fatal. Ventricular fibrillation, Pritikin said, is the number one cause of runners' death.

After *The Pritikin Promise* was published, Pritikin got a call from Jim Fixx, famed runner and author of *The Complete Book of Running* (Random House, 1977). Fixx complained bitterly to Pritikin, telling him he was scaring people away from running. He said that Pritikin's chapter on running, which was entitled "Run and Die on the American Diet," was hysterical in its tone and would surely frighten a lot of runners.

"That's my intention," Pritikin replied. He told Fixx that anyone who eats the American diet and runs is foolishly taking his life in his hands.

Pritikin told Fixx: "Too many men have already died because they believed that anyone who could run a marathon in under four hours and who was a nonsmoker had absolute immunity from having a heart attack."

Pritikin's views never carried much weight with Jim Fixx, despite the fact that Fixx used Pritikin as a resource for his second bestseller, *Jim Fixx's Second Book of Running* (Random House, 1980). Still Fixx remained personally unconvinced of Pritikin's ideas.

In 1984, Jim Fixx died of a massive heart attack. His cholesterol level at the time of his death was 253 mg.%, a level heart specialists say is eight times more likely to cause a heart attack than a cholesterol level at 160 mg.% or below.

Nathan argued that misconceptions had caused many athletes to fail to appreciate the advantages of a high-carbohydrate, low-fat diet. He maintained that complex carbohydrates provide the greatest endurance of any food since they are long-burning sources of energy, unlike simple sugars, proteins, or fats. Moreover, complex carbohydrates burn cleanly, leaving behind only water and carbon dioxide as by-products, both of which are easily eliminated by the body.

As usual, Nathan looked to nature to confirm science and his own ideas. As he put it in his book *Diet for Runners:* "Carbohydrates provide greater endurance for other species as well. Carnivorous animals can run with great speed but their endurance is minimal. Cats, for instance, have the ability to run faster than almost any other animal. The caracal lynx and the cheetah have been clocked at up to 65 miles per hour, but only for short distances. Cats are renowned for the inordinate amount of time they spend sleeping. However, herbivores, which make up the bulk of the animal kingdom, have far greater endurance. Giraffes and racehorses can not only run 45 miles per hour, but can sustain this speed for long periods of time."

Pritikin concludes this passage with his characteristic humor: "The endurance of man and pig, two of the few omnivorous animals, lies midway between that of the meat- and the plant-eaters."

Pritikin was never satisfied simply writing about his subjects or showing them to be scientifically true. He had to prove his ideas in real life. So in 1982, he sponsored a group of athletes who would compete in what has been called the most grueling of all competitive sports, the Hawaii Ironman Triathlon.

The triathlon requires that each athlete compete in a 2.4-mile ocean swim, a 112-mile bicycle race, and a 26.2-mile marathon run, each event taking place right after the other. Pritikin had a special kitchen set up in Hawaii six weeks before the event for his triathletes, including previous champions Dave Scott, Scott Tinley, and Scott Molina.

On October 9, 1982, the day of the event, the temperature was almost unbearable, reaching 115 degrees Fahrenheit on the blacktop of the streets. Nathan was very excited about his athletes' chances to do well. He believed fervently that under the most adverse conditions they would have the edge, since their bodies would have the most enduring fuel. And he was right.

Dave Scott placed first in the 1982 Triathlon, with a record-setting time of 9:08:23; Scott Tinley placed second, at 9:28:28; and Scott Molina placed fourth, with a time of 9:40:23. On the same high-carbohydrate, low-fat diet, Scott finished first again in 1983, with Tinley second. Scott finished first again in 1984, shattering his own course record with a new time of 8:54:20. Tinley again finished second.

"Nathan was overjoyed with the performance of the triathletes on his diet," recalled Ilene. "He wanted people to know that this was not just a diet for sick people, but for everyone, even high-performance athletes."

The idea of the high-carbohydrate, low-fat diet caught like wildfire among many top athletes. Tennis champions Martina Navratilova, Chris Evert Lloyd, and Ivan Lendl are just a few of the star athletes who excelled on diets based on whole grains, fresh vegetables, and fruits.

Pritikin Program Hospitalized

That fall Pritikin was also working feverishly on his new Pritikin Hospital Plan, which opened in November 1983 at Metropolitan Hospital in Springfield, Pennsylvania. The hospital provided an eight-day intensive Pritikin program of diet and exercise for inpatient care. The program addressed the same disorders as the other Pritikin centers, providing the same general diet and exercise program, but did it over a shorter period of time. In addition, all other patients at the hospital had the choice of eating Pritikin meals instead of the standard hospital fare.

While all of these projects were important to Nathan, their significance paled in comparison to his loftiest aim, which was his plan to conduct a study showing that atherosclerosis could be reversed by lowering blood cholesterol.

A year before, Nathan and Robert were sitting in the study talking about heart disease when Robert mentioned casually that it was too bad doctors couldn't take cholesterol out of the blood in the same way that dialysis can replace the kidney function and remove waste products from the blood.

The idea struck Nathan like lightning. While he firmly believed that diet alone could cause cholesterol to drop sufficiently to produce reversal of atherosclerosis, he grasped at the possibility that reversal could be expedited by filtering cholesterol out of the blood. Pritikin was already aware of a technology based upon plasmapheresis, the separation of plasma, the pale yellow fluid portion of whole blood from the cellular blood constituents, which was being used to separate blood constituents, such as immunoglobulins. Nathan wondered if this same technology–or a more efficient kind which would not require separating out the plasma– could be applied to test his most far-reaching hypothesis: that by lowering cholesterol sufficiently, atherosclerosis could be reversed. While he could also do this with diet alone, or diet and lipid-lowering drugs, he was excited by the technology because it could lower cholesterol levels so rapidly, and therefore could produce results in a much shorter period of time. Patients could have their cholesterol levels lowered dramatically in an hour; reversal of atherosclerosis–which might otherwise take eighteen months or longer–could be accomplished in less than a year.

Pritikin's idea was to place a group of patients with extremely high cholesterol levels on the Pritikin diet to keep their cholesterol levels from rising. They would simultaneously undergo regular blood-filtering treatments to remove LDL cholesterol for a year–long enough, he believed, to demonstrate reversal of plaques by angiogram. Once he showed that atherosclerosis could be reversed by lowering blood cholesterol, he would have provided the "final proof" that the underlying cause of heart disease could be eliminated. The method could also prove lifesaving for the occasional intractable cases where people with dangerously high cholesterol levels were not responding fast enough to diet alone.

The technology that made all of this possible–called LDL-apheresis, or selective removal of low-density-lipoproteins from the blood–was still in its infancy when Nathan became interested in it. Pritikin studied the work of the early researchers who were Canadian, German, and Japanese. He also telephoned, met, and corresponded with several of them. Eventually, he decided to continue working on and improving the existing technology. Meanwhile, he developed his own approach, in which the LDL-cholesterol would be filtered from the blood without separating out the plasma. To facilitate his efforts, he entered into an agreement with an American firm, Cobe Laboratories, and embarked on a joint development program with them. He also enlisted his son, Robert, and Dick Brotherton to work under his technical guidance on his experimental projects.

While developmental work was proceeding, Pritikin went to Rush Presbyterian Hospital in Chicago to work out details for a major study in which LDL-apheresis would be used to reverse atherosclerosis. The study never got off the ground at Rush, but Evanston Hospital, an affiliate of Northwestern University, called Pritikin and expressed interest in doing the study.

In the fall of 1983, Nathan met Dr. Peter Dau, a physician and expert in plasmapheresis at Evanston Hospital in Chicago. Over the next three months, the two worked out an extensive protocol. They then submitted it to the Food and Drug Administration for approval. It would take months before the protocol was even considered.

Nathan Scores a Personal Victory

In January 1984, Nathan got good news from an unexpected quarter. The National Heart, Lung and Blood Institute (NHLBI) announced the findings from its ten year Lipid Research Clinics Coronary Primary Prevention Trial (LRC). The study, which cost the American taxpayers $150 million, provided "final proof" that lowering blood cholesterol reduced the risk of heart attack and deaths due to heart disease.

The study was conducted over a ten-year period and involved 3,806 men between the ages of 35 and 59, all of whom had cholesterol levels of 265 mg.% or higher.

The men were divided into two groups. One group received dietary instruction meant to slightly lower cholesterol level, plus a placebo. The second, or experimental group, received the same dietary instruction and a drug called cholestyramine. Neither group knew whether they were receiving the drug or the placebo.

The drug plus the small changes in diet reduced the men's cholesterol levels by 19 percent to 28 percent, depending on how diligently the men took the drug. Many had to reduce the quantities of the drug because of its severe side effects.

After ten years of research, the study's results showed that the diet-and-drug group had fewer heart attacks and deaths due to heart disease than the diet-and-placebo group had. The study showed that a 1 percent reduction in blood cholesterol resulted in a 2 percent reduction in the risk of heart disease. That meant that if a person reduced his cholesterol level by 25 percent, his chances of having heart disease were cut in half.

For Pritikin, the LRC study was vindication. Nathan always had maintained that the scientific evidence outlined a simple equation: a high-fat, high-cholesterol diet raises blood cholesterol level, which causes heart disease. The opposite was also true: a diet low in fat and cholesterol results in a lower incidence of heart disease. Pritikin had seen this simple relationship between cholesterol level and degenerative disease for more than 30 years, but here, finally, was the so-called smoking gun.

"I'm glad the National Institutes of Health has finally realized that cholesterol has something to do with heart disease," he said later. "The only thing that's unfortunate is that it took them $150 million to discover it."

But Pritikin was not going to overlook the side effects of the drug, especially when diet was just as effective at lowering cholesterol level as drugs, but had no side effects.

When the study was reported in the *Journal of the American Medical Association* on January 20, 1984, the scientists noted, "Very early in the follow-up period, the number of CHD events [heart attacks, angina attacks, and other related incidences of coronary heart disease] was higher in the cholestyramine group, but by two years the two curves [between the drug and placebo groups] were identical."

The scientists further reported that "in the first year, 68 percent of the cholestyramine group experienced at least one GI [gastrointestinal] side effect, compared with 43 percent of the placebo group. These diminished in frequency so that by the seventh year, approximately equal percentages of cholestyramine and placebo participants . . . were so affected."

The kinds of side effects from the drug that the scientists were referring to were constipation and heartburn, belching or bloating, gas, nausea, a greater number of "operations or procedures involving the nervous system," a greater incidence of gallstones and gallbladder disease, a greater incidence of respiratory illnesses, and finally, "various GI tract cancers were somewhat more prevalent in the cholestryamine group."

Said Pritikin after reading the study: "The drug has so many side effects that you're not going to get many people to stay with that approach. In the first year, 68 percent of the drug group had severe abdominal pains; 39 percent had constipation; 27 percent had heartburn; 16 percent suffered from regular nausea. The drug group experienced 50 percent more ulcers than the placebo group; 140 percent more gastritis [inflammation of the stomach lining]; 175 percent more ulcers; 100 percent more gallstones; 300 percent more pancreas disease."

In fact, the scientists mentioned darkly that cholestyramine has been found to be a promoter of colon cancer in animal studies. The researchers suggested that further study should be done on the drug.

Pritikin pointed out that the reason the side effects dropped off after the first two years of the study was because the men couldn't tolerate the prescribed dosages of the drug and began to reduce the dosages on their own. The scientists noted that as well. In fact, 27 percent of the men taking the drug dropped out of the study.

Pritikin maintained that the diet used in the study was essentially the American Heart Association (AHA) diet. Since that diet could reduce the cholesterol level only 4 percent, it was essentially an ineffective treatment, thus guaranteeing reliance upon the drug for serious reduction of cholesterol.

"Since 1961, the American Heart Association diet has uniformly failed in having an effect on human heart disease," said Pritikin.

But what really riled Pritikin was the inference that cholestyramine was the preferred method of treatment , and that people with cholesterol levels of 265 mg.% or higher should go on drug treatment to reduce their risk of disease.

"The principal recommendation by the National Institutes of Health was this: That anyone in this country with a cholesterol level of 265 [mg.%]– and that's up to four million people–should immediately go on the drug on a daily basis for the rest of their lives.

"To recommend that kind of program for four million people is criminal."

Pritikin was familiar with cholestyramine, and had even recommended its use in the past for short periods of time for a handful of patients whose cholesterol levels were exceedingly high and could not be lowered sufficiently with diet. But to make a blanket assertion that the drug be widely pre-scribed was, for him, dangerous advice.

In a sense, Nathan was having it both ways: He had claimed a per-sonal victory on the basis of the raw data, but he also pointed to the scientific community's dependence upon drugs when diet could be more effective, and without the side effects. He was still pushing for the scientific establishment's complete acknowledgement that diet was the method of choice for most people in the treatment of heart disease.

Indeed, even Dr. Claude Lenfant, who took over for Dr. Robert Levy as director of the NHLBI, acknowledged that the new data suggested that many coronary bypass operations no longer were necessary.

Said Lenfant: "While underscoring the benefit of such surgery for many, the findings suggested that the medical management would be just as effective in about 25,000 cases during the next year that otherwise would result in bypass operations."

Though Pritikin continued to keep a lash to the back of the scientific establishment, he realized that this study had vindicated him. He was able to lower the average person's cholesterol level by 25 percent in four weeks' time–almost twice what the LRC scientists managed to do–without the use of drugs. Moreover, the long-standing criticism that he had not proven he was reversing atherosclerosis was suddenly full of holes. Pritikin was preventing heart disease and heart attacks. By the NHLBI's own standard, he was cutting the average Longevity Center participant's chances of having a heart attack in half in less than a month!

After the study results were in, Pritikin contacted the Mount Sinai Medical School and proposed that the school co-sponsor a medical conference with his Pritikin Research Foundation. Mount Sinai agreed. The medical school appointed Dr. Virgil Brown, chairman of the AHA's Nutrition Committee, to be the forum's director. All papers and speakers would be approved beforehand by him to ensure their medical veracity, a standard practice with such conferences. There was, however, one nonstandard request: that Nathan not use the conference to promote the Longevity Center, which was regarded as a business and therefore a partisan interest. He agreed. The conference was set for April 27.

In the eyes of the scientific establishment, Pritikin had arrived.

CHAPTER 21

Respect and Acceptance from the Medical World

By 1984, the work Nathan Pritikin had begun more than 30 years before was almost in full bloom. The LRC Study and the acceptance by Mount Sinai Medical School to co-sponsor a medical conference with him scientific evidence had convincingly demonstrated the basic soundness of his approach, and high-ranking scientists in the nation were acknowledging him as the leading exponent of the low-fat, low-cholesterol diet in the treatment of degenerative disease. As far as Pritikin was concerned, however, his greatest achievement lay just ahead. He wanted to prove that lowering blood cholesterol caused reversal of atherosclerosis. That proof was very much in sight with his cholesterol-lowering study at Northwestern University's Evanston Hospital, Pritikin believed.

All he needed was time. But time was becoming an increasingly questionable commodity. The lymph swelling and edema were getting worse. By March of 1984, he could no longer stand for more than 20 to 30 minutes without suffering extensive swelling in his lower legs and ankles. He wondered how much longer he could go on before he would have to begin treatment once again.

By the time the Mount Sinai conference arrived, nothing could dampen his spirits. He arrived in New York City on April 25, ready to take full advantage of the fact that some of the most powerful doctors and scientists in the country would be listening to him speak.

The one-day conference was to be held on April 27. On April 26, Pritikin hosted a preconference dinner for 35 conference participants. The menu included mushroom-barley soup, tossed salad, choice of dressings, chicken teriyaki with sauce, steamed snow peas, brown rice, fresh pineapple, and dinner rolls. For dessert he provided a "Pritikin carrot cake"–one of

Nathan's favorites–and Postum (coffee substitute) or chamomile tea. The meal was catered by the Longevity Center in Downingtown, Pennsylvania, and was an enormous hit. Those who ate the dinner realized that the Pritikin diet was not so ascetic after all.

The following day, Nathan gave his speech. The 400 doctors, scientists, and other health professionals who came to listen to his talk expected him to discuss the risk factors of adult-onset diabetes. That was the talk he submitted to Dr. Virgil Brown for approval, but Nathan had no interest in repeating basically the same speech he had given before countless audiences already. He began by relating the story of what Finland had done to correct the incredibly high heart disease rate among its citizens.

"The worst epidemic of deaths in the world from ordinary foods has been in east Finland," Pritikin began. "They have the highest cholesterol intake in this world, because they live on dairy foods. In fact, the ones who have the highest death rate are the lumberjacks in their thirties. Lean and strong, they eat 5,000 calories a day of cheese and eggs. As a result, the diet in east Finland makes that area number one in the world in heart disease deaths. Young men dying of cholesterol-clogged arteries were leaving widows, many with young children. Because of this enormous hardship, the widows in the North Karelia region petitioned the government to do something about the tremendous epidemic.

"The government decided to do something about it. They secured 28-year-old Dr. Pekka Puska, just out of school, and they said, 'Dr. Puska, here is a $150,000 budget. Go do something for the 180,000 people in North Karelia.' Do you know how far $150,000 goes in this country for health care? Our budget for heart disease in this country is $700 million a year–$150,000 is petty cash for postage. Dr. Puska had no preconceived notions and, not being taught anything about nutrition in school, said, 'Well, I'll go to the medical literature and learn what I can.' He concluded that excess cholesterol and fat seemed to be responsible for heart disease. And so he decided to follow that idea. He got the public health authorities in North Karelia to advocate the cutting down of fat and cholesterol. He decided to try to convince the people to stop eating so many eggs; he recommended low-fat instead of whole milk. He even took the lard out of their favorite sauna sausages and put mushrooms in instead. Now that was a sacrifice!

"In just five or six years, North Karelia, which had had the number one death rate from heart disease in east Finland, became number five in heart disease deaths. Dr. Puska was then about 33 or 34 years old, and he accomplished in Finland what our $700-million-a-year budget has not accomplished in this country simply because he took the available knowledge and applied it."

Pritikin then launched his attack on the American Heart Association (AHA) and its recommendations on fat and cholesterol.

"In 1956, Dr. Norman Jolliffe, Director of Public Health in New York City, decided to try the polyunsaturated fat approach [the kind of fats advocated by the AHA] and devised the Anti-Coronary Diet. He started with a 30 percent fat diet and about 300 milligrams of cholesterol [per day], which is the same as the American Heart Association 1984 recommendations. He personally closely adhered to it. Dr. Jolliffe died of a massive heart attack in 1960. Unfortunately, he died of moderation."

Pritikin outlined the results of the (MRFIT) and LRC studies, which showed the inability of the American Heart Association diet to lower cholesterol. The recommendation coming out of those studies was that if the diet did not lower cholesterol sufficiently, drugs should be used.

Such a recommendation, Pritikin said, would put many more millions of Americans on drugs in addition to the millions who are already on them.

For those with high blood pressure alone, the numbers are staggering. "Accordingly, 60 million people pay $30 billion a year for drugs. That's nothing compared to the side effects. On these drugs, for example, men after two years lose their sexual potency, but that's no problem. Planned Parenthood is thrilled about that. The Pritikin diet can get 85 percent of drug-taking hypertensives back to normal, off all drugs, in three weeks."

When he was finished with the AHA, he directed his attack to the American Diabetes Association (ADA). Pritikin pointed out that the ADA had just recently started a large campaign to diagnose and treat the existing ten million adult-onset, or type II, diabetics in the United States. Their method of treatment, however, is a diet that "has been used over a period of 20 or more years, and it does not get them off their medications. . . . "

The ADA booklet "tells physicians if they cannot lower blood sugar enough on the American Diabetes Association diet, then they must put the patients on drugs. They recommend the oral drugs for the whole ten million if they can't get their blood glucose down enough by the American Diabetes Association diet, a diet that has already failed. Would you like to know who is financing the total $4 million cost of this education program? It is Upjohn Pharmaceutical Company, the world's largest maker of oral hypoglycemic drugs for diabetics. . . .

"We [the Pritikin Longevity Center] report getting two out of four [adult-onset diabetics] off insulin in three weeks, and 90 percent of those on oral medications giving up their drugs. . . .

"I am a little bit upset, obviously, because I see three principal diseases all being directed towards drug therapy. Yet, scientific evidence is clear that the simple Pritikin dietary program, published in the medical literature, can eliminate the need for drugs in the high-cholesterol group, in the hypertension group, and in the diabetic group. . . . "

Pritikin concluded forcefully:

"I think it's ironic that the health agencies responsible for protecting our health are, in effect, destroying our health and shortening our lives. A million and a half people are dying each year prematurely because their food supply is poisoned with excess fat and cholesterol. Fifteen million people have suffered and died prematurely in the last ten years because vital dietary information has been withheld. We intend to correct that tragedy."

After Nathan finished his talk, Brown acknowledged the importance of Pritikin's criticisms of the AHA and the scientific establishment.

"I think it is very important for people such as Pritikin to hold us to task and say here is the ideal over here," said Brown.

Two years later, Brown would praise Nathan for his "total dedication" in "raising the awareness that the composition of diet plays an exceedingly important role in the etiology and treatment of heart disease." Brown stated that Pritikin's "influence was clearly felt throughout the world." As for Nathan's criticisms, Brown wrote that "I believe that by expressing this view, he furthered the goals of the AHA by helping to counter the opinion of those who wish to do nothing."

On April 28, the night after the conference, Nathan hosted a banquet at which Senator George McGovern talked about the enormous strides made in less than a decade in educating the public on the relationship between diet and health. "That's true," said McGovern, "to a considerable extent because of the tenacity and courage of Nathan Pritikin. . . . " McGovern stated that Pritikin was "preaching the truest gospel of good nutrition and the basis for a long and healthy life."

He told the packed banquet hall that "While he is small in physical stature, in my judgment Nathan Pritikin is a towering giant in intelligence, in imagination, and in courage."

A month later, Brown, Dr. William E. Connor of the Oregon Health Sciences University, and Pritikin were asked to write articles for the *New York Times* on the relationship between diet and health. Their articles ran side by side under the common banner: "Three Experts Discuss Cholesterol."

Still One Goal Short

Pritikin was now regarded as among an elite group of researchers in the country. Ilene recalled how "delighted" Nathan was with the kind of recognition he was getting. But none of the attention put him off his loftiest goal: proving reversal of atherosclerosis.

After the Food and Drug Administration gave its approval to use the proposed LDL-apheresis experiment to reverse atherosclerosis, Pritikin began pushing plasmapheresis expert Dr. Peter Dau hard to get the study under way. There were numerous holdups, however.

Dau had trouble getting patients to volunteer for the study. Patients had to undergo angiograms before and after the study to see if there was any reversal of plaque in the coronary arteries.

There were serious questions over how many plasmapheresis treatments each patient would receive per week. It was finally decided to give each patient one treatment weekly, though Nathan at first thought that two would be necessary to keep the cholesterol level sufficiently low. Finally, there were endless problems of getting the various hospital departments–cardiology, hematology, labs, and others–to work in a coordinated manner for the study. All of the study subjects were to follow the Pritikin diet as well, so Nathan had to teach the program to staff members and cooks at the hospital.

Nathan pushed through each of these problems with his typical determination.

"Nathan was a real driver," said Dau. "He would not take no for an answer."

In fact, the extent to which Pritikin was pushing himself caused Dau to watch in amazement.

"When I first started working with him, I just stood back and said, 'Wow, this is a motivated guy,'" said Dau.

"Nathan had a mania about heart disease. He was willing to pay the price in terms of commitment and energy to see that a cure was found for heart disease. Six hundred and sixty thousand people die of heart attacks each year, so the scope of the problem is enormous when you think about it. He would call up and say, 'Oh, you didn't have that done yesterday?' or 'Peter, if we have that piece of information now, why can't we begin today?' His temperament was always matter-of-fact. His attitude was that if this was given top priority, heart disease would be eliminated."

As much as he was driving himself, he was also trying to motivate the doctors and scientists who were participating in the study.

"He was leading us doctors down the road to regression. He was so well versed with the literature that he was not just competent with doctors, he was leaping past them. The reason Nathan was able to do all of this–and to lecture doctors on health–was simple: he was a genius. There's no other way to put it. He knew more than most doctors and that was convincing."

There seemed to be no end to the obstacles facing him and the study, however, and Dau finally projected that they wouldn't get their first patient started until the fall of 1984.

Nathan originally had planned that he and Ilene would live for several months at Evanston Hospital to oversee the study and the dietary program to ensure that it was carried out according to his specifications. He told Dau on numerous occasions that he planned to "move out to Evanston and set up shop." But as his illness got worse, it soon became impossible for him to spend more than a few days away from Santa Barbara. Pritikin needed time to rest and to study his disease if he was going to find a way out of his deepening problem.

In fact, after the Mount Sinai conference, Pritikin wanted to slow down. His body was demanding it, and–just as important–he was mentally weary of his relentless pace. He was looking for more peace in his life. He had been promising Ilene for years that he would slow down and that the two of them would spend more time together. As a result, he was regularly turning down invitations to speak publicly. Often, he would announce proudly to Ilene that he had just turned down another invitation to lecture. Nathan wanted Ilene to know that he was finally keeping his promise. On a little card that noted his upcoming talk at Louisiana State University (LSU), which was scheduled for September 21, he had written the words, "Swan Song." As far as he was concerned, the LSU presentation was to be his last.

Cutting back on his schedule was easier said than done, however. His commitments were enormous and no matter how much he tried to get free time, there was a whole machinery at work–particularly the Santa Monica and Downingtown centers–that was demanding his presence.

Terry Graves, who ran the Downingtown Center in 1984, remembers Nathan's attempts to reduce his workload.

"That whole year [1984] he would always call me up before he was scheduled to come out and try and get out of it," she recalled. "And I would always talk him back into it. . . . And then the Santa Monica Center would call him up and say, 'You're carrying Downingtown. Why aren't you here as much as you are there?' So it would force a double commitment for him."

No one outside his immediate family knew at the time that Pritikin was sick, but soon his son Robert began to step in and tell people his father just wasn't available.

But even Robert couldn't keep his father from maintaining a demanding work and travel schedule. Pritikin saw many of his commitments as personal promises to friends, people to whom he was loyal and could not let down. This was particularly true of Terry Graves, of whom Nathan was very fond. By September, he was still going monthly to Downingtown to talk to the center participants and local media people. That month, Ms. Graves had set up a demanding schedule of patient consultations and a television interview for him.

"I didn't know he was sick, but I knew he was looking worse and worse.

He used to wear a brown jacket a lot, but as he got more pale he didn't look good in it, so I told him not to wear it," she recalled. "When he arrived at the airport [in Pennsylvania that month] the first thing he did was stand there in his dark slacks and nice soft tweed jacket and say, 'Is this okay?' He looked so comical saying that, that I just stood there and applauded him."

Pritikin had turned 69 on August 29, and that September Terry Graves had planned a surprise party for him at the Downingtown Center. The party was to take place after he had seen patients and done a TV show.

"He was very pale when we were doing the TV show and they had to use a lot of makeup on him," she recalled. "He was also losing his voice consistently. He was putting in 12 to 14 hours a day working, but he became very insistent about the time he needed to sleep. He would always tell me he needed eight hours sleep, and if something didn't fit with eight hours sleep, he wouldn't do it. Before, he would stretch himself, but now he wouldn't."

The night he had completed his work at Downingtown, he sat in his room at the center reading. His son Ken was with him at the Downingtown center. Terry Graves and Ken had conspired to bring Nathan downstairs for a surprise party that evening. Nathan was wearing running clothes– even though he hadn't run in more than nine months–and Terry kept on sending word up to Ken to have Nathan change his clothes before he came downstairs. After he had been asked several times to change, he finally told Ken, "Tell Terry I can eat dinner in the clothes I am wearing." A few minutes later, he was escorted downstairs and as he walked into the large dining room of the center, a band struck up "Hail to the Chief" and about 100 people yelled "Surprise!" and "Happy Birthday!" Terry Graves was standing at his side applauding him. Nathan–holding back the tears– turned to her and said, "I should have changed my clothes."

A Battle for Life

In October, Pritikin's hemoglobin had fallen to a low 8.5 grams. He was now in desperate straits and had to concentrate on his disease. Dr. David Golde, his physician, had been pressing him to begin interferon treatments. The interferon had been successful in raising the red blood cell count for some patients with hairy cell leukemia. By this time, Pritikin was in a corner. With a hemoglobin of 8.5 and falling, he needed to do something immediately. Robert, Jack, Ken, Janet, and Ken's fiancée, Trisha Thompson, all were pressed into service to do library research for Nathan.

Desperate for a solution and believing that the interferon was harmless at worst and potentially life-sustaining at best, he agreed to begin the treatments. Nathan would administer the therapy by injecting himself with the dosages of interferon three times per week–Sunday, Wednesday, and Friday–over a ten-week period. The first treatment was scheduled for November 1, his and Ilene's 37th wedding anniversary, but the scheduled starting date had to be pushed up to October 29 because his hemoglobin was dropping so rapidly.

Despite the hopes his physicians had for the therapy, the interferon was the final straw. The drug began to destroy his red blood cells viciously and brought him to the very precipice of death.

Pritikin kept an ongoing and extensive record of his reaction to the interferon.

He took his first dose at 11:30 A.M. on October 29, and two hours later was in the throes of a raging fever. By 4:15 P.M., his normal pulse rate of 64 beats per minute had jumped to 100 beats. He suffered chills and convulsions. On October 31, he took an injection at 12:30 P.M. and by 4:00 he wrote, "sleep under max covers: 2 x comforter, robe on, and blue sweater and green blanket."

As each day of treatment passed, the symptoms only grew worse. The fevers typically got as high as 104 degrees Fahrenheit. The chills and tremors grew more violent. At night he would lie in bed with his teeth chattering, his body shaking wildly.

After taking an injection on November 4, he wrote, "Uncontrollable shaking; involuntary chills." He recorded his temperature over several hours until nearly seven hours after the dosage, it reached 104.5. By 4:45 that afternoon, he wrote: "Removed blanket, robe, and sweater about 3:30." He took Tylenol when he couldn't bear the chills any longer. He graphed his temperatures, the chills, and the dosages and the times he took the Tylenol. His body's reaction to the interferon was completely unexpected and he was trying desperately to understand it.

Worst of all, however, was the fact that his hemoglobin was dropping precipitously. On November 6, his hemoglobin had fallen to 7.4 grams, 7 grams below normal.

"He was getting very low dosages of interferon," recalled Dr. Ken Foon. "I have never seen anyone react as he did to such low dosages. His reaction was terrible."

Foon said that he knew of no scientific reason for Pritikin's "unusual reaction" to the interferon. "I would surmise that this was a man who took very good care of himself and was unusually sensitive. His body was finely tuned and you couldn't mess with that balance."

Nathan was literally incapacitated by the interferon on the days he took the drug. Ilene would screen people away from him on these days. She acted as gatekeeper now, even on the days he hadn't taken the interferon.

Terry Graves had returned to Santa Barbara that fall to work for Nathan at the Pritikin Research Foundation in his home.

"You just couldn't see Nathan on certain days," she recalled. "At first, I just accepted it, but it was unlike him to be unavailable to me. Something was up but no one knew what it was."

People assumed that Nathan was hard at work on one of his projects or that he was simply exhausted from his recent travels.

"We really didn't think it was anything more than exhaustion or a cold that Nathan was suffering from," recalled Stan Keller. "He was working so hard at the time that there was every reason to believe that he should be tired."

The family was protecting him as best they could, but he still wanted to do more than was possible. That November, he had scheduled a trip to the city of Quebec, Canada to talk to a Canadian researcher about his LDL-apheresis project. When Janet found out he was planning a long trip, she was horrified. She complained to Ilene and Nathan, but he insisted that if his blood count increased he was going.

"Dad wanted to go about business as usual, carrying on with the charade. I was angry and adamant that he not go, and in the end his poor blood count clinched the cancellation of the trip."

After Nathan's blood count fell to 7 grams in November, it never returned to normal.

One day that month, Terry Graves went into Nathan's study and saw that his skin color was unusually yellow. "I said, 'Nathan are you all right? Do you have hepatitis or something?' He just sloughed it off and went about his work."

By December 3, his blood count was at 6.5; on December 21, it was 5.6; and on December 27, it had fallen to 5.

"In December, Nathan started to talk in more urgent terms," recalled Dick Brotherton, who was working on Pritikin's LDL-apheresis design. "Whenever he'd call about the LDL-apheresis project, he'd say things like, 'We've got to hurry, we haven't got much time' or 'We're running out of time.'"

That month, he started to get periods of despondency, especially after experiencing a particularly bad day of side effects from the interferon.

"I remember going over to the house then," recalled Terry Graves. "And I was ushered into his bedroom, which never had happened before, and he was slumped in his chair and I could see that he was depressed. I had never seen him like that before. He didn't want to get up out of his chair. Something was wrong. Everything was halted then; he wasn't getting any phone calls; no publicity. I asked him, 'Are you all right?' And he said, 'I just had my phone unplugged so I should be all right. I could either unplug my phone or hire a psychiatrist, and I figured I'd unplug my phone because it's cheaper.'"

He was quickly losing weight. He looked gaunt and weak.

Inevitably, his spirits would bounce back. The morning news show

"Good Morning America" asked him to appear in January as part of a series on the people who had changed American life over the previous decade. And Nathan agreed to appear on the show, despite his condition and his obviously poor appearance. Ilene gently but firmly advised against it, telling him that he could not appear on television looking as he did. He agreed. Still, he valiantly tried to keep his spirits up while he coped with the brutal side effects of his disease and the treatments.

"He remained optimistic on the outside," Ilene recalled. "We all hoped the interferon would reach a turning point and bring his blood count back up, but by late December it was clear that the interferon had been just a terrible nightmare."

In December, Pritikin was diagnosed as having hemolytic anemia, a disease in which the red blood cells are destroyed by antibodies created by the person's own white blood cells. When Ilene asked him what hemolytic anemia was, his face clouded over and he said, "Oh, that's bad."

With the diagnosis of hemolytic anemia, Nathan knew that in all probability he faced a death sentence. For the next month and a half, he would resist the diagnosis, hoping against hope that he did not have hemolytic anemia.

He never told Ilene or the children what he suspected, however. It was only later that Ilene would learn his real concern about the anemia.

In December, he stopped the interferon.

On January 3, Pritikin's hemoglobin had dropped all the way to 4.5 grams and he was feeling faint and suffering dizziness.

By that time, he had already made plans to receive blood transfusions. But even that turned out to be more difficult than expected. For one thing, an adequate donor had to be found. Neither Ilene nor the children had his blood type, which was 0 positive. He did not want to resort to the UCLA blood bank because he was afraid of hepatitis and AIDS infection. Janet's husband, Steve Trent, had Nathan's blood type and was able to donate blood, but more donors would have to be found. Nathan and Ilene placed an ad in the *Los Angeles Times* and Ilene contacted the local YMCA in an effort to recruit potential donors, explaining that she was trying to help a friend.

Pritikin's leukemia made transfusions all the more difficult because the antibodies in his blood were antagonistic to the blood of several of his prospective donors. Finally, a series of appropriate donors was found. But blood transfusions were only a stopgap measure, since it was clear that his immune system was destroying his own red cells.

Golde prescribed steroids in order to slow the destruction of red blood cells, but this therapy backfired horribly as well. After Nathan took the steroids, the destruction of red blood cells became more rapid. The steroids also caused the onset of severe diabetes and very rapid weight loss.

He would need insulin now. The diabetes also caused a chronic thirst that he couldn't seem to quench.

Foon was still months away from having his antibodies ready as a therapy for Nathan's disease. Pritikin had read about another experimental therapy for leukemia, called Pentastatin, which was being used by Dr. Alexander Spiers at Albany Medical Center in Albany, New York. Pritikin had contacted Spiers in late December and made plans to go to Albany to receive the treatment under the doctor's supervision. Pritikin would not arrive in Albany until January 21. In the meantime, he continued to keep his illness a secret and tried to maintain some semblance of his schedule. (It was in connection with the Albany trip that Nathan had intended to appear on "Good Morning America," which airs from New York.)

With time running short, he pressed Peter Dau to move ahead on the atherosclerosis reversal study, but there were more delays and it would not be until later that January that the first patient would be enrolled in the study. Pritikin's own LDL-apheresis design was still in the development stages, but moving ahead under Robert's and Dick Brotherton's efforts. Brotherton went to Quebec to work with Lupien's staff and run some tests of the device. Nathan anxiously awaited word on his progress.

Meanwhile, the Longevity Center was in the midst of a new expansion effort. The center had plans to open several fitness centers around the country, the first of which was to open on January 19 in Pacific Palisades, just outside Santa Monica. The fitness centers were not live-in programs, but local health centers where people could come during the day or evening hours for exercise and advice about diet.

On that Saturday morning, January 19, Pritikin was on hand to open his new Palisades Fitness Center with a ribbon-cutting ceremony.

Nathan's voice was weak and, for many, could barely be heard. There was no microphone available and many of the 100 guests present for the ceremony couldn't hear most of what he said because it was simply inaudible.

After the ceremony, Stan Keller greeted him. The two shook hands, but Nathan didn't say a word. He just fixed Keller a look that froze in Keller's mind. "There was a look in his eye that I had never seen before," recalled Keller. "Looking back at that moment, I suppose Nathan was saying good-bye."

Wilma Keller had arranged to have a videotaped interview with Pritikin done at the center after the ceremony, but Robert stopped his father from doing it. It was obvious that Nathan was in no condition to do an interview, though Pritikin was refusing to acknowledge that.

After the ceremony, Nathan went home and prepared to go to Albany with Ilene. As Terry Graves would say later, the ribbon-cutting ceremony at the new Palisades Center was "his last hurrah."

CHAPTER 22

The Disease
He Couldn't Cure

*N*athan and Ilene left from Santa Barbara Airport for Albany on January 21, 1985. Pritikin was going to Albany because he hoped the Pentastatin would do three things: reverse the hemolytic anemia caused by the interferon, halt the muscle wasting and raging diabetes caused by the steroids, and, finally, treat the malignancy in his bloodstream.

They hoped that if the treatment in Albany was successful, Nathan could return home and continue taking the therapy on his own. He would administer it himself by injection, as he had the interferon.

Pritikin was extremely weak and could barely lift the smallest piece of luggage he and Ilene had brought with them. Ilene had to carry the larger, heavier bag. Before they left for their flight to Albany, a fellow passenger at the airport turned to his wife and made a joke about Nathan and Ilene and their incongruous burdens. Overhearing the man, Nathan started laughing as well. "Did you hear that guy?" Nathan asked Ilene. Despite his desperate straits, Nathan saw the humor in the incident, too.

When they arrived at Albany airport, a cab took them over the snow-covered streets to their roadside motel. Nathan noticed that the motel dining room was in an adjoining building some distance from the lodge. The parking lot and grounds were covered with snow and ice. When the cab driver was about to let them out, Pritikin said, "No, this won't do. Take us to the best hotel in town." He was too weak to deal with cold and the layout of the motel.

The cab driver brought them to the Albany Hilton. They signed in as Mr. and Mrs. Howard Malmuth, continuing the alias Nathan had earlier adopted. Not even Dr. Alexander Spiers knew at first that it was Nathan Pritikin he was treating. Eventually Nathan told Spiers, but asked him to keep the information private. Nathan had grown a mustache to further conceal his identity. Soon the weight loss would become so severe that his emaciated body would further hide any physical signs of the old Nathan Pritikin.

Once inside his hotel room, he resumed his meticulous recordkeeping. As the days went by, Spiers would provide him with extensive blood test records and Nathan could follow his depressed and fluctuating hemoglobin levels, as well as the reticulocyte count, which showed the rate at which new young red blood cells were being formed by his body. He recorded all his symptoms, the times they manifested, and their duration. He tried to correlate his symptoms to the life span of his red blood cells; the normal life span is 30 days. He was looking for clues, hoping for any sign that the treatment might be lengthening the life span of his red blood cells.

By the time he arrived in Albany, he had already lost 25 pounds and, since he had only 7 percent body fat to begin with, it was pure muscle mass that he was losing. The weight loss was caused largely by the steroids, but even after he stopped them he continued to waste away.

Over the next several days he underwent extensive examination and testing by Spiers at his office, which was in a wing connected to the Albany Medical Center.

He immediately began getting blood transfusions and, ironically, LDL-apheresis treatments, which were meant to remove the large protein molecules, or macroglobulins, from his bloodstream. Eventually he would receive three Pentastatin treatments as well, which also were administered by injection. .

He was getting progressively weaker and at times even faint. In one of his early meetings with Spiers, Pritikin went into the bathroom for a moment while Ilene waited for him outside in a reception room. After waiting several minutes, Ilene grew concerned and went toward the bathroom, only to find Nathan in an adjoining room lying on an examining table being looked over by Spiers and an attendant. When she talked to him, Ilene learned that Nathan had fainted in the bathroom and fallen face down on the tile floor, breaking his front tooth and splitting his lip. Spiers found that Pritikin's blood pressure was extremely low and gave him fluid intraveneously, which restored his blood pressure to normal. Spiers examined the tooth and noted that the remaining structure was still sound and that it could be capped easily. He even recommended a dentist for Nathan to see before he returned home to California.

Ilene was upset by the episode. She felt that Nathan's dangerously low blood pressure should have been recognized earlier during the office visit. In that way, he could have been protected from such falls.

"When I expressed my distress with this unnecessary added insult to all he was experiencing, he would make light of it, saying, 'Oh, it's nothing,' or 'It will help my disguise.' When I would say to him he'd have to have the tooth capped before he returned home, as it really ruined his appearance, he would indicate to me that he really wasn't vain and it didn't matter."

His deterioration was causing him increasing discomfort. The relentless thirst continued. He began drinking whole bottles of fruit juice, which was something he never did in the past. There were other problems. He complained that everything he drank, including water, tasted sickeningly sweet, which was another reaction from the diabetes. Eventually he found that the drinks didn't taste as sweet when they were cold, so he needed everything iced. His mouth was excessively dry, but none of his doctors could account for this symptom.

There were occasional breaks in the intensity of the situation, small oases of time for him and Ilene to be together and try to forget their crisis. Ilene recorded those moments in her diary months later.

"We did have a few normal meals together at the Hilton–almost our last," she wrote. "The Hilton has a beautiful intimate dining room and we had four or five dinners there. A very tall, blonde, friendly hostess would greet us evening after evening and direct us to a cozy niche.

"We felt quite the romantic couple. I would usually put on one or another of the two dresses I'd brought with me, plus the long pearls I'd taken to serve as my one piece of jewelry for the trip. Our meal was usually the poached salmon they featured, plus their good dinner salad. As they didn't have baked potatoes or an acceptable alternative, we'd usually carry down a loaf of Pritikin bread–which I'd found in a rather well-stocked health store in Albany–and Nathan would make sandwiches with the salmon.

"There was a nice-looking young man who played piano as we ate, rather ruining the music he played with his innately unmusical sense of rhythm. We moaned when lovely tunes were massacred by him, and laughed a bit, too."

After ten days at the Hilton, they moved to a one-bedroom suite at Jeremy's Inn in Albany, where Ilene could cook their meals in the small kitchen. Ilene bought some grains that she boiled on the stove, hoping to reverse the precipitous weight loss.

Albany was cold and dark that January. There was considerable snow and ice on the ground and the intensity of the winter seemed to shut them in all the more, closing them off from the brightness of the sun and the active lifestyle they had come to love in California.

Nathan's "sad, sad face replaced the animated, thoughtful, sometimes impish face I knew as my husband's," Ilene wrote later. "once, sitting in one of the two armchairs in our motel room–sitting side by side, holding hands–he looked at me and said simply: 'Look at you; you're in the prime of your life. And look at me.'"

He tried to bury himself in his charts and notes. For "light" reading, he had brought with him a medical book that he had wanted to read for some time. The book was a review of medical physiology he had purchased at the UCLA bookstore. He had also brought several other books that discussed his type of illness, which he thought might be helpful.

When he wasn't reading or resting, he was testing himself: taking his temperature, noting his symptoms, recording the blood test results Spiers had provided him. The fevers, chills, and tremors continued, though not as severely as they had during the interferon treatments.

He was getting weaker fast. He needed help to make it from their room to the cab that would take them to Spiers' office. By the time he got there, he was exhausted.

Spiers soon concluded that Pritikin in fact did not have hairy cell leukemia, but what he called a "splenetic lymphoma, macroglobulinemia, with circulating cells that looked like hairy cells but were not." In addition, Pritikin suffered from hemolytic anemia, which was destroying his red blood cells and would surely have killed him without blood transfusions.

The Pentastatin was designed for hairy cell leukemia, but after diagnosing Pritikin as having the splenetic lymphoma, Spiers consulted with the National Cancer Institute (NCI) to determine if Pentastatin would be useful in Pritikin's case. NCI scientists said that it might be helpful and Spiers administered small doses of the drug three times.

Eventually, Spiers stopped the Pentastatin and began regular dosages of another anticancer drug, called cyclophosphamide. Spiers found that Pritikin's condition made a slow improvement on the new drug. But he was battling so many other problems, most of which were side effects from the interferon, steroids, and the hemolytic anemia. The anemia caused liver and severe kidney damage–so severe, in fact that Pritikin needed kidney dialysis to survive and had to be hospitalized.

For the kidney dialysis, which he received every other day, a catheter tube was inserted into his leg. The tube caused slow bleeding in the area, leaving a large bloodstain in his bed beneath his leg. Once in the hospital, he continued to receive blood transfusions. He also received one more Pentastatin treatment.

It soon became apparent that he was being kept alive by artificial means.

Ilene valiantly tried to keep his spirits up by remaining optimistic herself. "I simply didn't permit myself to reflect on the possible seriousness of the situation," she wrote. "I lived from minute to minute like an automaton, trying to be cheerful and always optimistic. I tended to his needs cheerfully and briskly or to tasks that needed to be done, mentally preoccupying myself with reading. *The Stories of John Cheever* served me well, each story being brief but captivating. Earlier I would bring the *New York Times* into our room, but the rattling of the pages annoyed Nathan as his physical condition worsened, and he asked me to stop turning the pages. I read *The New Yorker,* too, and once read aloud to him a remarkable account of a blind boy from India, who at the age of 15 came alone to the United States to enroll at the Arkansas School for the Blind because his Indian father yearned to have the boy have a better education than available to the blind in India. His interest for a while was maintained and I was thrilled that he could for a few minutes be mentally removed from the miseries of the trap that circumstances had created for us.

"Earlier, before the noise of the pages turning bothered him too much, he would ask me to summarize for him the important news as reported in the *New York Times,* and I would do so. Even in those critical days, his interest in the state of the world burned brightly."

Pritikin refused to eat the hospital food. Instead, Ilene made him oatmeal at Jeremy's Inn and brought it to him in sufficient quantities each day. He had calculated how many calories he needed to sustain him in the hospital and what amounts he would need to eat at specific intervals. Sometimes Ilene had to feed him because he lacked the strength himself.

Each day, Nathan or Ilene would telephone the children. Usually they would call Robert or Ken, who would then relay the information on to the other children. Whenever she called, Ilene tried to put the best face on the facts, always ending with an optimistic note that Nathan would pull through.

The children wanted to come to Albany to support their father, but he refused to let them see him like this. He told Ilene that he did not want the children to come to the hospital; their presence would just distract him from studying his illness, he said. Ilene relayed Nathan's request and the children reluctantly respected his wishes. But it was clear that Pritikin was protecting his family and himself from the emotional burdens that would be created if his children were present at the hospital. He had always been the patriarch, the one who took it upon himself to find a solution to the major problems the family faced. But now he was wholly dependent upon Ilene. He could do nothing for his family or himself. His life was out of his control. This was not the way he wanted to be seen or remembered.

His body continued to waste away. By mid-February, he had lost nearly 40 pounds since he had begun the interferon more than two months before. Nothing broke his heart more than the weight loss.

"The gaunt body that confronted him in the mirror would bring him to tears," Ilene would write later. Because his case was so interesting, teams of young physicians on the hospital staff would come to his bedside and ask him to describe the history of his treatment. When he got to the part that involved the use of steroids and the consequent weight loss, he would inevitably be brought to tears.

"He compared himself to a German concentration camp victim," Ilene wrote. "And, in fact, the almost 25-pound weight loss in less than three weeks did make his already thin body look pitifully emaciated.

This was a particularly brutal punishment of his disease. The body he had studied so many years and taken such meticulous care of was being destroyed right before his eyes. He simply couldn't bear to speak about it.

Despite his weakness, he continued to work as long as he could on his notes. He was still trying to see a pattern in his illness that might lead him to a solution.

But the one fact that he could not reconcile was the hemolytic anemia. As Ilene wrote: "The almost fatal (in his mind) diagnosis of hemolytic anemia was one he fought against mentally. I think to him that was like admitting to himself: 'This is the end.' He carefully graphed his hemoglobin level, taking into account the drop to be expected as the transfused cells died off at their anticipated rate. Several times he told me that he thought he didn't have hemolytic anemia. He wanted so much to disbelieve that diagnosis."

He was not alone. Ilene, too, wanted to believe he could still find an answer. She remained sanguine, battling against the facts.

One of the doctors on the Albany Medical Center staff must have noticed that Ilene was not dealing with the perilous truth of her husband's circumstances. The doctor, who had seen Nathan earlier in the day, walked up to Ilene and told her flatly: "I think you should know that your husband's prognosis is terrible." His words shocked Ilene. She hurried to Spiers and asked him directly what he thought of Nathan's condition. Spiers equivocated, saying that Nathan's condition was guarded but that there were still lots of things that could be done.

Ilene accepted Spiers' pronouncement, but the cruel blow from the other physician brought her face to face with reality and was the first step toward preparing her for the worst. Months later, she would say that she saw a certain kindness in the doctor's crushing words, because without them she would not have been the least bit prepared for what lay ahead.

Still, the signs were there. It soon became apparent that Nathan's kidney damage was permanent and that if he did survive the immediate crisis, he would need kidney dialysis for the rest of his life.

In a soft, understated way, he started to complain about his suffering.

The fact that he understated his complaints seemed to make them all the more powerful to Ilene. He became increasingly weak and had to stop keeping his records.

No one outside his immediate family knew that Pritikin was at Albany Medical Center. When Nathan wanted to keep track of what was going on at the Longevity Center or elsewhere, he called or had Ilene call.

He had been in regular touch with Dick Brotherton to keep track of the progress of his LDL-apheresis design. Brotherton was running into snags. The delays kept him from conducting a series of important tests on the equipment that would let them know if it would work at all. On February 19, Nathan called Dick Brotherton in Quebec and asked him if he ran the experiment.

"No," Brotherton said. He told Nathan that he had run into some problems with the filtering device and that he thought he would be ready to run the experiment the following day. Brotherton noticed immediately that Pritikin's voice was extremely hoarse and almost inaudible.

"What's wrong with your voice?" Brotherton asked him.

"Oh, I've got a little laryngitis, that's all," Nathan said.

"I hope you're going to see a doctor," Brotherton said. There was a pause before Pritikin spoke again.

"Do you think it's going to work?" Pritikin asked. The question hit Brotherton like an electric prod. It was utterly unlike Pritikin to ask Brotherton if the device was going to work, since it was Pritikin who designed it and maintained such a faith in the device all the while. To Brotherton, being asked this question by Pritikin was like a general asking a foot soldier if he thought they could win the war.

"Of course it's going to work," Brotherton said, trying to reassure Nathan. "We'll make a few changes and it will work. It's just going to take some time, that's all. I'll run the experiment tomorrow and I predict we'll have good results."

Brotherton asked Nathan where he was. Pritikin said he would tell Brotherton what he was doing later. Suddenly, Ilene was on the phone and saying goodbye to Brotherton. Two days later, Pritikin's invention to remove cholesterol from whole blood worked. But he never heard the good news.

At this point, the very qualities that had propelled Nathan Pritikin to accomplish so much now conspired to bring about his end. His overwhelming need to be in control of his life was in complete conflict with his current circumstances. He could no more tolerate being kept alive by a dialysis machine and drugs than he could being chained to his bed. The life he loved–with all its freedom and activity, his daily runs and his crusade for good health–was gone.

Nathan told Ilene that he wanted to begin working on his notes again. He wanted to cut up and reassemble parts of his charts and add new data. He told Ilene he would need a razor blade or an Exacto knife to do the job. She suggested he use a scissors, but Pritikin said that scissors wouldn't work, since he would have to poke a hole in the paper in order to cut out tiny sections that were part of his charts and graphs. He told her he also would need some tape in order to paste the chart back together.

Ilene purchased a throw-away shaver with a razor blade, but when she showed it to him, he rejected it. Nathan was becoming increasingly irritable, a characteristic so unlike him that he began to upset, and even frighten, Ilene. A nurse overheard him complaining about the razor and asked what he wanted. Ilene explained. Trying to be helpful, the nurse offered Nathan a scalpel. His eyes suddenly became wide with recognition.

He took the scalpel and placed it in an inside folder of his notebook, which contained his many graphs and his notes on his symptoms and blood tests.

Apart from his periodic bouts of irritability, Pritikin's demeanor did not change very much. "He was very courageous," said Spiers. "He knew how bad things were and he never manifested fear or panic at any time." Nathan remained as pleasant as possible to those around him, which was now as much his nature as his guise. He did not want to alert anyone to a change in attitude. "No one suspected what he might do," Spiers recalled.

Nathan particularly wanted to keep Ilene in the dark and told her nothing of the plan he was working out in his mind. As always, he was taking full responsibility for what lay ahead, and once again he was in control.

Ilene slept on a cot in the hospital room. When she awoke on the morning of February 21, her spirits were immediately buoyed by the soft, warm smile that radiated from him when he looked at her. "Look at Mr. Sunshine," Ilene said when she saw him.

They spent the day as if in a warm embrace. For the first time in weeks, Nathan seemed at peace. He smiled often. Several time, tears came to his eyes when he looked at Ilene. There was a glow about him, Ilene recalled, as if he had turned a corner.

"I remember saying about his smiling, 'You're smiling so much, it's like sunshine,'" recalled Ilene. "But it was really more like a sunshower, for there were his misty eyes, too."

Late that afternoon, Nathan told Ilene that he would like to be alone between 7:00 and 8:00 P.M. to rest. Ilene should go down to the coffee shop and have some dinner, he said. At 8:00, they could begin working together on his notes. Ilene agreed, knowing how exhausted he became at the end of the day.

In the late afternoon, his manner changed. He asked the nurse to put a sign on the door telling people he did not want to be disturbed between 7:00 and 8:00 P.M. After the sign was placed there, he asked Ilene if the nurse had signed her name on the order. Ilene looked at it and said that it had not been signed. Nathan became insistent. Tell the nurse to sign it, he said.

Reluctantly, Ilene went to the nurse and said, "Will you please sign the 'Do not disturb' sign on my husband's door? He's being very difficult."

The nurse obliged with a smile. Ilene and the nurse both realized that he was not feeling well and that they should placate him. Ilene went back into his room and sat down next to him.

"Let's just sit quietly and look at that wall," he told her. There was a wall opposite Nathan's bed and he fixed his gaze on it.

There was a moment of calm now; the parade of doctors, nurses, and technicians who seemed to be ever-present had retreated from them.

"Why don't we call the children?" Ilene said, grateful for the quiet but baffled by his strange suggestion.

Nathan agreed. He had spoken to Ken earlier that day so he tried to call Jack and Janet, but neither one was home. Then he called Ralph. Nathan asked Ralph about his wife, Shelley, and their one-year-old son, Willie. Ralph assured him that everyone was well. Ralph asked him how he was doing.

"The surf is going down, Ralph," Nathan said.

"No, Dad, the surf's coming back up, it's coming up," Ralph said, trying to reassure him. Nathan did not comment and Ralph continued to try to reassure his father.

The cryptic message hung uncomfortably in Ralph's mind.

After talking to Ralph, Nathan called Robert, with whom he had spoken the previous day. Robert said he had never heard his father depressed as he had been the day before.

"I was out of it yesterday," Nathan replied.

Robert told his father that he wanted to tell key people at the Longevity Center something about his father's condition. Nathan said he should wait a little longer.

"What are you going to do if something happens to me?" Nathan asked his son.

Robert assessed the Longevity Center's current business status, which he concluded was fine, but he didn't know how the public would react if something happened to his father.

"But what about all the scientific papers we've published?" Nathan asked.

"That's the scientific community, Dad," said Robert. "We're fine there. But I don't know how the rest of the public would react to us. But you're not going to die. You're going to make it. Your doctor tells me that your kidney and liver functions are improving." A pause followed. "Dad, we really love you and we're all pulling for you," said Robert. "Don't go trying to find out if there's a heaven up there."

"I know," Nathan said. "I really appreciate that." After another pause, Nathan said, "What if someone pulls the plug?"

Haltingly, Robert said: "It'll be a whole new world without you, Dad."

"Yeah," Nathan said. "It'll be a whole new world, a whole new world."

He asked to speak to Robert's wife, Christine, but she wasn't home at the time, so he asked Robert to say hello for him. With that, the conversation ended.

At 7:00 P.M., Nathan reminded Ilene that it was time for her to go to the coffee shop. He told her that he was tired, but that he would be ready to start working at 8:00.

Ilene's spirits were lifted by his attitude during the day. His renewed interest in studying his illness seemed to signal a return of his will to live. Before Ilene left, Pritikin insisted that she place his notebook on the table that straddled his bed directly in front of him. Ilene resisted. She saw no reason why he should need the notebook on his table now. He became firm and insisted. Once again, Ilene placated him.

His irritable flare-up was altogether unlike him. Ilene didn't like the sound of his voice; there was something there that she couldn't make out, something that perhaps she wouldn't dare let herself think.

"Sometimes you frighten me," she said.

Once the notebook was on his table, he seemed to relax and resumed his air of peace. They sat together for a few more minutes. In a reassuring tone, Nathan told Ilene to go and have a nice dinner. The tension had gone out of both of them. Just before Ilene got up to go, Nathan asked that she pull the privacy curtain closed. He thought he could rest better that way. Ilene pulled the curtain shut and left him, feeling reassured once again.

She spent an hour eating dinner in the hospital cafeteria. After dinner, she called Janet again and gave her an optimistic report. "Things are looking better," Ilene told her daughter. "Dad is taking an interest in his condition again, and in following his treatment," she said, referring to his desire to work on his notes. Nathan was rallying once again, she reported.

After she hung up, she returned to Nathan's room.

His body was sitting up in bed, gray and lifeless, in a pool of blood. He had cut his arteries at the elbows.

Ilene screamed. A team of doctors and emergency medics rushed into his room and began to administer emergency care, but he was already gone. There was no note. He had said all the good-byes he had wanted to say.

Later, after the cause of death had been established by the coroner and the sheriff's office, a nurse approached Ilene and offered to go into the room with her to bid Nathan a last good-bye. Together they went in and Ilene stroked Nathan's hand and tearfully kissed him good-bye.

Robert and Ken took the first plane to New York and arrived at 10:00 A.M. the following day, February 22.

That day, Dr. Jeffrey D. Hubbard, pathologist at Albany Medical Center, performed an autopsy on Nathan's body.

Hubbard believed that he was performing an autopsy on Howard Malmuth, and it wasn't until later that he learned it was Nathan Pritikin.

In his autopsy report, Hubbard wrote that the patient "has been followed since 1958 for lymphoproliferative disease having features of lymphoma and macroglobulinemia."

After examining Pritikin's heart and coronary arteries, Hubbard noted, "Coronary arteries show minimal yellow discoloration of the intima [inner lining of the artery wall] but there are no plaques and the lumens are widely patent [open and smooth]."

In his summary, Hubbard concluded, "Absence of atherosclerosis, except for small fatty streaks, is unusual in a man of this age."

Letters from scientists all over the world poured in to the Longevity Center praising Pritikin for his contribution to the health and well-being of an entire generation.

Dr. George Sheehan, a medical advisor to runners, wrote in the March 1 edition of the *New York Post:* "Pritikin was a major force behind our national fitness craze.

"Nathan has gone away, but his theories aren't going to go away. A combined program of exercise and diet is here to stay. He started it."

Dr. Ernst Wynder, president of the American Health Foundation and one of the premier cancer researchers in the world, wrote that Pritikin's "major scientific discoveries will withstand the scrutiny of time and above all, if properly applied, provide so many of us with a healthier and more useful life."

On February 28, a memorial service was held in Santa Monica at which George McGovern provided the eulogy.

"What is the mark of a great man?" McGovern asked. "A great man is one who commands the resources of his body, mind, and heart to a worthy purpose. Who has met that test better than Nathan Pritikin?

"When a reporter asked me if Nathan were controversial, I laughed and said, 'Of course he was controversial. So was Louis Pasteur, and Thomas Edison, and Madame Curie. You show me an original thinker with a mobilizing vision and I'll show you a controversial figure.' That is another mark of a great man."

The July 4, 1985 issue of the *New England Journal of Medicine* contained a complete report of Pritikin's coronary autopsy. The article reviewed Pritikin's history of heart disease dating back to 1955, when Dr. Lester Morrison first discovered his coronary insufficiency, and Pritikin's long battle with leukemia, dating back to 1958. After reviewing the data of his disease and the state of his coronary arteries at his death, the report noted that "in a man 69 years old, the near absence of atherosclerosis and the complete absence of its effects are remarkable."

Following Nathan's death and the publication of his autopsy results, many of the nation's leading newspapers and magazines ran articles reporting the remarkable state of Pritikin's heart. *USA Today* ran the head-line: "Did Pritikin's Low-Fat Diet Save His Heart?" *Medical World News* ran its story under the headline: "Pritikin: Vindication from the Grave?" Beneath the headline, the magazine reported: "The diet guru's autopsy results reveal a 'remarkable' cardiovascular system." The *Los Angeles Times* stated in its headline: "Autopsy of Pritikin May Renew Debate." The *Times* began the story with, "Nutrition guru Nathan Pritikin met his death by suicide in the face of two different kinds of leukemia last February with arteries like those of a child and a heart like that of a young man, according to results of his autopsy being published today for the first time."

By May 1985, Pritikin's study at Northwestern was officially under way. Patients were enrolled in the study to see if lowering cholesterol levels could reverse atherosclerosis. It would be a full year before preliminary results were in, but the doctors who worked with Nathan were hopeful that it would provide final proof that the underlying cause of the most heart disease could be reversed.

But in the end, Nathan Pritikin, and the thousands of men and women he helped restore to health, were the best proof of what his diet and lifestyle could do against the most widespread disease of modern times.

PART 2

Pritikin—The Program

CHAPTER 23

The Diet
that Fights Disease

*T*o a great extent, your health is in your own hands. You can make yourself healthier or sicker, depending on the foods you eat and the exercise you do or fail to do.

Since it was first introduced in 1976, the Pritikin Program has been effective in helping tens of thousands of people improve their health. Many of those people in ill health had been given a poor prognosis for recovery by their physicians; still others were given up for dead. And yet they were able to regain their health by following the simple program Nathan Pritikin created.

Today, many physicians are recommending the Pritikin Program as a safe, sane, and effective way to fight heart disease, promote health, and lose weight. Each year, thousands of people are converted to the Pritikin lifestyle.

If you, too, would like to improve your health or lose weight, the Pritikin Program can be your ally. It is a simple, easy-to-follow guide to better living.

Before you begin, however, you should understand the important role diet plays in causing and preventing disease. Following is a discussion of major diseases that afflict many people today–the same diseases that the Pritikin diet has been successful in fighting. Whether you have one or none, you should read about them all. It just may give you the incentive to change your eating habits for the better.

Before you go on this diet or begin an exercise program, however, you should consult your physician. Those who are ill should continue to follow the advice of their doctors. This guide is not meant as a replacement for a physician's care.

Now let's begin with a lesson on heart disease.

264

Diet and Artery Disease

Heart disease is deadly. It is the leading cause of death in the Western world. Illness of the heart and arteries, collectively called cardiovascular diseases, causes one out of every two deaths in the United States, accounting for 1 million deaths annually. Another 40 million Americans suffer from cardiovascular diseases, including angina pectoris and high blood pressure.

The underlying cause of most cardiovascular disease is atherosclerosis, a condition characterized by cholesterol plaque clogging the arteries to the heart, brain, and tissues throughout the body. Approximately 800,000 Americans die each year from illnesses related to this disease.

The process of atherosclerosis often begins in childhood, and sometimes even in infancy. It is a disease that progresses gradually throughout life until it eventually kills, usually by blocking blood flow to the heart or brain and causing a heart attack or stroke.

Studies of humans and animals, as well as human population research, have found a definite link between a diet high in fat and cholesterol and the development of atherosclerosis. Conversely, research has shown that a diet low in fat and cholesterol is a protective factor against the onset of heart disease, including high blood pressure. Here's why.

Scientists have shown that when you eat a diet rich in fat and cholesterol blood cholesterol rises, causing plaque, or cholesterol "boils," to form in the arteries.

As your cholesterol level rises, so too do your chances of having a heart attack or stroke. On the other hand, as your cholesterol level lowers, your chances of suffering a heart attack or stroke decrease. The American Heart Association says that a 1 percent drop in cholesterol equals a 2 percent drop in your chances of having a heart attack.

Most Americans–in fact, most of the Western industrialized world–eat much too much fat. It's estimated that some 40 percent or more of their daily caloric intake is consumed in the form of fat. Many people also consume far too much cholesterol–as much as 400 to 600 mg. each day.

Where does this fat and cholesterol come from? Animal foods, mostly. Red meat, eggs, and dairy products are all rich sources. The white meat of poultry and many fish–such as halibut, cod, flounder, and others–are moderate to low in fat. Plant foods have no cholesterol, but some, such as nuts and avocados, are high in fat. If your favorite foods fit into these high-fat categories, you can figure you're a candidate for high cholesterol. And it's this high consumption of fat and cholesterol that begins the process of atherosclerosis.

The early stages of the illness begin when large quantities of fat get into the bloodstream, causing the red blood cells to adhere to one another, or clump together. This condition is referred to as "rouleaux formation," because the red blood cells cling together to look like a "roll of coins" (or, in French, a "rouleaux").

Even a single high-fat meal can produce this clumping of red cells. After a fatty meal, large quantities of microscopically small, sticky, fat balls (called chylomicra) pour into the blood, causing red blood cells to clump together.

These clumps of red blood cells are too large to pass through tiny capillaries. Normally, a red blood cell in 7.5 microns in diameter. A capillary is 3.5 to 4 microns wide, but the normal disk-shaped red blood cell can pass through this tiny passageway by bending or folding in half at the center. But when they are clumped together, this flexibility is gone. It's as if a roadblock has been set up. It makes passage to the tissues–which need the oxygen and nutrients carried by the blood for survival–difficult or even impossible.

The cells that do manage passage get through carrying a diminished oxygen supply, the same as you would if you had to leave a backpack behind to squeeze through a narrow space. The tissues fed by such sludged-up blood end up being oxygen-deprived. If the condition persists, cells throughout the body can die of "starvation."

One of the organs that is affected the most is the brain. The reduced supply of precious oxygen causes the brain to become sluggish and tired. Thinking becomes cloudy and slow. This is why you may feel fatigued and lethargic after a high-fat meal. This lack of energy can become chronic when high-fat foods are consumed regularly.

But this isn't the only bad side effect of a high-fat diet. The high level of cholesterol that fatty foods contain puts you at risk for plaque buildup in the arteries. The excess cholesterol needs a place to go as it rolls through the bloodstream. It's eventually dumped in various organs, such as the spleen, liver, kidneys, heart, and lungs. This is the beginning of what we know as atherosclerosis.

Cholesterol builds up because it cannot be burned by cells, although small amounts are eliminated each day through the bowels. Under optimal conditions, the body can cause a net loss of up to 100 mg. per day, thus creating a condition whereby the body is actually eliminating more cholesterol than it is taking in. But that amount of cholesterol loss can only happen when *minimal* amounts of cholesterol are consumed each day. For most people, however, this is not the case. They eat too much cholesterol. So, instead of the body efficiently eliminating this potentially harmful substance, it starts to collect it, storing it in the "best" spots–the tissues and bloodstream. As cholesterol accumulates in the blood, it begins to form plaques in the arteries.

The process begins as the cells within the inner lining of the artery become engorged with cholesterol, thus causing them to swell. At this point they are called "foam cells."

As the foam cells multiply, they form a "fatty streak"; eventually they grow to form a full-fledged plaque, which appears similar to a boil. The plaque, which is full of ever-expanding foam cells and dead cellular material, grows and begins to obstruct the flow of blood through the artery. Eventually, the plaque itself bursts, sending debris into the bloodstream. Blood rushes to the ruptured area and forms a clot, which may further narrow the channel of the artery, producing total or partial blockage which—if it's a coronary artery—can cause a heart attack. Meanwhile, the escaped debris (called emboli) may block the flow of blood where they finally lodge, with such dire consequences as loss of vision, stroke, or even death.

The body can grow new blood vessels to the clot in the ruptured area to maintain a blood supply, but the damage is already done. The new vessels are weak and prone to hemorrhaging.

If fat and cholesterol levels in the blood remain high, plaques will continue to grow, threatening to close off the flow of blood in the arteries everywhere: to the heart, which leads to a heart attack; to the brain, leading to a stroke; or to other parts of the body, causing death to tissues elsewhere.

Advancing atherosclerosis and the continual production of foam cells within the arteries is the condition taking place in most people today. Too much fat and cholesterol leads to too much plaque. Too much plaque leads to a health crisis. Or even death.

There are many studies that show that the process of atherosclerosis is preventable—and, perhaps, even reversible. Prevention and recovery of health are accomplished by reversing the process that causes disease. Instead of a diet high in fat and cholesterol, you should eat a diet low in fat and cholesterol. And there are populations of people who prove it can work.

Many traditional and primitive populations, such as the Japanese, the Tarahumara Indians, and others, enjoy a life of little heart disease and few other degenerative illnesses—as long as they maintain the low-fat, low-cholesterol diets of their ancestors.

The Japanese, for example, didn't suffer from coronary heart disease until some of their people adopted an American-like diet. As long as the Japanese remain on their traditional diet, they are fine; when they come to the United States and begin to eat more fat and cholesterol, they suffer much higher rates of heart disease, diabetes, and cancer.

Certain American populations, such as the Seventh-Day Adventists, who eat low fat and cholesterol diets, also have a much lower incidence of coronary disease, cancer, and other degenerative illnesses.

Research also indicates that those with heart disease can recover their health and may be able to reverse the underlying cause of the illness. Studies done on monkeys have demonstrated repeatedly that atherosclerosis can be eliminated from the coronary arteries by eating a diet low in fat and cholesterol.

In 1970, M. L. Armstrong and his associates showed reversal of atherosclerosis in the rhesus monkey. Armstrong fed 30 monkeys a high-fat diet for 18 months. At the conclusion of this period, he examined the coronary arteries of 10 monkeys and found that their arteries were 50 percent closed from plaque. This first group of 10 monkeys he called the "baseline group."

Armstrong then took the remaining 20 monkeys and placed them on two different diets–10 of the monkeys were fed a low-fat diet with no cholesterol and the other 10 ate a 40 percent unsaturated fat diet (using vegetable oils) and no cholesterol. He fed the two groups of monkeys these separate diets for 40 months. He then examined the arteries of both groups.

Armstrong found that the monkeys on the low-fat and no-cholesterol diet had reversed their plaques by a fourth of that shown by the baseline monkeys. In short, they had eliminated much of their artery plaque.

The monkeys on the high unsaturated fat, no cholesterol diet had also reversed their atherosclerosis, but not as much as the low-fat group; the high unsaturated fat monkeys reversed their plaque by about 20 percent of the baseline group.

The study showed that both a low-fat diet and a diet of unsaturated fats reversed atherosclerosis in monkeys, but of the two, the low-fat diet had a much greater reversal effect.

Armstrong's work has been repeated again and again, most notably at the University of Chicago by Dr. Robert Wissler, who has shown atherosclerosis can be created and reversed in monkeys using diet alone.

In 1977, Dr. David Blankenhorn at the University of Southern California demonstrated reversal of atherosclerosis in the femoral arteries (located in the thighs) in humans. Blankenhorn brought about reversal of atherosclerosis simply by lowering cholesterol levels. Reversal of atherosclerosis in the coronary arteries in humans has not yet been proven, but many leading scientists believe that the evidence shows it can be done.

Monkeys have a metabolism similar to that of humans, and they react to a high-fat, high-cholesterol diet as humans do: their blood cholesterol levels increase, plaque forms in the arteries, and eventually they suffer heart attacks or strokes. The disease process appears to be the same in both monkeys and humans. In the same way, when people adopt a low-fat, low-cholesterol diet, they experience a striking improvement in health; their blood pressures and cholesterol often drop, and overall vitality, mental clarity, and endurance increase. While scientists don't know as yet what exactly is taking place within the coronary arteries of people, all the signs point to reversal of atherosclerosis, as it does in monkeys.

Nathan Pritikin found that in order to cause the greatest loss of cholesterol from your body, your daily cholesterol consumption should not exceed 100 mg. per day. The total calories of fat in your diet should not exceed 10 percent. Translated into lay terms, this means no more than three ounces per day of low-fat animal foods. The rest of the diet should consist of whole grains, fresh vegetables, and fruit. These are the basics that make up the Pritikin diet.

When a diet low in fat and cholesterol is consumed, the cholesterol content of the blood is reduced and circulation improves. Cells that were starving for oxygen and nutrients are now nourished. Circulation increases to the heart, brain, and tissues throughout the body.

Most of the heart patients who follow the Pritikin Program experience a remarkable restoration of health. The symptoms of heart disease are reduced and often eliminated. Blood cholesterol levels go down and blood pressure improves. It all adds up to a reduced risk of heart attack and stroke, an abundance of vitality, mental clarity, better sleep, optimal weight, improved bowel function, and many other positive side effects.

After studying the effects of the Pritikin Program on the first 893 patients to come to the Pritikin Longevity Center, Loma Linda University found that the average drop in blood cholesterol after only four weeks was 25 percent. Of those who arrived with cholesterol levels between 260 mg.% and 279 mg.%—a cholesterol level that puts a person at extremely high risk of having a heart attack—the average patient's cholesterol level at the conclusion of the program was 190 mg.%, which put them at very low risk of having a heart attack.

The Pain Known as Angina

Angina pectoris is a characteristic pain that settles in the chest around the heart area. It can range from mild to severe. It is a condition associated with insufficient oxygen to the myocardium, the cardiac muscle that comprises the heart wall. Pain occurs because the heart is being suffocated.

Studies show that a reduction of oxygen to the heart is caused by a high-fat, high-cholesterol diet. Lipids, or fats, reduce the amount of oxygen in red blood cells by creating the rouleaux formation mentioned earlier. In addition, atherosclerosis reduces the amount of blood and oxygen to the heart and other tissues. Together, they sharply reduce the quantity of oxygen available throughout the body, including the heart, causing angina pain. They also reduce the quality of life.

Studies have shown that a single high-fat meal will bring on the symptoms of angina among people who already have the illness. The tiny fat balls called chylomicra that pour into the blood as a fatty meal is digested cause even greater red blood cell clumping, thereby further lessening their oxygen-carrying capacity.

In animal studies, this drop in oxygen level in the blood has been shown to be as high as 35 percent. The action of the fat influx may be all that is needed to trigger angina symptoms; you don't have to be under physical or emotional stress.

Simple carbohydrates, such as sugar, can have the same effect if ingested in sufficient quantities, because they increase triglycerides, a type of blood fat. The chylomicra, which are the primary cause of the angina symptoms, are composed substantially of these triglycerides.

Triglycerides, Pritikin maintained, independently raise the risk of both heart disease and angina pain.

The treatment Pritikin recommended for angina is the same as that for atherosclerosis: a low-fat, low-cholesterol diet, emphasizing complex carbohydrates found in whole grains and vegetables. This would increase the amount of oxygen available to the heart and other organs, thus eliminating the pain that results from coronary insufficiency, or inadequate oxygenation of the cardiac muscle.

Better Blood Pressure

High blood pressure, or hypertension, is the most common cardiovascular disease in the United States. It is a major risk factor in the development of atherosclerosis, and often leads to heart attack or stroke. Studies show that as blood pressure increases, so too does mortality. It's doubly dangerous because you can have it and not know it.

High blood pressure can cause a number of severe disorders, including damage to the kidneys, pancreas, and the retina of the eye. Coupled with atherosclerosis (as it most often is), high blood pressure can cause aneurysms, or "blowouts," of arteries leading to the brain; this results in a stroke.

Blood pressure is considered "high" when it exceeds 140/90. Many insurance companies state that blood pressure is high when diastolic pressure–the second of the two numbers–is above 85.

Blood pressure is caused by the beating of the heart. The diastolic phase occurs when the heart is expanding in order to become filled with blood. At this point, the heart relaxes, but pressure remains in the arterial system. The systolic phase occurs when the heart contracts, forcing blood to pass rapidly throughout the body.

In the United States and much of the Western world, blood pressure increases with age. But it appears that it doesn't have to be this way. By the time Americans reach the age of 65, three-quarters of them have elevated blood pressure, but in nonindustrialized societies older people show the same blood pressure as infants. In other words, high blood pressure is not a natural consequence of aging.

Studies show there are three causes of high blood pressure: atherosclerosis, excessive intake of salt, and diseases of the kidneys and adrenals. Of these, atherosclerosis and excessive salt intake are responsible for about two-thirds of all high blood pressure victims. A high-fat diet causes blood pressure to increase in a number of ways. First, rouleaux formation, or aggregation of red blood cells, increases blood pressure by causing blockages at the tiny passageways of capillaries. The clumps of red blood cells cannot pass through the capillary and thus create a bottleneck, or blockage, preventing blood from passing freely along its way.

Atherosclerosis increases blood pressure by reducing the diameter of the blood vessel, thus causing pressure to build within the vessel–much like squeezing a hose when the water is running. Atherosclerosis also causes blockages in the renal vessels within the kidneys, thus preventing blood from flowing freely through the kidneys' tiny filters.

A high-fat diet also causes blood platelets to secrete the hormone thromboxane, which causes arteries to constrict, further elevating pressure within the arterial system.

The presence of high levels of sodium from salt, causes water retention in the body, thus increasing the presence of water in the tissues and blood stream. This increases the plasma volume and thus increases blood pressure.

Salt and fat act together to increase blood pressure, but either one alone can cause the disease.

Populations that do not suffer from atherosclerosis are also free of high blood pressure. The only exception to this may be the Japanese, who consume large quantities of salt. Among them, programs to reduce salt intake in the population have effectively reduced the blood pressure of the participants. Foods high in fat, cholesterol, and salt are therefore the most dangerous for those concerned about lowering blood pressure.

Loma Linda University found that 85 percent of those who arrived at the Pritikin Longevity Center taking medication for high blood pressure left the center off all medication and with normal pressures.

Diet and Diabetes

Diabetes is an extremely serious disease. It afflicts between 11 million and 12 million Americans and is the third leading cause of death in the United States, following heart disease and cancer. Diabetes is associated with a wide range of other illnesses, including atherosclerosis and other forms of heart disease, blindness, gangrene, progressive loss of hearing, impotence, and palsy. Under certain extreme conditions diabetes can cause coma and death.

If you have diabetes, it means you cannot adequately utilize blood sugar, which is needed as fuel for the functioning of cells. Without fuel, cells die. Because diabetics cannot make sugar available to cells in adequate amounts, the sugar level rises in the blood stream and is filtered out through the kidneys, resulting in sugar spilling into the urine.

There are two types of diabetes: juvenile, or type I, and adult-onset, or type II. Juvenile diabetics produce inadequate amounts of insulin, or lose the ability entirely. Insulin is the hormone used by the body to convert blood sugar to energy. Juvenile diabetics experience rapid weight loss and require insulin injections in order to metabolize sugar. One out of every ten diabetics in the United States is a juvenile diabetic.

The vast majority of diabetics–about 11 million in the United States–are adult-onset. This disease occurs in adulthood and is associated with obesity, though many adult-onset diabetics are lean. Adult-onset diabetics run all the same risks of contracting related illnesses as juvenile diabetics; they are prone to heart and vascular disease, poor circulation, blindness, gangrene, and diabetic coma.

Juvenile diabetes is much harder to treat successfully than adult-onset diabetes. The Pritikin Program helps to stabilize sugar levels and reduce insulin requirements in juvenile diabetics, but it cannot rescue the juvenile diabetic from his or her daily need for insulin. Adult-onset diabetics, on the other hand, have been successfully weaned from drugs and insulin with the use of the program.

For many years, researchers believed that diabetics simply could not produce insulin. As a result, insulin was administered–and still is–to many diabetics, while others, with less severe cases, receive oral drugs.

Around 1970, it was discovered that adult-onset diabetics actually produced more insulin than nondiabetics. This was a surprising discovery because it had long been thought that the problem with diabetics was they did not produce enough insulin, and therefore could not utilize existing blood sugar as a fuel for cells. Research, however, showed that the insulin produced by these diabetics is ineffective in making sufficient quantities of glucose, or blood sugar, available to the body's cells. Something in the complex chain of events that enables the body to turn sugar into fuel for cells goes wrong.

Scientists are still not sure what exactly causes diabetes. When you eat a meal containing carbohydrates, either from unrefined plant foods or simple sugar (such as a candy bar), the body produces insulin, which travels through the bloodstream and attaches itself to cells at certain sites, called insulin receptors. The insulin then signals the cells to produce glucose transporters, which are protein molecules that transport the glucose into the cell. The cell uses the glucose for fuel to carry on its myriad functions.

Nathan Pritikin created an analogy for people to visualize what is taking place in sugar metabolism. He said that the cell was like a room with many doors, some of which were meant to allow sugar to enter. Insulin was the gatekeeper to the cell, allowing sugar to enter as it was needed.

Research has shown that fat in the diet somehow prevents the insulin from doing its job. Fat causes this process of sugar metabolism to break down, though exactly how it does this is still unknown. Pritikin theorized that fat may be interfering with these insulin receptor mechanisms (there are many sites for potential problems along this delicate chain of events in sugar metabolism). He speculated that the fat gets to these doorways of the cell first, thus preventing the insulin from acting as a gatekeeper into the cell.

He recognized that there are many possible ways that fat may interfere with the mechanisms of sugar metabolism. Perhaps it affects the cell's ability to produce glucose transporter molecules, or changes the transporter molecules themselves, making them unable to bring glucose into the cell. There are other possibilities, which scientists, including those currently at the Longevity Center, are studying.

What is known is that as the fat content of the diet increases, so too does the body's inability to metabolize sugar. The more fat one eats, the more likely one is to contract adult-onset diabetes.

For centuries, and up until very recently, however, diabetic diets were based on a high-fat content because it was thought that it was necessary to restrict carbohydrates. This notion was derived from the early observation that sugar was present in the urine of diabetics. Therefore, it was reasoned, diabetics cannot metabolize sugar or foods from which sugar is derived, that is, carbohydrates. Restriction of carbohydrates in the diabetic diet required that fat content be increased.

Research done in the early 1900s showed that many healthy people could be made to test diabetic simply by placing them on a high-fat diet. Yet, people put on a low-fat diet could not be made to test diabetic even if fed a pound of sugar a day. Other studies showed that high-carbohydrate diets in which fat was restricted had been successfully used to treat diabetics during the early part of the 20th century.

In one study done in 1935, Dr. H. P. Himsworth found that when he placed healthy young men on a high-fat diet for a week, they tested diabetic; however, after he took the same young men off the high-fat diet and placed them on a low-fat regimen for a week, they tested normal.

These studies largely had been ignored until Pritikin rediscovered them and began to apply their findings to those with adult-onset diabetes. He showed that a diet made up mostly of complex carbohydrates could eliminate the symptoms of diabetes.

There is an important distinction to be made between complex carbohydrates, found in whole grains and vegetables, and simple carbo-hydrates, such as table sugar or honey. These two different types of carbo-hydrates have vastly different effects on the body.

A complex carbohydrate molecule consists of a large group of sugar molecules, all bound together. These large molecules require enzymes in the intestines to break them down and make them available as blood sugar for fuel for cells. The process is a gradual one, in which sugar is made available to the cells in a steady flow. As a result, on a complex-carbohydrate diet there is a continuous supply of energy over a longer period of time.

Simple carbohydrates, on the other hand, are composed of one, two, or just a few sugar molecules. They do not require the work of intestinal enzymes to break them down to become available as blood sugar. Simple carbohydrates, such as those in a candy bar, begin to pour into the bloodstream the minute they enter your mouth. You experience a burst of energy. However, the available sugar is burned quickly, which can cause a sudden drop in blood sugar to below normal levels. The sudden absence of available blood sugar, or fuel, may leave some people feeling fatigued, lethargic, and even dizzy. This condition is called hypoglycemia.

Once they are in the bloodstream, simple sugars are converted to triglycerides, or blood fats, if they are not burned as fuel or eliminated through the urine.

Simple sugars thus contribute to the diabetic state, though not nearly as much as fat.

The effects of complex carbohydrates versus simple sugars are drasti-cally different. Complex carbohydrates, found in whole grains, vegetables, and fruits, create long-term energy and endurance, while simple sugars give rise to quick bursts of energy that do not sustain themselves, but quickly burn and result in lower than normal amounts of energy. Simple sugars combined with a high-fat diet increase the risk of adult-onset diabetes by raising blood levels of fats.

Loma Linda University reported that half of all those who arrived at the Longevity Center taking insulin for their adult-onset diabetes left the center off insulin and free of diabetic symptoms. Fully 80 percent of those taking oral drugs for their type II diabetes left the center off all drugs and symptom-free.

Reduce the Risk of Cancer

Studies long have shown that a diet rich in fat, cholesterol, and fiber-deficient foods is a leading cause of common cancers: colon, breast, and prostate. In 1979, the Surgeon General published *The Surgeon General's Report on Health Promotion and Disease Prevention*, stating that the typical American diet, rich in fat, cholesterol, and sugar and lacking in fiber, was responsible for most of the cancer in the United States. In 1982, the National Research Council of the National Academy of Sciences published *Diet, Nutrition, and Cancer*, a review of the evidence demonstrating the dietary factors that cause cancer. The National Research Council stated that a causal relationship does exist between high levels of fat in the diet and the incidence of prostate, breast, and colon cancer.

In the case of colon cancer, the combination of fat and lack of fiber (refined grains, such as white bread and other refined flour products, have the fiber removed during processing) produce the perfect conditions within the intestines for the onset of cancer. Fat increases bile acids, which in turn creates the environment preferred by anaerobic bacteria. The bacteria then convert bile acids into carcinogens.

Lack of fiber lengthens intestinal transit time, the time required for ingested food to move through the intestinal tract, increasing the amount of time that toxins are present in the system.

Population studies in Japan and in Africa have shown repeatedly that people on diets low in fat and rich in fiber from whole grains and vegetables suffer almost no sign of colon cancer. Breast and prostate cancer are equally rare among people who consume this low-fat, low-cholesterol diet.

In the case of breast cancer, high levels of fat in the diet increase hormone levels, especially that of estrogen and prolactin in women. Estrogen levels have been found to be high in women who eat a high-fat diet. Bacteria, which thrive on bile and fat, produce estrogen, which in turn seems to adversely affect reproductive organs, create cysts, and increase prolactin levels.

Prolactin is the hormone responsible for the production of milk. Women on high-fat diets have been found to have abnormally high levels of prolactin, even when not lactating.

Children on high-fat diets also show high levels of prolactin and estrogen. Researchers have shown that high prolactin levels create imbalances in breast tissue and the endocrine system early in life, perhaps predisposing young women to cancer later on.

Prostate cancer is also a fat- and hormone-related disease. In countries such as Japan, prostate cancer was unheard of prior to the 1950s. Research has shown that as meat consumption increased in Japan during the 1950s and 1960s, prostate cancer increased with it. Many studies have shown that diets rich in fat and cholesterol are directly associated with higher rates of prostate cancer.

What it all boils down to is this: There is no genetic immunity among the people who traditionally have been free of the common cancers. When the Japanese migrate to the United States and adopt more American-like diets, their rates of colon, breast, and prostate cancer all rise to the levels approaching that of Americans.

Animal studies have shown that low-fat, low-cholesterol diets seem to protect against cancer, even when a known carcinogen is injected into the bloodstream.

Dr. Jeremiah Stamler, of Northwestern University in Chicago, studied the relationship between lung cancer and smoking. Stamler discovered something that at the time seemed peculiar. Although smoking is a known carcinogen, a powerful indicator as to whether the smokers in the study got cancer was the amount of fat and cholesterol in the diets.

Stamler found that in smokers with cholesterol levels of 220 mg.% and below, only 5 in 1,000 smokers got lung cancer. However, in smokers with cholesterol levels between 220 mg.% and 250 mg.%, 18 per 1,000 got lung cancer. In smokers with cholesterol levels over 275 mg.%, 37 per 1,000 contracted lung cancer. In other words, a "straight-line relationship" appears to exist between the amount of fat and cholesterol in the diet and the incidence of lung cancer. This and other research indicate that fat and cholesterol seem to make other carcinogens more powerful.

Research done by W. Addelman and published in the *New England Journal of Medicine* in 1972 reported that four patients, all of whom had cancer–three with prostate cancer and a fourth with an ovarian tumor–all experienced complete remissions of their cancers after dramatically reducing their cholesterol levels.

The diets of traditional populations–low in fat, cholesterol, and sugar and rich in whole grains, fresh vegetables, fruit, and fish–long have protected people from the widespread incidence of cancer that is common today in our modern, industrialized society. The Pritikin diet is a replica of this traditional regimen.

Scientists now say that such a diet may do much toward preventing cancer.

Relief from Gout and Other Forms of Arthritis

Gout is a painful joint problem that usually settles in the big toe. It was a raging problem in sixteenth- and seventeenth-century England, where the aristocracy ate meat three times a day. Twentieth-century America has also suffered from the illness because, like the rich of Shakespeare's England, most Americans can afford to eat meat in great quantities.

The villain associated with this painful inconvenience is uric acid, a product of protein metabolism. Blood levels of uric acid increase in people who consume a diet rich in animal protein, especially organ meats.

When uric acid is elevated, it collects around the joints and crystallizes. White blood cells eat the crystals in an effort to eliminate them from the body. This is one of the normal functions of white blood cells: to eliminate unwanted substances, including pathogens and bacteria, from the blood itself. These white blood cells have "stomachs" called lysosomes, which attempt to digest the uric acid crystals with their powerful digestive juices. The digestive juices of lysosomes are more powerful than the acids of the human stomach. Uric acid crystals, however, are indigestible and, once inside the lysosomes, puncture the stomachs of the white blood cells. This causes the digestive juices to spill out of the cells and into the spaces between the joints. Pritikin said that these acids attack the joints and bring on the painful symptoms of gout. The disease actually is brought on by the high protein levels. Treating gout requires eliminating typically high levels of animal proteins, especially organ meats.

Many of those who have suffered from other forms of arthritis, including rheumatoid arthritis and osteoarthritis, and who have adopted the Pritikin Program have experienced remarkable reduction and even cessation of the symptoms of the disease.

Scientists are still studying why a low-fat, low-cholesterol diet may be effective in the treatment of arthritis. There are several logical reasons that may explain why such a diet improves arthritis pain. For one, the Pritikin Program has been proven to dramatically improve circulation throughout the body, including the joints. This increases the flow of oxygen to the affected areas of the body and helps reduce edema, or swelling from body fluids, which tends to reduce oxygen levels in the tissues and increase pain.

High levels of fat in the bloodstream cause red blood cells to sludge and block capillaries. This creates swelling in the joints and prevents oxygen from reaching these areas. Lack of oxygen causes tissues to become inflamed and painful. Swelling also causes stiffness in the joints.

The presence of uric acid crystals from high protein intake may also play a role in the onset of rheumatoid arthritis and osteoarthritis, as they do in gout. The crystals cause the white blood cell to become punctured and spill acid in the joints. Swelling may further affect the white blood cell by causing it to exist in an oxygen-depleted environment, thus causing the white cell to burst open and spill its digestive juices into the sensitive synovial lining of the joints.

These illnesses need more study, but people who have suffered with arthritis and have adopted the Pritikin Program have consistently reported improvements in their conditions after going on the program.

Improve Poor Hearing

Hearing gradually deteriorates with age in the United States and in much of the Western world. Most people accept the loss of hearing as an aggravating side effect of aging. Nathan Pritikin did not. He maintained that aging is not the cause of most hearing loss. He claimed that diet is.

To back up his belief, he pointed to studies comparing the hearing of United States citizens with that of Africans. They consistently showed that African tribespeople possess better hearing at the age of 70 than the average American at 20. An interesting observation, without a doubt. How can this be?

Researchers compared the hearing capabilities of people living in Wisconsin–the dairy-producing capital of the United States–with the African tribespeople, the Mabaans. The researchers found that a random sampling of 30- to 35-year-old Wisconsinites showed such hearing loss that not one Mabaan at any age could be found with comparably impaired hearing.

Similar studies were conducted comparing the hearing capabilities of Finnish people with those of Yugoslavians. Finland has the highest per capita rate of coronary heart disease in the world; the average cholesterol level in Finland is 290 mg.%. The average cholesterol level in Yugoslavia is approximately 180 mg.%. Researchers found that Finnish children begin to suffer hearing loss at the age of 10 and by 19 have distinctly impaired capacity to hear the 16,000 to 18,000 cycles per second range of sound. No such hearing loss existed among Yugoslavians.

Other studies have shown that by reducing fat and cholesterol intake, hearing capabilities markedly improve. Pritikin argued that many types of hearing disorders were due to poor circulation in the hearing organs. Plaque development in the blood vessels to the inner ear limits blood and oxygen to the hearing organ and reduces its sensitivity to sound.

Pritikin found that a low-fat, low-cholesterol diet would restore hearing capability enormously.

Guard against Eye Disease

Fifty percent of all blindness is the result of impaired circulation, Pritikin believed. And the usual cause of the poor circulation is a high-fat, high-cholesterol diet. The degree of blindness depends largely on how badly the circulation to the eye has been affected.

Pritikin called the eyes the windows of the body. "Through them the internal circulation and most of the vascular problems arising in the body can be studied with minimal danger and discomfort to the patient," he wrote.

A striking example of how the eye serves as a window to the body is the emergence of an opaque or grayish circle or semicircle around the iris of the eye. Physicians refer to this abnormal condition as the "arcus senilis" (arc of age), and those who develop it suffer a much higher rate of coronary heart attacks than those who do not.

Arcus senilis emerges in men and women older than 40, when great quantities of cholesterol have been consumed, causing plaque development in the coronary arteries and elsewhere in the body and the development of this visible deposit of cholesterol, triglycerides, and phospholipids in the cornea of the eye. One out of three people older than 40 have this telltale semicircle around the iris, reflecting their advanced atherosclerosis.

The atherosclerotic process developing throughout the body may harm the eyes in several ways. Very often, fragments break off from atherosclerotic plaques elsewhere in the body, finally lodging themselves in and around the eyes, reducing blood flow to them. These can be seen by an ophthalmologist as crystals of cholesterol floating within the eye itself. Very often the crystals cut off blood to a part of the eye, resulting in partial blindness. Sometimes, large fragments of plaques can break off and block the large vessel in the eye called the central retinal artery; when this is blocked completely, there is total loss of sight.

Glaucoma is a very common eye disorder among older people and is the chief cause of blindness among U.S. adults. Glaucoma is caused by vascular changes in the eye, a symptom of which is elevation of the normal pressure within the eyeball, called the intraocular pressure. This pressure is kept constant by fluids within the structure of the eyeball, but blood that has a high fat and cholesterol concentration can cause the pressure to rise. Elevation of intraocular pressure is usually accompanied by visual field changes limiting the range of vision and even producing total blindness.

Plaque buildup in the vessels of the eye causes a reduction of blood flow and an increase in pressure within the eye. When the retina, the photographic plate of the eye, is affected by a reduction of blood flow, less blood reaches the optic nerve, to which it is connected. The optic nerve sends impulses from the retina to the brain, so when less blood reaches it, visual changes characteristic of glaucoma result.

Pritikin believed that the high-fat, high-cholesterol diet consumed in Western societies is the basic cause of most glaucoma, and described a number of complicated mechanisms that he believed were responsible for the raising of intraocular pressure. One of these has to do with the interference of the continuous fluid drainage from the eyes. The fluids in the eyeballs must be drained and replenished at a constant rate to maintain the necessary intraocular pressure, as well as the cleanliness and health of the eye. This fluid is filtered by a meshlike tissue in the eye. If an accumulation of tiny particles of fat and cholesterol blocks the drainage outlet in the meshlike filter, the fluid backs up and pressure builds within the eye.

Another related factor, Pritikin said, had to do with the reduced oxygen content of fat-laden blood. This causes a corresponding increase in the blood's carbon dioxide content, resulting in dilation of the blood vessels of the eye, increasing the pressure within the eye, and, in turn, raising intraocular pressure.

Still another mechanism is the elevation of cortisol levels due to the high fat content of the blood on a Western diet. Cortisol, chemically classified as a steroid (like cholesterol), is normally produced by the body. Pritikin maintained that increased amounts of cortisol is produced in the body on a high-fat diet. The cortisol, he said, affects the meshlike filter in the eye, causing it to swell and become blocked, thus increasing intraocular pressure.

In his extremely detailed and heavily documented argument, Pritikin showed that the high incidence of glaucoma or of cataracts, common eye diseases in the West is tied to our high-fat, high-cholesterol diet.

Obviously, diet isn't the only answer for blindness. There are many reasons why eye diseases may occur. But by reducing the amount of fat and cholesterol in the diet, the symptoms of glaucoma and other forms of blindness caused by poor circulation can be prevented, Pritikin believed.

Pritikin's answer to a range of degenerative diseases–heart disease, adult-onset diabetes, arthritis, cancer, diseases of sight and of hearing– was his low-fat, low-cholesterol diet, which he devised based on his understanding of nutrition and the diets of peoples who do not suffer from these diseases. He found it to be remarkably effective in the thousands of people who turned to his program to turn away from disease.

CHAPTER 24

Watch Your Weight Go Down

*W*eight loss comes naturally on the Pritikin Program. That's because it spotlights tasty, nourishing foods, such as whole grains, fruits, and vegetables and snubs the typical American diet that has been a menace to our health.

Where in the world is obesity most prevalent? Right here at home! We in the West suffer from widespread obesity, while people who live in nonindustrialized nations and consume a diet made up primarily of whole grains, vegetables, and fruit–in other words, "starchy" foods–have little or no incidence of obesity. The American diet, rich in fat, refined foods, and sugar, is the ideal regimen for causing overweight. Let's see why this is the case.

Food is used by the body as fuel. Weight gain occurs when we eat more than the body needs as fuel. The surplus is stored as fat. Exercise burns fat, but too many of us lead relatively sedentary lives and, therefore, need even fewer calories than we are consuming.

Ideally, you should eat foods that provide only enough calories to meet your energy requirement. If you are overweight, you'll need to eat fewer calories than you now do, so that your body can burn the surplus fat that you have stored.

Still, diets that require you to go hungry for any length of time are difficult if not impossible to maintain. Pretty soon, you're eating everything in sight because you simply cannot fast forever. What you want is a diet that you can eat until you are satisfied, but one that does not provide an excess of calories that ultimately would be stored as fat.

The only way this can be done is to eat a diet that is rich in bulk–to create a feeling of fullness–but relatively low in calories, in order to avoid weight gain. This is precisely what the Pritikin Program provides.

The stomach has a volume of about four cups. When it is filled, the stomach signals the brain to stop eating. The stomach doesn't know how many calories are in a specific food, nor does it care. What matters is whether there is a sufficient quantity of food to create the feeling of fullness.

Fats and oils are calorically dense: a tablespoon of fat has twice the calories of the same tablespoon of brown rice or a slice of whole wheat bread.

One of the most common and destructive myths in controlling weight is that whole grains and vegetables–foods commonly called "starchy"– are higher in calories than animal foods such as dairy products, eggs, and meat.

Many people think that they should avoid foods such as brown rice or whole wheat bread in order to avoid calories. Instead, they mistakenly eat cheese, steak, pork, or some other high-fat food. And they get several times the calories they need.

An eight-ounce cup of cooked brown rice, for example, has about 232 calories. The same size serving of romaine lettuce has 10 calories, Brussels sprouts 56, and collard greens 63. The equivalent size hamburger has about 648 calories, while an eight-ounce cup of cheddar cheese has 450 calories.

The same is true for desserts. Fruit has nowhere near the calories of sugary desserts. An apple has about 73 calories; an eight-ounce serving of ice cream has about 330.

Whole, unrefined foods are ideal for losing weight or maintaining optimal weight. Unrefined foods are rich in fiber and water. Fiber provides bulk, giving the feeling of being full after eating.

Refined foods, on the other hand, are disastrous to those who want to lose weight. Refined foods have the vitamins, minerals, fiber, and protein removed during processing. What is left behind is the calorie-rich, refined carbohydrate. If you were to compare a given volume of natural, unrefined food to a refined food, you would see that the whole, natural food is made up of fiber and other nutrients which provide bulk but minimal calories, while the refined food has these constituents stripped away and ends up calorie dense.

For example, the average whole sugar beet, rich in fiber and water, weighs about two pounds and has about 500 calories. However, when the sugar is extracted from the beet during processing, what is left is a high-calorie food product: two pounds of sugar now contains 3,500 calories!

Generally, the more refined a food is, the more calories it contains. This is especially true when such foods are combined with fats in the form of cheeses, cream, butter, and oils, as in many prepared foods.

In order to avoid an abundance of unnecessary calories, you must avoid fatty foods and highly refined foods. Natural foods, or what Pritikin used to call "food as grown," are rich in fiber. This provides bulk and feelings of satisfaction, signaling the brain that we are full, without loading us down with calories in the process.

The Pritikin diet is ideal for losing weight and keeping it off. For one thing, you can eat as much and as often as you like; you don't have to starve yourself in order to lose weight. Once you are down to your optimal weight, your body stabilizes and your weight tends to remain fairly constant.

Those who are already at their optimal weight will stay there on the Pritikin Program. There are enough calories in the Pritikin diet to maintain optimal weight and provide an abundance of long-lasting energy.

In addition to the diet, the Pritikin Program encourages you to take brisk, daily walks, which will speed up the process of weight loss, improve muscle tone and cardiovascular fitness, and help to prevent many serious illnesses.

To find out how it all works, turn to the next chapter.

CHAPTER **25**

The Pritikin Diet
for Optimal Health
and Weight Loss

*T*he Pritikin diet has come a long way since Nathan Pritikin first served his version of a healthful meal to his first patients at his Longevity Center in January 1976.

As sick as they were, many of the people at that first session found a bit of humor in what they were expected to eat. One man joked that Nathan's chicken soup was so chickenless that it was made by waving a chicken over a pot of water warming in the sun. By anyone's admission, the food was bland and uninspiring. But there was a reason for it. Nathan's primary goal at the time was healthfulness, not taste. Pritikin maintained (correctly, as his patients found out) that taste is learned, not inherited. New tastes can be developed. As these people felt themselves growing stronger and healthier, they found the reason for it all–the food–wasn't all that hard to swallow.

But that was more than a decade ago. Over the years, professional chefs and nutritionists have taken Nathan Pritikin's basic food principles and cultivated them into a taste experience. They experimented with the sauces, spices, and condiments of other cultures–Mexican, Chinese, and Italian, for example–to add flavor and bring out the maximum taste of natural foods. Today, when patients check into a Pritikin Longevity Center, they experience the Pritikin Program at its best. Though the basic guidelines have never changed, new research has prompted adjustments in serving size, such as for fruits and shellfish. You should find it much to your liking. Today's Pritikin diet not only fosters health and vitality, it is also delicious and satisfying.

You, too, can experience the same healthfulness by following the principles of the Pritikin diet, which follow. Some ideas on how to prepare

284

interesting and tasty dishes are given. But don't hesitate to experiment with them yourself. The idea is to take healthful foods and turn them into something *you* can enjoy. The payoff is optimal health and weight loss.

The Diet Basics

1. Whole Grains. Do you love to eat bread? Pasta too? Such things are the backbone of the Pritikin diet.

Two or more servings of whole unrefined grains–brown rice, wheat, millet, barley, oats, and buckwheat–should be part of your daily diet. They can all be found in such things as whole grain breads, pastas, cereals, and rice dishes. They are important because they contain appropriate amounts of fiber, vitamins, minerals, and protein. They also contain an abundance of complex carbohydrates, which give long-term energy.

2. Vegetables. You can eat vegetables to your heart's content on the Pritikin diet. The one exception is olives, which are excluded because they are high in fat. In the early days, Pritikin would joke that a person could safely eat one olive per day, and his staff carried the joke on by creating a recipe for a one-olive tamale pie.

The Pritikin-recommended vegetables are the leafy greens. This includes romaine lettuce, mustard and collard greens, spinach, kale, broccoli, and other dark greens. Your vegetable selections don't need to be exclusively green, however. Potatoes, yams, carrots, and squash are all nutritious and are encouraged eating. You should eat at least one six- to eight-ounce raw salad daily. Try to prepare the rest of your vegetables in a variety of ways to avoid monotony.

3. Fruit. All fruits are permitted on the Pritikin diet with the exception of avocados, which are high in fat, and dried figs and dates, which are high in simple sugars. Three to five pieces of fruit should be included in the daily diet. Fruit, however, should not comprise more than 20 percent of your daily calories.

Fruit is limited because it contains both complex and simple carbohydrates. Simple carbohydrates can elevate triglycerides, or blood fats, meaning that an overabundance of fruit in the diet could raise the chances of heart disease and diabetes.

Pritikin himself loved desserts, and he became a whiz at whipping up tasty fruit desserts with a blender or food processor. Nathan found out how to create smooth and creamy fruit desserts to replace his former love–ice cream.

4. Meat, Poultry, Fish. The Pritikin diet recommends restricting flesh food to no more than 3½ ounces each day.

Pritikin himself preferred lean fish and the white meat of poultry, because of its lower fat content, and encouraged the same habit in his patients. He allowed patients to eat range-fed beef; unlike the marbled or fatty beef found in most supermarkets, it's fat content is comparable to fish and the white meat of poultry.

Shellfish and shrimp, which are higher in cholesterol, are permitted only in small quantities (meaning not every day) as a substitute for other cholesterol-containing foods.

Three ounces of fish, chicken, or range-fed beef per day should keep your total cholesterol intake below 100 mg., the upper limit the body can tolerate before plaque begins to form in the arteries. This is because the body is built to eliminate up to 100 mg. per day of cholesterol. What isn't sent from the body is distributed through the bloodstream.

5. *Milk*. Milk products–even skim milk–should only have a limited role in the diet, Pritikin believed, because of their high protein content. The view that large amounts of protein are needed in the diet was assailed by Pritikin as a great myth. He pointed out that at the period of greatest growth in the human life cycle–infancy–the protein content of breast milk is only 6 percent. Nathan argued that milk was an inappropriate food for human consumption after weaning. He pointed out that most of the human population around the world does not drink milk after weaning, but these people suffer no mineral deficiencies.

Nonfat milk products, however, are permitted on the diet in limited quantities. Low-fat yogurt and certain cheeses made with skim milk can be eaten sparingly.

6. *Beverages*. Coffee, tea, and alcohol are not recommended on the Pritikin Program. Pritikin viewed caffeine and alcohol as drugs and believed they have adverse effects on health.

Fruit juices are permitted in limited quantity, for the same reason fruit is limited–to keep triglycerides down. The best drink is water, Pritikin maintained, but need be consumed only when you're thirsty. He said you get plenty of water in the fruits and vegetables you eat. Also, the fact that the diet is naturally low in salt reduces your need for water.

7. *Supplements*. Pritikin was opposed to taking nutritional supplements. He considered them an artificial way to nourish the body and felt they were potentially dangerous when consumed in amounts that are excessive. He maintained that a diet like his, one that contained whole foods, can supply all the vitamins and minerals a person needs if followed properly.

What all this breaks down to is a diet that's composed largely of complex carbohydrates–some 80 percent of your daily calories on the Pritikin diet–should come from whole grains, fruits, and vegetables. Protein constitutes 10 to 12 percent; fat 10 percent or less. This is the diet that populations such as the Tarahumara Indians, the Japanese, and certain African nations–people who have been spotlighted in this book–successfully eat without showing signs of any degenerative diseases. On the contrary, it *promotes* optimal health and *prevents* major illnesses.

Foods to Avoid

Some foods are totally prohibited on the Pritikin diet because they contain too much fat and cholesterol, which contribute to disease. These include:

1. *Red Meat.* Lamb, pork, duck, goose, grain-fed or fatty beef (the type typically sold in supermarkets), and organ meats are all off-limits.

2. *Whole Milk Products.* This includes most cheeses, whole milk, creams, powdered milk, and butter. Nonfat milk products, as mentioned above, can be eaten in limited quantity. Nondairy creamers are also prohibited because they are high in fat.

3. *Desserts and Snacks.* Included in this category are all puddings, sherbets, ice cream, canned fruit in syrup, gelatin desserts, fried foods, including potato chips, all bakery products containing shortening and sugar, candy, and soft drinks, especially colas which contain caffeine.

4. *Nuts and Seeds.* Nuts and most seeds are, in general, off-limits on the Pritikin diet, due to their high fat content. Chestnuts, which are low in fat are permitted; and ground seeds can be used in small quantities as seasonings.

5. *Salt.* All table salt and all salty foods, such as crackers, pretzels and smoked fish, should be avoided.

How to Follow the Pritikin Program

Let's assume that you wish to start the Pritikin diet tomorrow. What should you do?

A good first step would be to clear out all the forbidden foods from your refrigerator, freezer, and pantry. Your goal is to eliminate foods high in fat, cholesterol, refined sugar, and salt. It may hurt a bit, but be relentless; if it's bad for you, get rid of it. Throw out all the no-no's–the butter, margarine, cheeses, cream, oils, salad dressings with oils, peanut butter, salty crackers, and the frozen, canned, and packaged foods laden with harmful ingredients. Out goes the ice cream. Out goes the whole or low-fat milk. Out go the potato chips and cookies. Out go the buttery crackers. And so on. Check the foods listed above under "Foods to Avoid" and make sure you banish them from your kitchen.

Now here's the good part. Start building your healthy kitchen with the vast array of foods that are good for you. The idea is to stockpile healthy foods and make them appetizing and pleasing, so when you're hungry you'll *want* to reach for them.

Start first by purchasing nonperishables, such as grains and grain products: brown rice, whole rolled oats, whole grain pasta, whole grain bread and crackers without fats, oils, and sugar, and so on. Choose salt-free or low-salt products whenever possible.

Next, the perishables. You'll be shopping for provisions from the produce section for a variety of vegetables and fruits and from the refrigerator section for nonfat dairy goods, if you wish to include milk products in your diet. Permitted dairy foods include nonfat or skim milk, nonfat yogurt, hoop cheese, cottage cheese under 1 percent fat, and green or sapsago cheese (a skim milk hard cheese).

Frozen foods you may wish to purchase include vegetables without sauces, and fruits and fruit juices without added sugar. You may also want to stock up on herbs and spices to add interest to your meals.

You now have a model Pritikin kitchen, or something close to it. Perhaps you aren't quite ready to give it all up–like your morning cup of coffee or a single personal evil like an after-dinner cookie. That's all right. Once you get started on the Pritikin diet and start feeling the benefits in terms of your energy and well-being, you'll find total conversion to the program much easier.

Planning Your Meals

To get your program off to its best start, you should make every effort to work out a way to spend some time preparing your daily meals.

If you are satisfied with simple foods and like to keep your kitchen time to the minimum, you can keep your menu plain. A little poached fish, some steamed vegetables, and a potato is a good example of a typical plain Pritikin dinner. But if you enjoy working with food and have the time to experiment and prepare, then please do so. Just remember to keep within the guidelines mentioned above. You may even decide to alternate your attention on the food depending on your mood and inclination–one day plain, one day fancy. But let's face it: a small amount of cooking is unavoidable.

An important rule is this: Don't just think three meals a day. The best way to keep away hunger is to eat every few hours. This means keeping plenty of snacks on hand. Low-calorie snacks are best, especially if weight loss is your goal. For weight watchers, sliced raw vegetables, a small green salad, or a bowl of soup, especially thin soups, are ideal. A few whole grain crackers can be used to accompany these foods. For active people who do not need to lose weight, bread makes a convenient snack food, but it will tend to increase your daily salt intake somewhat if consumed in excess. Raw fruits are good snack foods for everyone, as long as recommended fruit allotments are not exceeded.

If your goal is to lose weight, eat a raw salad and low-calorie soup at your main meal each day. This will help make you full without loading up on some of the higher-calorie foods, such as beans, peas, potatoes, and corn.

Prepare and Experiment

Keeping a few cooked staples, such as brown rice or beans, on hand in your refrigerator will help make meal preparation faster. If you've never cooked brown rice or beans, now is the time to learn how. You may use long-, medium- or short-grain brown rice (the cooked texture of the long-grain is preferred by some), and any of several different kinds of dried beans. Pinto, red, or kidney beans are all favorite choices. Cook large batches that can be kept in the refrigerator for three to four days, or even longer. Cooked beans and rice may also be frozen, then defrosted before using.

Potatoes, too, are a good cooked staple. Cook unpeeled red or white potatoes; peel while hot, if desired, and cover and store in the refrigerator for use alone or in salads or soups.

In a pinch, you can heat and use the rice and beans as is, seasoning the beans with a little commercial taco sauce. Or you can add the rice or beans to various dishes you make. The potatoes, too, can be eaten as is, perhaps sliced and topped with an instant dressing made by mixing nonfat yogurt with a little Dijon mustard. Or you can place the slices on a Teflon pan and bake them until browned to make mock french fries, eating them with the yogurt-mustard dressing if you wish.

You can use the combination of nonfat yogurt with a little Dijon mustard in so many ways that you may want to prepare a quantity and keep it on hand as one of your refrigerator staples. Not only is it excellent on any kind of potato, including baked potatoes, it is also delicious on such steamed green vegetables as broccoli, green beans, cabbage and artichokes. You can use it, too, as "tartar sauce" for poached, broiled, or baked fish, as a sandwich spread, and as a dressing for a fish salad.

Soups are another good thing to keep on hand. If you have been a soupmaker, you can easily adapt many standard recipes by simply omitting ingredients that are Pritikin no-no's and supplementing flavor, if necessary, with permitted seasonings. If you've never cooked soups, try your hand at some simple recipes, like split pea or lentil soup. You can turn leftover vegetables into a quick soup by adding the vegetables and the liquid in which they were cooked to a soup base of canned, chopped tomatoes or tomato purée (preferably unsalted), thinned with water, then seasoned to taste.

Now let's take some of the imagination we have just inspired and see how you can use it during mealtimes.

Breakfast–Think Big

If you are in the habit of eating a small breakfast or none at all, you're in for a great big change. On the Pritikin Program, a filling breakfast is important.

The very best breakfast is a hot cooked cereal, such as old-fashioned rolled oats or a good-quality wheat cereal. It stays with you for hours, keeping you from temptation when the doughnuts or croissants call out to you during your midmorning break.

Being too busy in the morning is no excuse for missing out on a cooked breakfast. If you plan it into your schedule, it doesn't take that long to prepare a cooked cereal in the morning. A cooked cereal is routinely served at the Pritikin centers in the morning because it provides such excellent nourishment and prevents blood sugar from dropping quickly. Give it a try. You can cook it with a little chopped fruit (apples, pears, peaches, bananas, nectarines, and so on) or raisins, and serve it with nonfat milk and cinnamon, if you wish.

What if you hate cooked cereal? There are alternatives. You can have an acceptable packaged dry cereal (look for high fiber, low fat, and no sugar on the label), eating it with sliced fresh fruit, nonfat milk, and a few raisins. Or you may opt for cold cooked brown rice that has been stashed in your refrigerator, topping it with sliced fresh fruit and a dash of cinnamon. In fact, cold cooked brown rice with a sliced banana was Nathan Pritikin's favorite breakfast.

If you want another course with your breakfast, toast (made with a good whole grain bread) is a fine accompaniment to your cooked or dry cereal. For a spread, layer it lightly with an acceptable (no sugar) jam, or some home-cooked chopped or puréed fruit. Or thinly slice a banana lengthwise on top of your toast, mash it a bit, then sprinkle on some cinnamon.

Pancakes and waffles made with whole wheat flour and topped with fresh fruits or low-fat cottage cheese are another option.

Lunch Choices

Your meal design for lunch may vary, depending upon whether you eat at home, pack a lunch for work or school, or eat in a restaurant. (Dining-out suggestions are given later in this chapter.)

Think of lunch as your vegetarian meal. If you're like most people who wish to eat some animal foods, you'll want to save it for your evening meal. But don't feel you're missing out. Vegetarian lunches can be interesting and appealing.

Let's say you haven't done any cooking in advance, so there are no beans, rice, potatoes, or soup on hand, and you don't want to do any cooking. In that case, you can still make a perfectly acceptable lunch consisting of a few slices of a good whole grain bread or some whole grain crackers, some raw vegetables, such as cut-up, raw carrots, celery sticks, tomato, cucumber, or other choices, and some fresh fruit. You can even slice a banana lengthwise on some bread for a banana sandwich. You may want to add a little nonfat yogurt or a skim-milk cottage cheese.

With a little effort, you can improve on this basic lunch considerably, especially if you have some of the recommended cooked staples on hand.

If it's a salad you'd like, you can quickly make many different kinds. Fix a tossed or green salad with a variety of raw vegetables, using lots of dark green lettuce, such as romaine, then give it more substance, if you wish, by tossing in two of your cooked staples–a handful of beans and some chunks of cold potato. Dress the salad with a nondairy, no-oil commercial salad dressing, or make your own by combining a good-quality vinegar with a little frozen apple juice, water, and some seasonings. If you'd prefer a Russian-style dressing, make your own by combining nonfat yogurt with a little tomato purée, using dried herbs for seasoning.

Or make a bean or rice salad with the cooked beans or rice you have on hand. Chop up some celery, green onions, and green pepper, mix with the beans or rice, and dress with a nondairy, no-oil dressing.

Another good luncheon dish made with the cooked beans is a bean dip. Mash the cooked beans, season well with chili powder, cumin, onion powder, and other seasonings of choice, and serve with oven-toasted corn tortillas, made by baking corn tortillas on an oven rack until lightly brown, then broken into chip size, if desired.

You can also use the bean dip as a sandwich spread. And here are a few more good sandwich ideas. Slice red onions and tomatoes, layer on bread with lettuce and spread the bread with a dressing of nonfat yogurt mixed with a little Dijon mustard or tomato purée.

If you wish to have some animal food at lunch, add a few thin slices of white meat of chicken or turkey. Or make a tuna salad sandwich. To make the tuna salad, mix some chopped celery and green onions into water-packed tuna, adding a little cooked rice as a filler to reduce the amount of tuna needed. Dress the salad with nonfat yogurt that has been mixed with a little Dijon mustard. Or make an egg-white sandwich by cooking an egg white in a no-stick pan. Serve on bread along with sliced tomatoes, lettuce, and a little Dijon mustard.

Dinner Possibilities

If you're going to eat animal food, save it for your evening meal. Chicken or fish is your best bet. A simple plan not involving any advance preparations would be to broil, bake, or poach a fish fillet or half a chicken breast. Accompany the meal with a baked or steamed potato or yam and steamed vegetables. Greens, such as mustard greens, collards, and kale, are highly recommended on the Pritikin diet because of their nutritional value, and are especially important if you are not eating dairy foods (they provide needed calcium).

When broiling fish, baste it with a little lemon or tomato juice instead of butter. You can also use these liquids in baking fish, or you may prefer to top the fish with sliced tomatoes and onions and some dried herbs or other seasonings. White wine, orange juice, and unsweetened pineapple juice are also excellent used sparingly to add flavor to some fish and chicken meals.

Before cooking chicken, always remove the skin and any adhering fat. When broiling it, baste with defatted chicken stock, if you have it. (Many Pritikin cooks like to prepare chicken stock in quantity and keep it on hand in the freezer in ice cube trays as a staple. It has other uses, too, such as in stir-fry cookery.) You can also baste chicken with vegetable stock or vegetable juices.

There are many delicious recipes for baking chicken Pritikin style, and you may be able to adapt others from standard recipes by simply deleting ingredients that are not permitted.

Other favorite dinner entrees are based on pasta dishes. Some people find whole wheat pasta unpalatable at first, but most grow to prefer it. You can prepare a simple spaghetti sauce by simmering canned tomato products, such as tomato sauce and tomato paste, with a little Burgundy wine, chopped onions and mushrooms, and seasonings, including several bay leaves. You can also use a little ground beef or turkey in the sauce. Before serving, sprinkle the pasta with sapsago cheese. Some standard spaghetti sauce recipes can readily be adapted to Pritikin guidelines, eliminating oil, butter, or cheese. Spaghetti sauce is a good recipe to prepare in quantity and freeze for future meals.

If you have cold rice or beans stored in the refrigerator, you have still other interesting entrée possibilities for your dinner meal. Make "fried rice" by cutting up a variety of vegetables, Chinese style, and cooking them briefly in a *small* amount of liquid, such as nonfat chicken stock or vegetable stock or even water, adding chopped fresh garlic and other seasonings, such as grated fresh ginger or a little soy sauce. When the liquid is evaporated and vegetables are tender-crisp, stir in lots of cooked rice. Heat gently and stir until rice is warmed through.

Make your beans into a quick oven casserole, adding lots of chopped vegetables and Mexican-style seasonings, or use this bean mixture for taco dishes. Simply oven-heat corn tortillas until warm, then fill with the warm bean mixture. Serve the bean dishes with rice that has been heated.

There's Room for Dessert

Fruits, raw and cooked, are the traditional Pritikin dessert. But be sure not to exceed your daily recommended amount of fruits. For variety, cut up an assortment of fruits to make a fruit salad, mixing in a little frozen fruit, such as blueberries or cherries, and topping it with a little nonfat yogurt. You can also mix fresh and frozen fruit with some cold cooked rice for an unusual but tasty dessert.

Favorite snacks are air-popped popcorn and fruit smoothies, made by blending a frozen banana, a little sweet liquid, such as frozen apple juice or frozen fruit and berry juices, and other frozen fruits, such as cherries or strawberries.

Do's and Don'ts of Dining Out

When dining out you need to be careful–chefs have ways of sneaking things you've never dreamed of into your dishes. Since your options are often limited in a restaurant, you can stretch your limits a bit–as long as you don't do it too often. For example, you can't ask the waiter to give you only three ounces of fish, but you can ask him to keep it simple and free of butter and other fats. Since a typical serving of these foods in most restaurants in six to eight ounces or even more, you can divide the serving with your dinner partner or take the surplus home in a doggie bag.

Good "safe" accompaniments in a restaurant would be a plain baked potato (order two if you're hungry) and a green salad, served with lemon or red-wine vinegar. Some people who follow the Pritikin diet carry their salad dressing with them in a small sealed container for use at restaurants.

At lunch, you can order a breast of turkey sandwich, without butter or mayonnaise, on sourdough bread or a whole grain bread. Request that the chef be light on the turkey and heavy on the lettuce and sliced tomatoes.

Often you can find a suitable soup (vegetable with a broth base) in a restaurant. If you are eating in a natural foods restaurant, you also may have the choice of many vegetable- or grain-based dishes. Chinese restaurants offer the possibility of ordering mixed vegetables, cooked without oil, with or without a little chicken or seafood, and a large bowl of rice.

Put Walking into Your Life

On the Pritikin Program, an eating program isn't complete without its traditional accompaniment–exercise.

Nathan recommended that his patients take up walking as a form of therapeutic exercise. It's something just about everyone can do and it is the least likely of all exercises to create problems. While he himself loved running, and many of those who follow his program jog or run, he cautioned against running for several groups of people. For those who are considerably overweight, running can cause bodily injury because of the extra stress on the weight-bearing joints; and for those not following a healthful diet or those in the high-risk category for cardiovascular disease, it can even result in sudden death.

To be effective, walking needs to be nonstop and done at a reasonably brisk pace for a minimum of 20 minutes. A total of 60 minutes of walking per day five to seven days per week constitutes a reasonable walking program. The daily walking can be done at one time or in several sessions.

A ten-minute warm-up walk at a slow pace should precede the brisk walk. Conclude your exercise period with a five-minute slow cool-down walk. The warm-up and cool-down periods are important because they allow the heart rate and blood pressure to increase and decrease at safe rates, reducing the chances of cardiovascular problems.

If you have been diagnosed as having heart disease, high blood pressure, high cholesterol, and/or are over the age of 36, you should get your doctor's approval before embarking on an exercise program.

There is the program in a nutshell. It's easy to follow because there's no ironclad prescription to eat a certain food on a certain day at a certain time. By sticking with the healthy foods–the whole grains, vegetables and fruits–and avoiding the bad foods–the high-fat, high-cholesterol foods–you'll automatically be on a scientifically valid program to improve health and promote wellness. Add a little exercise and you're on the Pritikin Program.

And on your way to better health.

Books by Nathan Pritikin

If you want more information about Nathan Pritikin's ideas on diet and health, you can refer to any of his books. They are:

Diet for Runners. New York: Simon & Schuster, 1985.

The Official Pritikin Guide to Dining Out. Indianapolis, N.Y.: Bobbs-Merrill Co., 1984. (Coauthored with Ilene Pritikin.)

The Pritikin Promise: 28 Days to a Longer, Healthier Life. New York: Simon & Schuster, 1983.

The Pritikin Permanent Weight-Loss Manual. New York: Grosset & Dunlap, 1981.

The Pritikin Program for Diet and Exercise. New York: Grosset & Dunlap, 1979. (Written with Patrick M. McGrady, Jr.)

Live Longer Now. New York: Grosset & Dunlap, 1974. (Written with Jon N. Leonard and J. L. Hofer.)

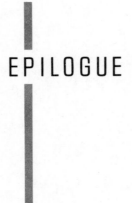

EPILOGUE

*O*n June 19, 1987, just two years after Nathan Pritikin's death, the *Journal of the American Medical Association* announced a study that showed regression of atherosclerosis in the coronary arteries of humans. The two-year study was done by Dr. David Blankenhorn and his associates at the University of Southern California in Los Angeles. Blankenhorn got his results by reducing the blood cholesterol of his patients by 26 percent, a drop similar to the one achieved at the Pritikin Longevity Centers. The scientists lowered blood cholesterol by using diet and drugs. However, the study made clear that a low-fat, low-cholesterol diet alone could achieve the same results.

Blankenhorn's study provided the long-awaited "final proof" that atherosclerosis could, in fact, be reduced and even eliminated from the coronary arteries of people simply by lowering blood cholesterol.

The study made front page headlines around the country because, for the first time, it showed that the underlying cause of most heart disease could be cured.

In 1966, Nathan Pritikin made the same claim that coronary atherosclerosis could be reversed by lowering blood cholesterol. Pritikin based his premise on the available research–most of which had been done on animals–and the fact that he was able to cure himself of coronary insufficiency with his own low-fat, low-cholesterol diet and exercise program. Pritikin made the claim again in his book, *Live Longer Now,* which was published in 1974. A year later, he believed that he had demonstrated regression of coronary atherosclerosis in two men who participated in Pritikin's Long Beach Study.

Nathan was widely criticized for his statements. Many scientists believed that his thesis was so far-fetched that they used it to dismiss him.

Twenty years later, Nathan Pritikin has been vindicated.

296